The Rise and Fall of the Age
of Psychopharmacology

The Rise and Fall of the Age of Psychopharmacology

EDWARD SHORTER, PHD

*Professor of Psychiatry, Professor of the History of Medicine,
Faculty of Medicine, University of Toronto*

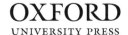

OXFORD
UNIVERSITY PRESS

OXFORD
UNIVERSITY PRESS

Oxford University Press is a department of the University of Oxford. It furthers
the University's objective of excellence in research, scholarship, and education
by publishing worldwide. Oxford is a registered trade mark of Oxford University
Press in the UK and certain other countries.

Published in the United States of America by Oxford University Press
198 Madison Avenue, New York, NY 10016, United States of America.

Library of Congress Cataloging-in-Publication Data
Names: Shorter, Edward, author.
Title: The rise and fall of the age of psychopharmacology / Edward Shorter.
Description: New York, NY : Oxford University Press, [2021] |
Includes bibliographical references and index. |
Identifiers: LCCN 2021016419 (print) | LCCN 2021016420 (ebook) |
ISBN 9780197574430 (paperback) | ISBN 9780197574454 (epub) |
ISBN 9780197574461 (Digital-Online)
Subjects: MESH: Psychopharmacology—history | Psychotropic Drugs—history |
Drug Industry—history | Mental Disorders—drug therapy | Drug Development—history |
Physician-Patient Relations | History, 20th Century | History, 21st Century | United States
Classification: LCC RM315 (print) | LCC RM315 (ebook) |
NLM QV 11 AA1 | DDC 615.7/8—dc23
LC record available at https://lccn.loc.gov/2021016419
LC ebook record available at https://lccn.loc.gov/2021016420

DOI: 10.1093/med/9780197574430.001.0001

In memory of
Barney Carroll
Don Klein
Mickey Nardo

Contents

Preface   ix
Abbreviations   xi

PART I: GETTING GOING

1. Introduction   3

2. Before Psychopharmacology   15

3. The Rise of Psychopharmacology   27

4. Things Get Rolling   43

5. Depression and Schizophrenia   59

6. Industry: Early Days   77

PART II: WORSENING

7. DSM   101

8. Science   123

9. KOLs   139

10. Trials Begin   163

11. Trials: Fantasy Patients for Fantasy Diseases   177

12. Trials: Industry Takes Over   189

13. Marketing   195

14. Journals   223

15. FDA   231

PART III: SCIENCE DISASTER

16. Prozac and Its Cousins   243

17. Sally   265

18. Atypicals   275

19. TMAP   299

20. The Fall of Psychopharmacology   305

21. Conclusion   323

Acknowledgments   327
Notes   329
Index   411

Preface

The Lord hath created medicines out of the earth; and he that is wise will not abhor them. —Ecclesiasticus, 38:4

As I was at the Y talking to my buddy, who is 55, he reached for a pill bottle, took out a 2-mg tablet of Abilify, a psychiatric drug, and swallowed it. "This has changed my life," he said.

By 5 PM each day he used to storm around ready to hit someone, loud, full of fury, and he experienced several arrests and an inability to keep himself from yelling at the cops. Now, he says, "This has given me my life back. I'm normal again."

So, treating mental illness with drugs—psychopharmacology—really can work. The drugs are often highly effective.

But what did my friend have? Mania or hypomania? He wasn't euphoric, had no flight of ideas, no hyperactivity, and certainly no psychosis. He was just chronically angry and agitated. That's not in the DSM, the diagnostic bible of psychiatry. And chronic anger is not one of the official indications for Abilify either, which was launched as an "antipsychotic." Abilify is now also indicated for "bipolar disorder." My friend had neither psychosis nor bipolar disorder. Yet, his clinician had the good judgment to prescribe the drug.

So, in my friend's case, psychopharmacology was effective, but the official side of it—diagnoses and treatments—was nonsense.[1] This is not the way medicine is supposed to work. People still take drugs for the brain and mind that often work, but the science has gone out of it. Neither the diagnostics nor therapeutics of psychiatry today may be said to have a scientific basis. The idea that you are better because Prozac has somehow restored your level of serotonin is just baloney.

There have been many books on how the pharmaceutical industry has taken over academic psychiatry, but what interests me is how things have declined over the years, from the relative dignity of the arm's length relationship between industry and the academy in the 1960s, to the invasion and capture of academic psychiatry by industry in the 1990s and after. How did this decline happen? Nobody has written about that.

I am not belittling the studies documenting the parlous state of affairs today. These are written by investigative reporters and indignant scholars who have done their homework, and what they say is sadly true. But how about the status quo ante? Was it equally bad, or was there some kind of "Golden Age"? I am deeply suspicious of Golden-Age rhetoric, as it usually reflects a nostalgic smear of Vaseline on the rearview mirror. But medical ethics do tend to crumble under the pressure of the profit motive.

The rise of psychopharmacology was a brilliant scientific event. Its fall has resulted from the triumph of commerce over science. These have been among the most important events in medicine—and in people's lives—over the last half century. Millions of Americans take psychiatric drugs, and patients have been given such ersatz diagnoses as "major depressive disorder" and "adult ADHD," which have made mental semi-invalids of them. This is not a victory of science in psychopharmacology. It is a perversion of science in the interest of commerce.

The story of the successful treatment of madness has been very positive, and we should not forget that as we navigate the tangle of scams, jury-rigging, and distortion that lurk beneath the surface of the field. Alec Coppen, a pioneer in British neuroscience who practiced at West Park Hospital for many years, told David Healy in 1996, "People today don't realize what a tremendous impact the antidepressants, neuroleptics and lithium have had on the terrible morbidity of mood disorders and schizophrenia. . . . When I go to West Park now I find about 400 patients suffering from dementia. What a contrast to forty years ago, when there were 2,000 very disturbed young and middle-aged patients, many of whom are now leading ordinary and rewarding lives thanks to these advances."[2] This is worth something.

Abbreviations

ACNP	American College of Neuropsychopharmacology
ADAMHA	Alcohol, Drug Abuse, and Mental Health Administration
ADHD	Attention-deficit/hyperactivity disorder
AIC	Academic–industrial complex
AMA	American Medical Association
APA	American Psychiatric Association
CDER	Center for Evaluation of Drug Research
CINP	International College of Neuropsychopharmacology
CME	Continuing Medical Education
COMT	Catechol-*O*-methyltransferase
CROs	Clinical research organizations
CSR	Corporate social responsibility
DBSA	Depression and Bipolar Support Alliance
DESI	Drug Efficacy Study Implementation
DHEW	Department of Health, Education and Welfare
DSM	*Diagnostic and Statistical Manual of Mental Disorders*
DST	Dexamethasone suppression test
EBM	Evidence-based medicine
ECDEU	Early Clinical Drug Evaluation Unit
ECNP	European Congress of Neuropsychopharmacology
ECT	Electroconvulsive therapy
EEG	Electroencephalography
EKS	Expert Knowledge Systems
EPS	Extrapyramidal symptoms
FDA	Food and Drug Administration
FGAs	First-generation antipsychotics
GSK	GlaxoSmithKline
HARKing	Hypothesizing After the Results are Known
ICI	Imperial Chemical Industries
IITs	Investigator-initiated trials
IND	Investigational new drug
IRB	Institutional Review Board
KOLs	Key Opinion Leaders
LSD	Lysergic acid diethylamide
MAO	Monoamine oxidase
MAOIs	Monoamine oxidase inhibitors
MBM	Marketing-based medicine
MECCs	Medical education and communication companies

MRC	Medical Research Council
NDA	New Drug Application
NIH	National Institutes of Health
NIMH	National Institute of Mental Health
NNH	Number Needed to Harm
NNT	Number Needed to Treat
OCT	Office of Clinical Trials
PDAC	Psychopharmacologic Drugs Advisory Committee
PDR	*Physicians' Desk Reference*
PhRMA	Pharmaceutical Research and Manufacturers Association
PHS	Public Health Service
PI	New York State Psychiatric Institute
PSC	Psychopharmacology Service Center
PSSD	Post-SSRI sexual dysfunction
QEEG	Quantitative EEG
RCTs	Randomized controlled trials
RDC	Research Diagnostic Criteria
RDoC	Research Domain Criteria
SAMHSA	Substance Abuse and Mental Health Services Administration
SDA	Serotonin-dopamine antagonist
SGAs	Second-generation antipsychotics
SKB	SmithKline Beecham
SKF	Smith, Kline & French
SNRIs	Serotonin-norepinephrine reuptake inhibitors
SSRIs	Selective serotonin reuptake inhibitors
STI	Scientific Therapeutics Information
TCAs	Tricyclic antidepressants
TD	Tardive dyskinesia
TMAP	Texas Medical Algorithm Project
VA	Veterans Administration
VNS	Vagus nerve stimulator
WBSTs	Worldwide business strategy teams
WHO	World Health Organization
WSJ	*Wall Street Journal*
Y-BOCS	Yale-Brown Obsessive-Compulsive Scale

PART I
GETTING GOING

1

Introduction

Psychopharmacology . . . is compelling chemistry, for the first time,
to look behavior in the face.—Joel Elkes (1965)[1]

John M. ("Mickey") Nardo, in his retirement, practiced psychiatry in a volunteer clinic in the Appalachian hills of Georgia. "I worked in the clinics today," he
wrote in 2012. "In the morning, I saw adults—a lot of them. I had three patients
where the central issue was unrecognized antidepressant withdrawal syndromes.
I had three patients who'd been told they were 'bipolar' (who weren't)." But the
high point of the day came that afternoon. His last patient was an adult woman
"with persistent PTSD from a terrible event eight years ago that involved the
death of her son. The tension of undoing bad diagnoses and bad treatments all
day just disappeared as I talked to this woman about her illness. I felt like a doctor
instead of someone putting out brush fires, a case-worker in a social agency, or a
med-check doctor."[2]

There are, said Nardo, plenty of psychiatrists out there, "doing what
I did, trying to help people with their mental illnesses, the systems they have
to negotiate, their misdirected treatments, their iatrogenic symptoms, their
medications . . . and sometimes even those afflictions of the mind brought on by
life experience in childhood and beyond."[3] There are many such clinicians. This
book is not about them.

This book is about the physicians who created the mass use of antidepressants
and antipsychotics and the industry that whispered in their ears. In the United
States in 2015 to 2016, almost seven adults in ten (69.0%) had used a prescription
drug within the past 30 days. In adults 40 to 59 years old, the most frequently
used drugs were antidepressants (prescribed to 15.4% of the entire population
in that age group).[4] This means that if you go to the supermarket, one in seven
of the middle-aged shoppers you encounter will have taken an antidepressant within the past month. In other words, a seventh of your fellow shoppers
are "depressed." Moreover, almost all of them (84.3%) have been taking their
antidepressants long term.[5] Nardo was amazed to find that his poor working-
class patients were all on prescription drugs. He was familiar with the statistics
I've just cited. "All of this has happened in a period where psychiatry has been

telling itself that it's *medicalizing*, but there's nothing about those figures that's *medical*."[6]

An Age of Psychopharmacology? Yes, indeed, because psychopharmacology turns out to be as much a cultural concept as a medical concept. Treating patients with psychoactive drugs has always been with us. There is nothing wrong with this. Psychopharmacology means investigating systematically the different effects of drugs on different mind and brain diseases. This, too, in unproblematic. But the "Age of Psychopharmacology" implies that an entire medical culture, indeed a whole popular culture, has been wrapped around a concept so that it has become an "age."

Psychopharmacology was a kind of cultural style within neuroscience. Soon abducted and corrupted by industry, it ceased to be a rigorously scientific discipline of its own, becoming instead a commercial trope for selling drugs. Wide-eyed speculations about neurotransmitters and receptors and jury-rigged drug trails replaced scientific evidence.

Yet, psychopharmacology was not entirely unscientific: Important questions about the impact of pharmaceuticals on the brain were investigated and in some cases resolved. But in retrospect there was an Age of Psychopharmacology, comparable to the Age of Anxiety or the Age of the Railroad. A culture of psychopharmacology arose in the 1950s and 1960s, and today it is dissolving.

In making this case, I often quote Mickey Nardo (and, yes, I refer to him by his universal nickname, Mickey). He was a psychiatrist with earlier training as an endocrinologist, who was on the faculty at Emory University for years, then in private practice in Atlanta. After Atlanta, he retreated to the hills of Appalachia in Georgia, where he volunteered his time in a local charity clinic and wrote a blog, "One Boring Old Man," which is among the most productive sources for this period—from roughly 2011 to his death in 2017. He was a kind of James Boswell acting as a chronicler to the latter-day Samuel Johnson, who in this case was Bernard ("Barney") Carroll, one of the great scientific figures of late twentieth-century psychiatry. Carroll led the Mood Disorders Unit at the University of Michigan for years, then was chair of psychiatry at Duke University, then moved to California to compose his own blasts against the "Key Opinion Leaders" (KOLs), a synonym for what he and others perceived as the sell-outs of today's psychiatry.

A theme: The last 30 years have witnessed the degradation of psychiatry as a clinical discipline. The two great arms of medicine are diagnosis and treatment, and the psychiatric diagnoses in the DSM (*Diagnostic and Statistical Manual of Mental Disorders*) turn out not to correspond to real diseases at all. The treatments are mainly ineffective (the SSRIs), or effective but toxic (many of the antipsychotics) and inappropriate in patients.

One problem is that psychiatry has been devoured by "depression." The only two adult diagnoses left standing are depression and schizophrenia. You don't need an MD degree plus 4 years of postgraduate training to say, "You're depressed" and prescribe Prozac. A garage mechanic could do it. A comparable degradation has happened to no other medical specialty. Psychiatry is unique.

Mark Kramer, head of clinical psychopharmacology at Merck for 13 years (between 1989 and 2002) put this failure of science in slightly different terms: The real problem, he said, is "that in one half century the best minds have not provided a compelling pathophysiological basis for most people with stereotypic syndromal phenotypes who are flagrantly disabled."[7] In other words, in the "show-stopping" illnesses of psychiatry, such as chronic social withdrawal ("schizophrenia"), psychotic depression, melancholia, and catatonia, we still have no idea what is going on. These are all disabling illnesses. It is said that in medicine that only illness worse than psychotic depression is rabies. But what happens in the brain to produce this degree of disablement is still entirely unclear.

I am scarcely the first to have chronicled this discouraging progression from decades of discovery and excitement to the pall of corruption and stagnation that latterly has beset us. Barry Blackwell, a pioneering psychopharmacologist (he discovered the "cheese effect" in the monoamine oxidase inhibitors), contrasted the "Pioneer Era" of the years 1940 to 1980 with the "Decades of Stagnation" of the years 1981 to the present.[8]

I realize that this critical approach skirts nihilism, as though psychiatry were bankrupt as a clinical discipline and ineffective in office practice. No! This is not the impression I wish to convey. Many psychiatrists are highly effective as healers, and this is for two reasons.

One is that the old hands do develop a sense of which drugs work on which patients. The official indications and diagnoses are rarely helpful, but experience speaks volumes, and the feeling that an unhappy and agitated patient might respond to a drug initially marketed as an antipsychotic is what clinical experience is all about.

Second, in psychiatry the trust built up in the doctor–patient relationship counts for a lot. Hungarian psychoanalyst Michael Balint called this the doctor using him- or herself as "a pill."[9] And there is a good deal of evidence that the personality and commitment of the physician make as much difference as the medication that he or she prescribes.[10] The resources of psychopharmacology, if they work at all, may well be secondary. Mickey Nardo reminded us that, "At its core, the patient–physician relationship involves a mutual commitment between a patient and her physician to her own well-being. We psychiatrists call this the therapeutic alliance and have plenty of evidence that it is the source of healing."[11] Roger Greenberg, a psychologist at Upstate University Hospital in Syracuse, attributed the small therapeutic success of the "antidepressants" to this doctor–patient relationship: "Creating a strong collaborative treatment alliance with a clinician who is viewed as caring, empathic, open, and sincere augurs well for a positive outcome. . . . These qualities are as important for patients receiving drugs as they are for those involved in psychotherapy."[12]

It is the therapeutic alliance that is part of the secret of effective healing in psychiatry, the deep intrinsic confidence of the patient that, in these skilled hands, he or she will get better. Psychopharmacology, if anything, detracts from this intrinsic power of the doctor–patient relationship. Yet many of the drugs *are* effective, and in serious illnesses, life without them can be a horror story.

The Big Picture

After the Second World War, the scene shifted from the Old World to the New World. Europe, in ruins, dropped out of the forefront of research, and the Continent not only was strapped for funds, but also had lost its Jewish investigators and clinicians, who previously had often been its most brilliant scientists, to New York and Los Angeles. The New World swung into leadership because Washington had money for pricey equipment, such as PET scanners, and for large trials. Heinz Lehmann, who left Germany in 1938 as a young MD to migrate to Canada, said, "I think that's where America has stolen the edge." "German medicine," he said, "was an impressive thing and there's no doubt about it. When we all went away [meaning the Jews], I don't think this tradition was transferred to America, but it was abolished in Germany."[13] For a few brief decades, the United States was the legitimate world leader in psychiatry. The 1950s were the golden age of drug discovery, and although the drugs were not necessarily discovered in the United States, they were developed there and were turned into successful commercial products.

By the 1970s, the old psychoanalytic psychiatry was stumbling toward the tar pits. Freud's doctrines, the backbone of Main Street psychiatry, had started to encounter widespread disbelief. Likewise, the old custodial psychiatry was doomed. The asylum, which previously had been the epicenter of biological thinking in psychiatry, was rapidly being dismantled.

A new psychiatry lay in its hour of birth, incorporating the huge advances in drug treatment that had occurred since the 1950s, but creating as well new thinking about diagnosis. The hope, largely unfulfilled, was that the new treatments would turn out to be specific for new diagnoses, and it was around diagnosis that the new psychiatry of the 1970s and after coalesced.

At the beginning, there were such hopes! In testimony before the Senate in May 1958, Nathan Kline, who had a private psychotherapy practice on Park Avenue and directed research in the New York State asylum at Orangeburg, said he hoped that psychopharmacology would pass from "the correction of mental aberrations" to "improving the functioning of healthy individuals, which I think is the next great step to be taken after the present one."[14]

Then the successes largely came to an end. Older psychiatrists like Nardo were often astonished at the deterioration of the field they were once so proud of. These men and women typically began as young clinicians and scientists in the 1970s, full of excitement about the ability of psychiatry to actually relieve the suffering of patients with severe illnesses and thrilled at shoving off from the psychoanalytic wharf. Then the savor of the moment turned to ashes as the useful drugs were abandoned for mediocre patent-protected ones, and the discriminating diagnoses—such as melancholia—were abandoned for such gross catch-alls as "major depression." Yet most of all, what astonished the veterans of another era, of a golden age, was how industry invaded the field, turning many colleagues from reflective clinicians into shills. The term is not too strong. The toxic term "Key Opinion Leaders," or KOLs, came to characterize many of the most prominent figures in the field as sell-outs.

There have been two derailments.

One is the DSM calamity, which began in 1980 with the DSM's third edition. The sturdy classical diagnoses of yore, many of which really did "cut Nature at the joints," as they say, were replaced by the DSM confections, a monstrous compilation of artifacts and half-diagnoses.

The second derailment was that the therapeutics of the years before 1970—which included some highly effective drugs, such as the amphetamines, the benzodiazepines, the classical "tricyclic" antidepressants, and such all-purpose agents as chlorpromazine (which was later defined as an "antipsychotic")—have been replaced by the less effective but relentlessly marketed SSRIs and "second-generation" antipsychotics.

These first two derailments are perhaps remediable. But a third, which may be harder to turn around, was the destruction of the field's intellectual autonomy after the invasion of the pharmaceutical industry.

Despite this intellectual disaster, psychiatrists remain highly effective as clinicians. So, this is where psychiatrists stand: their medications are, at best, non-specific feel-good agents and, at worst, placebos. Their diagnoses are an inchoate hodge-podge of meaningless labels. Thus, wherein lies the secret of psychiatry's success? It is largely in psychiatrists' one-to-one relationship with their patients, the therapeutic alliance. And there is a good deal of evidence that this alliance is the main source of healing. Robert Cancro, a resident at Kings County Hospital in New York in the late 1950s, was treating "a severely regressed psychotic young man" who would come to their sessions, turn his chair away, "and stare into space with a silly smile on his face, and talk in a totally disorganized fashion." It wasn't evident to Cancro that the patient was even aware of his presence. Cancro found the exchanges "meaningless."

One afternoon, the patient

> told me that the "medication" was helpful [he was in a trial], but that he really looked forward to "our little talks." I was stunned. How could he look forward to "talks" that had no theme, started no place, and went nowhere? It began to dawn on me that he valued the human contact, despite my inability to comprehend the nature of the contact. I then had a further revelation that it took him over an hour and several bus transfers to get to the clinic. He paid a high price for that brief human contact, and obviously valued it more highly than I realized. The lesson of all this was that being a psychiatrist meant being a healer. Healing involved not only medication, but the relationship.[15]

This one-to-one relationship is precisely what makes psychiatry different from neurology, although in theory both treat brain illnesses. As Nardo put it in 2014, what separates psychiatry from neurology is the "interpretation and 'making sense' of the personal struggles of our patients. When we put the word 'mental' in front of the word 'illness,' we are demarcating a territory of human suffering that has issues of meaning at its core."[16] This is a noble enterprise: helping suffering humankind to come to grips with the meaning of their suffering, and to hope that restoration may eventuate through understanding the circumstances that have made them ill, rather than through Prozac. This approach will not work with the show-stopping illnesses, such as catatonia and psychotic depression. Yet most patients do not have these illnesses; they have vague and nonspecific feelings of demoralization, fatigue, anxiety, and not being at ease in their skin as a result of their life circumstances. This is called "dysphoria." Here, meaning is everything. Will medications and DSM-style diagnoses help us here?

Two Cycles

Psychiatry has always been buffeted by "cycles." Sometimes, the dominant paradigm changes quite dramatically, as in the shift from psychoanalysis to biological psychiatry, and sometimes the shift creeps in on little cat feet, as it did in 1850 in the world of Samuel Woodward, former superintendent of the Massachusetts State Lunatic Hospital. He noted that treatment was turning away from "depletion" (bleeding), from external irritants, drastic purges. and starvation. Instead, coming in now were "baths, narcotics, tonics, and generous diet." "Not less to be appreciated in the improved condition of the insane," he said, "[is] the change from manacles, chains, by-locks and confining chairs to the present system of kindness, confidence, social intercourse, labor, religious teaching and freedom from restraint." How salutary, he thought, that in this "age of improvement," the lot of the insane should have been so improved.[17] Thus did one cycle end and another begin.

The long view shows that there are causation and treatment cycles. In causation, the nineteenth century once had, as Ralph Gerard put it in 1956, a fascination with "material causes of psychiatric disorders. . . . With the advent of modern 'dynamic' views in psychiatry, the pendulum swung in the other direction; sociological, psychological and interpersonal factors in the etiology of mental disturbance were much emphasized. Now the pendulum is swinging back a bit toward the importance of material biological factors." Indeed, Gerard said there had been a bit of an "overshoot." "We have all wished mental disease to be determined mostly by sociological causes, because this situation seemed more hopeful from the therapeutic standpoint. If the individual had been broken by the group he could be healed by techniques of interpersonal interaction, but if he had bad genes, effective treatment was far in the future."[18]

And then there are treatment cycles. In the 1880s and 1890s, a great cycle began, as the patent-medicine industry flooded the world with drugs of dubious safety and utility. Still, people were just accustoming themselves to the idea that the highway to good health lay in pharmaceuticals, and these products were enormously profitable. But industry's invasion of medicine, so evident around 1900, subsided. George Simmons, who was instrumental in creating the AMA Council on Pharmacy and Chemistry in 1905, wrote, "Since the Council began its work . . . there seemed to be no statement too silly, no claim too extravagant, and no falsehood too brazen for use by those who wrote the advertising literature that physicians were asked to read and to believe." He lamented above all, industry's corruption of the journals and textbooks: "This commercialized materia medica has blighted our literature by debauching our medical journals and even by tainting our textbooks."[19]

To be sure, the age of patent pharmaceuticals did not sweep all before it. For the next 40 years, drugs that physicians prescribed (called "ethical specialties"), having at least some evidence of safety and efficacy, were the order of the day. Almost none of the drugs of that era were hugely effective, with the few exceptions being insulin, the opiates, and the barbiturates.

Nonetheless, this cycle had ushered in a time of almost frenetic treatment. In 1909, William Osler, professor of medicine at Johns Hopkins University, cautioned colleagues that, "The literature that comes to us daily indicates a thralldom not less dangerous than the polypharmacy from which we are escaping. [Osler believed the fewer drugs, the better.] I allude to the specious and seductive pamphlets and reports sent out by the pharmaceutical houses, large and small." He absolved Parke-Davis in the United States and Burroughs Wellcome in

England as "pioneers in the science of pharmacology." But the rest "traded on the credulity of the profession, to the great detriment of the public."[20]

By 1929, the Council, as Paul Nicholas Leech of Chicago said, had "more than 100,000 index cards dealing with drugs and drug therapy" in its files.[21] One observer, commenting in 1929 on this profusion, said, in a statement entirely applicable to our own times, "The almost daily announcement of new discoveries has produced a national state of mind in which we are surprised at nothing and, too frequently, are willing to accept at face value anything presented with the merest semblance of truth."[22] But pharmaceutical science was ending this credulity. In that file box with its 100,000 index cards lay the death knell of the cycle: the age of patent psychopharmaceuticals ended.

So, we should not imagine that industry's invasion of the practice of medicine is a recent phenomenon. At an AMA symposium on drug therapy in 1929, "emphasis was given to the need to replace the detail man [drug rep] as the main source of instruction in the use of medicines."[23] This cycle ended with the AMA's cold-eyed assessment of patent remedies, discarding most of them. As mentioned, in 1905 the AMA's Council of Pharmacy and Chemistry was founded, and it systematically evaluated new compounds. Simultaneously, Arthur Cramp became director of the AMA's Bureau of Investigation from 1906 to 1936 (it was originally called the Propaganda Department); his three-volume *Nostrums and Quackery and Pseudo-Medicine*, published between 1911 and 1936, makes riveting reading for students of the history of gullibility.[24] In the section on "female weakness," we learn that Lydia E. Pinkham's Vegetable Compound, a market-beater around the time of the First World War, was the remedy of choice for "tired nervous mothers."[25]

Thus ended the cycle. This is not to deny that effective agents for mental disease were not introduced: they included niacin for cerebral pellagra, penicillin for neurosyphilis, chloral hydrate for sedation—but they were few and far between and in no way gave rise to a specific science of treating diseases of the brain and mind.

The second cycle, the Age of Psychopharmacology, began around 1954, with the introduction of the antipsychotic chlorpromazine (Thorazine). For the first time, truly effective drugs became available for the treatment of serious mental illness.

However, a hallmark of the second great cycle was the invasion of psychiatry by industry. Yet, as stated, it would not be correct to think of this as a new problem. Around 1900, observers called attention to physicians who endorsed products for money. In 1907, Simmons said, "An honest, conservative statement about the merits of a proprietary preparation is as rare as are sweet violets in Ireland."[26] So again, the tendency of clinicians to sign off on products for pay is not new—but in those earlier days the purveyors typically did not have academic appointments nor were they regarded as leaders! The point is that the invasion of psychiatry by industry that bedevils us today is not recent—merely extraordinary in that it is physicians at the top of the heap, rather than those at the bottom, who are the perpetrators.

Thus, after 100 years, unscrupulous manufacturers would once again etiolate the evidence base of medicine, and as a result, our own days have seen the end of the Age of Psychopharmacology, the completion of this most recent great cycle. This time, there was no guardian at the ports; the FDA proved incapable of preventing the jury-rigging of the evidence of drug safety and efficacy, and, it would be fair to say, the pharmaceutical industry invaded and took possession of the practice of clinical psychiatry.

Thus, this book is about the rise and fall of the second great cycle, the Age of Psychopharmacology. The fall? Psychiatric drugs are still prescribed today in massive numbers. Yet the frame is shifting. Observers increasingly recognize that the intellectual paradigm of "neurotransmitters and their reuptake" has been exhausted, that there are no new drugs in the pipeline, and indeed that no new drug classes or novel mechanisms have been conceived for decades. The field's professional literature, at least that regarding drug trials, has been hopelessly corrupted, and the prescribing of an endless chain of SSRIs (Prozac cousins) is something you don't actually need specialty training in psychiatry to do. Nor, for that matter, as the psychologists increasingly clamor, do you need a medical degree to do it.

So, the next big thing will soon come along. We cannot yet know what it will be, but the second-generation antipsychotics that now clutter the treatment of depression are increasingly recognized as grossly inappropriate, and the prescribing of these powerful drugs for children is seen as a form of child abuse. The SSRI "antidepressants," as they are cleverly termed, are now viewed as drugs that suppress emotion rather than relieving depression. Their metabolites currently pollute our lakes and streams—and soon the Green New Deal will cry "Enough!"

Teasing Society from Biology

We live in a society where the belief is encouraged that one of four people in your subway car has a mental illness. A government survey for 2008 to 2012 found that "Among adults aged 18 or older, an estimated 22.5% (51.2 million adults) had in the past year at least one of the diagnoses [that interviewers assessed]; that is, almost a quarter of adults in the United States had one or more mental disorders (including adjustment disorder and substance use disorders) in the past year."[27] A quarter of the population do not have diseased brains. This extraordinary figure is possible only with the aid of culture.

Mind versus brain is often presented as a dichotomy. In figuring out why people become ill, you have to choose one or the other. But the two positions can exist side by side, depending on what illnesses one is discussing.

By the 1970s, there was a consensus outside of psychoanalysis that a "medical" psychiatry existed in which the major illnesses—melancholic depression, catatonia, and schizophrenia—were brain diseases that responded to the new drugs and to ECT (electroconvulsive therapy). The psychoneurotic disorders, by contrast, were considered psychogenic illnesses that responded to antineurotic medications, or nerve pills, such as meprobamate in the 1950s or the benzodiazepines in the 1960s and 1970s. In the 1990s and the new century, the SSRIs attempted to fill this role, but with little efficacy. Psychiatry thus followed the "medical model," in the sense that the major disease entities were considered to be brain diseases that could be individuated following the tenets of the medical model: (1) identification of a disease entity on the basis of specific signs and symptoms; (2) verification of the entity on the basis of biological tests; (3) validation of the entity on the basis of response to treatment. By the 1970s, there were two diseases that had been thus identified: melancholic depression and catatonia. Schizophrenia as a distinctive disease entity—an improbable assemblage of various disease conditions—was beginning to deconstruct itself. British psychiatrists Ida Macalpine and Richard Hunter epitomized this "brain" perspective in the *Times Literary Supplement* in 1974: "The abnormal mental state," they said, "is not the disease, not its essence or determinant, but an epiphenomenon. This is why psychological theories and therapies, which held out such promise at the turn of the century . . . have added so little to understanding and treatment of mental illness. . . . Type and degree of mental disturbance are determined by type and seat of brain disturbance."[28] This is a provocative statement of a highly reductionist position: mind disease reduces to brain disease. It would have sat well at the neurological National Hospital in Queen Square in London, where Hunter was physician in psychological medicine.

By contrast we find Mickey Nardo, practicing psychiatry in a charity clinic in the backwoods of Georgia, who emphasized disorder of the mind rather than brain disease. To be sure, he said, there were show-stopping illnesses, such as melancholia and schizophrenia. "In the 1970s, there was something of a growing consensus that Melancholic Depression and the Depressions associated with Manic Depressive Illness were prime candidates for biological research. The genetics were right. The clinical syndrome was unique. There were promising biomarkers: DST [the dexamethasone suppression test] and REM latency [rapid eye movement latency]." So that was the biological side.

But then, continued Nardo, there was another side. "When I see patients in the clinic tomorrow, I'm not likely thinking that many of them have brain diseases. The colossal failure of the research enterprise to find anything may be that there's not anything to find."[29] On another occasion, he said, "I worked in two clinics yesterday and I saw only one patient [who] might fit such a [biological] model—a sixteen-year-old with attention deficit disorder with hyperactivity (diagnosable from 100 yards). Everyone else had the kind of confusing complex of problems that afflict real people—no [diagnostic] entities noted. Some got medicines. Some got taken off medicines. Some were helped. Some weren't." Nardo then turned upon psychiatrists who insisted on reducing everything to specific diseases, "determined to make psychiatry 'evidence-based'—more like the rest of medicine with distinct disease categories, structured interviews, and treatment protocols. The focus was on treatments rather than on broad-based attempts to understand the breadth of the problems—more on neurochemistry than people."[30] Here was a seat-of-the-pants articulation of the difference between brain diseases, such as melancholia with the dexamethasone suppression test for it, and the riot of stress, distress, and unhappiness that Nardo saw on a daily basis in the charity patients. This is a differentiation that brain biologists like Richard Hunter missed.

Clearly, not all psychiatric disorders are brain diseases. Yet some are. The failure of the psychopharmacological paradigm lay in expanding the biological sort to encompass virtually the entire field. This expansion was accomplished by declaring that basically everything was treatable with drugs. It wasn't a random observation, born of an idle Tuesday afternoon seminar. The relentless expansion of indications was essential in the cut-throat commercial competition between companies: expanding indications meant expanding sales. This was commerce, not science.

How to find a golden mean between the biological and the social? Joseph Zubin, who founded the biometrics research program at the New York State Psychiatric Institute in 1954 and ended as professor of psychiatry in Pittsburgh, said at the 1988 meeting of the American Psychopathological Association, "The biological variables we talk about have primarily been wired in through evolution. The psychosocial variables came much later, when culture took over. Cultural transmission is not as efficacious, not as direct, and not as built-in as the biological, and yet it represents a very basic underpinning of total behavior."[31] Here, biology and culture are clearly juxtaposed, although it would be difficult to sort these out in dealing with patients.

Psychopharmacology and its diagnoses swam even further out of view in the mid-1950s when Frank Berger, a Czech-born psychiatrist, introduced meprobamate (Miltown), the first blockbuster drug in psychiatry. So, you'd think Berger would have bought into the biological model of specific medications for specific diseases? Not at all. This is what he told Leo Hollister (who was the éminence grise of US psychopharmacology) in an interview in 1995 about his arrival in the United States just after the war. Berger's first job was at a psychiatric clinic of the

University of Louisville: "My feeling was that most people we saw had really no psychiatric disorders. They were people, in my opinion, with problems of living, people who did not get along with their spouses, did not get along with their children, did not get along with their boss, and had not been taught, had not been educated, had not been prepared to handle all the crises of life. So they got stressed, broke down, and had to see a doctor, and the doctor did not know what to do. So he put one of the psychiatric names on them."

Hollister: "That's right. You are absolutely right!"[32]

2

Before Psychopharmacology

I used cold sheet wraps on agitated patients when I was a resident, and they were great. Of course they did not make money for Pharma, and they required trained nurses to apply correctly and continuously monitor the patients, but they sure were effective, and no side effects. So was chloral hydrate effective for sleep. And work therapy for depressed patients. Some of the old-fashioned remedies were useful, but not patentable and monetizable, so they faded away.—Robert Rubin, retired head of psychiatry, Los Angeles Veterans Administration Hospital[1]

Drugs for the Mind Go Way Back

Every culture has had drugs that treat disorders of the mind. This goes back to opium for melancholia in classical Greece. Ida Macalpine and Richard Hunter commented, "Each age indulges in the conceit that nervous disorders are on the increase because of the complexity of its civilization with its discontents. The seventeenth century had its 'sleepers,' and 'pills to purge melancholy,' the eighteenth its 'pacifick medicines' and the nineteenth its 'composing pills' and 'herbaceous tranquilizers.'"[2] Most of these decoctions were mixtures of alcohol and a laxative.

Yet not all. A researcher at the World Health Organization (WHO) commented in 1958 on, "a vast, old stream of experience of the race which, essentially unrecorded yet ever-present, has penetrated and dyed deep the varied fiber and pattern of many cultures. It is a humbling thought that mescal, cohoba, morphia, marijuana, and reserpine owe their discovery to chance rather than active search."[3] So, in a sense, there is nothing new about psychopharmacology. It is among the oldest of cultural acquisitions.

Pharmacology itself dates back to Germany in the 1880s. In 1912, Torald Sollmann of Western Reserve University in Cleveland, probably the Dean of American pharmacology, wrote, "This, then, is one of the most important fields of experimental therapeutics—the carefully planned, accurately executed, and intelligently digested study of the effects of drugs on human patients."[4]

It was in the mid-nineteenth century that biological thinking in psychiatry began to accelerate (it had always been present). In 1852, Heinrich Laehr, who at the time headed a provincial asylum in Halle and was considered a leader in the field, said, "Insanity is nothing else than a disease which only medical means may combat, and that, accordingly, it must be seen as a sin if the admission of an insane person to an asylum is hindered." (By playing on the concept of "sin," he was fencing with an older school of psychiatry that saw psychiatric illness as a kind of moral punishment.) Laehr said that a disturbance in brain substance caused a disturbance in thought.[5] Henry Maudsley, superintendent of the West London Hospital and benefactor of the psychiatric hospital named after him, was the forward scout of biological thinking in England. In 1874, he said, "The aim of the physician in the treatment of insanity is to bring the means at his command to bear, directly or indirectly, on the disordered nerve-element."[6] There were many such biologically thinking figures in the last third of the nineteenth century.

"If French is the language of diplomacy, then German may be said to be the language of psychiatry," as one sage put it.[7] European names dominate the older narrative. The many German-language psychiatric journals and the 16 university psychiatric hospitals where German was spoken provided a very fine layer of clinical description. English psychiatrist Malcolm Lader said, "We always used to say if you go back far enough and look at German literature at the turn of the century you're sure to find that someone described panic disorder and everything else."[8] The big manuals of diagnosis and treatment were written by highly experienced German and French clinicians, who often lived in service apartments in the mental hospitals and knew the patients closely.

The literature of psychiatry in those days was heavily in German. In a reference work called the *Surgeon General's Catalogue* of the US Army, in the series for the first third of the twentieth century, the bibliography for "hypnotics" goes on for three pages of small print; the names of the contributors are heavily German, indeed Jewish-German; and investigators such as Hans Hoff and Ernst Peter Pick, both of Vienna, are among the hundreds of names. By contrast, the English names are few and the American names vanishingly small. So scientific psychiatry was very much centered in Central Europe, and in the asylums, rather than on Main Street.[9]

This kind of senior experience is enormously important. Mickey Nardo tried to explain why results were often good in pilot studies but then washed out when the study was expanded to a number of centers. It was, he said, because the pilot studies were conducted by seasoned "experienced clinicians," and the expanded protocols by juniors. "The experienced clinicians are in on the ground floor and are diagnosing these patients intuitively based on long experience with schizophrenic people. As more (and less experienced) clinicians get involved in the studies, the intuitive factors fall out of the equation and their success rate falls with the change. So the old guys . . . can't take the show on the road. They can't pass on their intuition."[10] If Nardo is correct, this intuition factor would partly explain why the Germans and French ruled psychiatry for 100 years. Part of our narrative in the United States is that our senior figures seem to lose this kind of contact, and instead go on the industry-sponsored lecture circuit or idle their time away at conferences and do not really see much of patients.

As Frederick Goodwin, an old hand at NIMH, pointed out in 1987, "The great European tradition of descriptive psychiatry virtually died out in this century— consumed on the continent by two world wars and in the United States, diverted by efforts to extend psychoanalysis to the major disorders."[11] It is germane to our story that psychiatry's most promising effort at science failed to cross the Atlantic.

Science in Psychiatry Begins

> Very few take the path of scientific investigation, the only path that can lead us to a rational and positive explanation of man and sur-rounding nature. I hold that this ambition is one of the worthiest and most laudable that man can pursue because perhaps more than any other it is infused with the fragrance of universal love and charity.— Santiago Ramón y Cajal (1897)[12]

There is science as well as clinical medicine here. In terms of investigation, biological approaches to psychiatry (aside from postmortems) really began in 1928 at the Stadtroda Mental Hospital in Thuringia with Walter Jacobi and Helmut Winkler's "encephalographic studies of schizophrenia." The major finding: the cerebral ventricles are enlarged in schizophrenia.[13] This was the first important discovery related to schizophrenia as a brain disease, in the midst of psychoanalytic enthusiasms about the "unconscious." In 1979, Daniel Weinberger and colleagues at NIMH confirmed the finding using modern techniques.[14]

Investigators have sought to discern differential biochemical profiles of the various psychiatric illnesses. In 1892, Johannes Vorster, director of the Stephansfeld Asylum in the newly reconquered province of Alsace, reported blood findings in 112 patients: At the height of melancholia, periodic mania, and "acute insanity," all three groups of patients experienced falls in the specific gravity of the blood and in hemoglobin content. In the course of recovery, values for all three rose. But, at the onset of melancholia, yet not in the other illnesses, there was "a considerable increase" in both blood values.[15]

Based on similar blood findings, in 1931 the Nordmark Company in Hamburg introduced "Photodyn (Hämatoporphyrin)" for melancholia and migraine. It assumed changing blood chemistry, and it turned out to be an indifferent treatment.[16] Yet it is a nice illustration of the powerful reach of German psychiatry, then at the height of its influence. Later, all the work on biochemistry was forgotten.

There were other early scientific efforts to limn the differential impact of drugs on the mind, which is the essence of psychopharmacology. Among the efforts was the research in 1869 by Claude Bernard, professor of physiology in Paris, showing that different alkaloids of opium had opposing soporific and activating effects.[17] In Italy in 1884, Bartolomeo Bergesio and Giuseppe Musso at the Turin asylum studied, in a patient missing a piece of his cranium, the effects of alcohol, morphine, and paraldehyde (a foul-smelling synthetic sedative) on the cerebral circulation. They concluded that the drugs affect consciousness not by altering cerebral blood pressure but by unspecified changes in the "cells of the cerebral cortex."[18] This pioneering work remained widely unrecognized, but it may be considered a landmark in early psychopharmacology.

As an aside: neurochemistry is not psychopharmacology. There is a deep French tradition of neurochemistry going back to Michel-Augustin Thouret in the 1790s. Jean-Pierre Couerbe, at the Parisian School of Pharmacy, associated different mental conditions with different levels of phosphorus in the brain—and in 1834 expressed the hope that his research would soon "aid the therapeutic task of relieving certain maladies of the brain that are so horrible in man."[19] Yet none of the brain chemistry work really foreshadowed psychopharmacology, which studies the *differential* impact of medications.

Yet, French psychiatry also has a nineteenth-century record that is replete with physicians using medication in the treatment of mental illness, indeed of using agents like hashish experimentally. Jacques-Joseph Moreau (de Tours) is credited for introducing hashish into clinical science in 1845. It was Moreau's work on the psychological effects of different agents that earned him (in France in 1962) the sobriquet "the veritable founder of psychopharmacology."[20]

An important early American contribution to this international narrative was the pellagra story: Joseph Goldberger of the US Public Health Service reported in 1915 that the disease was caused by a dietary factor, and in 1937 Conrad Elvehjem, an agricultural chemist at the University of Wisconsin, found that the symptoms were reversible with nicotinic acid. Given that one of the symptoms of pellagra was dementia, preventing this condition may be seen as helping to create a psychopharmacologic tradition in the United States. In 1919, Columbia psychologist Albert Poffenberger reviewed the literature on the effects of intoxicants and pharmaceuticals on such functions as reaction times.[21] So it was not all just rank empiricism.

Long before psychopharmacology jelled as a field, psychiatrists dubious about psychoanalysis were toying with biochemical ideas, speculating that drugs specific for various illnesses of the mind must be possible. Walter Freeman, the Washington DC psychiatrist who shortly would originate "lobotomy," dilated on "psychochemical factors in mental disorders." At the "Section on Nervous and Mental Diseases" of the American Medical Association (AMA) in Philadelphia in 1931, he said, "The failure of microscopy to demonstrate structural alterations in the so-called functional psychoses is driving the investigator into new channels of research." Underlying the major illnesses there must be, he said, "structural deviation." He concluded that, "There are certain biochemical processes associated with disorders of behavior. . . . The psychochemist has a large order."[22] The "psychochemist" would shortly be rechristened "the psychopharmacologist."

These insights penetrated a good deal of clinical medicine. In 1936, William Houston, professor of medicine at the University of Georgia (and a pioneer in the therapeutic use of the doctor–patient relationship), wrote, "Out of a recognition of the relationship between the psyche and the soma, modern biological psychiatry has come into existence. As an obvious consequence there has been added a biological psychopathology."[23]

These early figures had a profoundly scientific orientation. Nothing could have interested them less than collecting speakers' fees from drug companies. Joel Elkes wrote of his days in medical school—he graduated from St Mary's Hospital Medical School in London in 1943—"I had a consuming curiosity about the molecular basis of immunological memory."[24]

Despite this budding science, psychiatry in these years still stood much in the shadow of neurology. Eliot Slater, head of psychiatry at the English national neurology hospital Queen Square, wrote of the early 1930s, "At that time neurologists were the most prestigious of all medical specialists owing to great advances recently made in the anatomy and physiology of the nervous system. . . . All the psychiatric training which was given to the London medical student was to take him for half a dozen visits to one of the small private mental hospitals, where he was shown a selection of patients far advanced in lunacy."[25] Thus, the mighty neurologists towered over the quivering psychiatrists. This would change with the arrival of psychopharmacology, when the psychiatrists would stride as primus inter pares onto the stage of medical practice.

Commerce

Yet treating the mind with drugs has a commercial side as well. Before 1900, almost no real treatments were available of a psychoactive nature, at least very few that were effective. There were a couple of exceptions to this. At Northampton

State Hospital in Massachusetts, "the whole therapeutics of insanity" included morphine, introduced in 1865, administered with a hypodermic syringe (which had just been invented). Clinicians noted this to be "a resource of great value in hospitals where many of the patients refuse to swallow any medicine." In 1866, potassium bromide was introduced to Northampton for epilepsy, and in 1870 chloral hydrate, an effective sedative.[26] That was the end of that hospital's list.

But going back in time, other preparations had an almost mystical effectiveness. English family doctors widely prescribed "the green medicine," a mixture of the barbiturate phenobarbital and the solanaceous-plant derivate hyoscine (scopolamine). Hyoscine has a latter-day reputation as a date-rape drug, but it is also prescribed for motion sickness and has a range of central nervous effects that are not well understood. Yet patients loved it. Ian Tait, who entered family practice in Sussex in 1959, said "Long after the early antidepressants became available the green medicine was often used as a first treatment. It very often worked," he said, "for mild to moderate emotional disorders."[27] Note that the word "depression" had not yet entered family medicine. Ultimately, the antidepressants carried the day because they were prescribed in hospitals, and when the patients returned to the family doctor, the green medicine seemed pokey and provincial. But, isn't this interesting?

Many other supposedly psychoactive preparations were just placebos and used not in hospitals but in family practice. Daniel Cathell, a Baltimore physician whose wit was as sharp as that of his neighbor, newspaper editor Henry L. ("H L") Mencken, said in 1893, "A mental agent should, as a rule, be small and easy to take; the bromides, the valerianates, mild tonics, and other harmless remedies are sometimes given." In any event, he considered their effect largely that of a placebo. "Should you ever have recourse to remedies intended to act chiefly through the mind, if you will take care to look your patient earnestly and steadily in the face, and give precise instructions concerning the time and mode of using them they will do double good. You will not only find that almost anything will relieve some of these mental cases, but will be further surprised to learn that it has evoked their enthusiasm, and that they are chanting its praise and vowing that they were cured of one or another awful thing by it."[28] That such behavior would be seen as unethical today does not make it any less effective.

After 1900, some effective treatments were introduced and scientific evaluation of them began. The barbiturates occupy center stage here. Entering clinical use in 1903, Bayer's Veronal (generically barbital) was first. The barbiturates went on to become an enormously popular drug class and figured in many "combo" treatments as well as in pure form. To be sure, they can be accumulated by suicidal patients for purposes of self-destruction, but this is true of many agents in the pharmacopoeia. (Of 18,600 suicide deaths in the United States in 1959, 1,073 were caused by barbiturates—thus, not a lot.[29]). But it was not true that they caused depression, and English psychopharmacologist Max Hamilton brushed this canard aside: "A long time ago it was said that barbiturates caused depression; this is simply due to the barbiturate removing the anxiety [in mixed anxiety-depression], with the result that the depression becomes manifest. If that should be so, then I would certainly give an antidepressant."[30]

The concept of a "clinical trial" was adumbrated in these years. In 1929, Albert Young, a pharmacologist at the University of Michigan, reported on "the sad experience of attempting to get other people to give it [a drug he was introducing] it a thorough trial before presenting it to the [AMA] Council. In this particular instance, we spent considerable money in having the drug made and sent it to about fifteen of the leading internists of the country, all of whom had previously said they would be glad to try it out. I believe about 5 per cent actually gave it a trial, and the others placed it on the shelf or put it in the wastebasket." So he had little info to give the Council.[31]

The great Berlin pharmacologist Louis Lewin is acknowledged as the godfather of toxicology, but he could as easily count as the most important founding figure in psychopharmacology, for he recognized the impact on the brain of pharmaceuticals for pleasure and for recovery from mental disease. He wrote in 1924, "Of the countless chemical agents in the world, none have a more intimate connection to the life of all humanity than those whose history and impact are described in this volume. I have given them the name 'phantastica.' . . . In all of these agents there is a direct impact on the brain, which in all of its forms is enigmatic and incomprehensible." These new agents, he said, transformed life itself. "They liberate the mentally tortured from their burden, give hope to those wracked by pain or doomed to death, give new energy to those enervated by work—a feat impossible even with strong will—and grant to those who are antisocial and deadened after work an hour of inner comfort and satisfaction."[32] The book, however, gave itself over mainly to the evils of addiction and chronic use. Yet Lewin's *Phantastica* is the first comprehensive effort to link drugs to behavior.

Patent Medicines

But the barbiturates were overwhelmed by the "patent medicines"—noted in the introduction—proprietary preparations whose ingredients were a secret.[33] This flood gave rise to scandalous abuses, and, as we have seen, in 1905, the American Medical Association, to break the back of this great upswing of popular remedies, founded the Council on Pharmacy and Chemistry. Through its publication *New and Nonofficial Remedies*, it exercised roughly the same function as the FDA today: vetting drugs so that only those of probable efficacy and safety reached the market. (It ceased certifying drugs in 1955.[34]) That reduced the use of "patent medicines" (the Council failed, alas, to abolish credulousness). In 1929, two executives of the AMA Council on Pharmacy said, "It is not safe to use in the human body a preparation of unknown composition, of unknown potency or of doubtful dosage or a preparation the claims for which have not been established by scientific unbiased evidence." They noted the "commercial domination of therapeutics" as the main reason for the creation of the Council.[35]

Morris Fishbein worked for the AMA Council. His job was to expose quackery, and the quackery of the era gives us some idea of how welcome the early science of pharmacology was. "To sell patients on cures is not difficult," he told a later interviewer. "[There was] Professor Samuels who used to take tap water and put in some salt and sell it for $5.00 a bottle to cure tuberculosis. You anointed yourself on each breast and the navel; you made the sign of the Cross. You only used five drops at a time for tuberculosis. We exposed him. He made millions of dollars. He used to come to Chicago before automobiles and had a tremendous carriage with black horses." Then, continued Fishbein, "There was Snake Oil Cooper even before that. He used to have a long, frock coat with five-dollar gold pieces for buttons, and he used to ride a carriage around the monument in Indianapolis. He had a big bag with nickels, dimes and quarters and he threw out handfuls and hundreds of kids fought for that money in the streets."[36] So, there was money in the early days of the drug industry, or at least in this version of it.

A food and drug inspection agency called the Bureau of Chemistry had been lodged within the Department of Agriculture. It changed its name in 1927 to Food, Drug, and Insecticide Administration, shortened in 1930 to Food and Drug Administration (FDA); in 1940, the FDA was placed under the Federal Security Agency, which in 1953 became the Department of Health, Education, and Welfare. It The FDA would be a major player in the story, and from the get-go the Bureau of Chemistry had normal relations with industry. The big companies were organized in the American Association of Manufacturers of Medicinal Products. (The smaller ones were in the American Pharmaceutical Manufacturers Association.) Robert Fischelis, who fronted for various industry associations, recalled of the 1920s and 1930s, "This was a period in which there was a good deal of cooperative effort, in connection with developing drug problems, about standardization of. ampoules, and what kind of tests ought there to be. . . . A joint contact committee, indeed, was set up, with members from the two manufacturing trade associations and dealt with the Food and Drug Administration."[37] But there is a difference between this kind of respectful collaboration, which nurtured psychopharmacology in its rise, and the regulators' waving through ineffective drugs, which had a role in the decline of psychopharmacology.

Getting Set

Antidepressants, known as such, began to be marketed. In 1936, the amphetamines, introduced several years previously for asthma, started to be indicated for depression. It is unquestionable that Benzedrine and Dexedrine, the first amphetamines, are effective in mild to moderate depression, and it is probably a loss that they have now vanished from view. Indeed, in 1938 the first controlled trial in US psychiatry employed Benzedrine successfully in the treatment of the "depressed phase" of a number of female patients whose main diagnosis was their psychotic illness[38] (see Chapter 3).

Alongside these two classic agents, a variety of other remedies for "schizophrenia" and other conditions flourished. In 1932, Constantine Pascal, at the asylum Ville-Evrard in Paris—one of the first academic female psychiatrists—proposed a kind of "progressive dynamogenesis," including ether in progressive doses, cocaine, hashish, peyote, and strychnine.[39] It was Pascal who introduced the concept of "shock treatment" into psychiatry, and she clearly had obtained results with some of these remedies—which today have not entirely lost currency. (It has been customary among historians of psychiatry, many of whom are committed to talk therapies, to speak disparagingly of these early treatments as examples of desperate empiricism. Yet some of these clinicians were experienced investigators; their work was blotted out in the triumph of psychoanalysis, and it is conceivable that they have things to say to us today.) In any event, by the end of the Second World War, a psychiatric armamentarium was budding.

A Golden Age

In some ways, the years from 1930 to 1960 constituted a kind of "Golden Age," with pharmacology rocketing forward as a science. Early on, industry scientists began collaborating with regulators and standards agencies in the form of the "Combined Contact Committee" of the American Drug Manufacturers' Association and the American Pharmaceutical Manufacturers' Association,[40] which merged in 1958 to become the Pharmaceutical Manufacturers Association. The content of the meetings the collaborations was more on forms of preparations and drug purity than drug discovery—and university scientists were, apparently, not involved.

After the late 1940s, drug discoveries were the order of the day. Talk of a golden age is of course always suspicious, a reflection more of nostalgia than of a real past. Yet looking back at psychiatric drugs and relations with industry, it does seem like a different world. Is "high-minded" too strong? As Torald Sollmann said in 1930 on the subject of trials: "Therapeutic remedies certainly need evaluating; hospitals furnish generally the best and often the only opportunity for critical therapeutic tests, and in return the hospital should profit not merely by the consciousness of doing its moral duty but also by the more healthy attitude of its staff which critical work engenders, and by the greater and more scientific interest in the treatment of its patients." Sollmann closed with a warning about industry: "Collaboration with commercial firms who do not fully understand the professional attitude and obligations involves great risk of damage to reputation."[41] Sollmann lived in a world where a doctor's "professional attitude," or reputation, was worth gold, and certainly could not be purchased for money. Hospital physicians would conduct trials as part of their "moral duty," and patients would participate in them from a desire to further science, not because they had responded to a newspaper ad and were being paid.

After the 1960s, placebo-controlled randomized controlled trials (RCTs) became the gold standard of evidence (see Chapter 10). It was the ability of industry to corrupt such trials—and the willingness of academic psychiatrists to accommodate this corruption—that greased the downhill scientific slide of psychiatry. Yet even before the Second World War, the concept of placebo controls was quite accepted, although the whole apparatus of randomized double-blind placebo-controlled trials had not yet evolved. Sollmann continued, "Apparent results must be checked by the 'blind test,' i.e., another remedy, or a placebo, without the knowledge of the observer, if possible. The placebo, in expectant treatment [a trial over time], also furnishes the comparative check of the natural course of the disease; comparison with another remedy helps toward a just perspective."[42] Lest we congratulate ourselves too heartily on our modern system of trials, bear in mind that this was said in 1930.

Diagnoses

The Age of Psychopharmacology wrapped itself tightly around two diagnoses, schizophrenia and depression (see Chapter 5). Yet both diagnoses had long histories, before the introduction of chlorpromazine in 1952 marked the beginning of the psychopharmacologic era. Psychiatry had always known psychotic illness in its acute and chronic forms. Loss of contact with reality is part of the human condition, and religious transcendence forms just as much a part of the experience as does the ingestion of psychedelics.

A shadowy figure in the background of this story is Emil Kraepelin, a professor of psychiatry in Heidelberg and Munich. In 1893, Kraepelin famously popularized the term "dementia praecox" and in 1899 made it—along with "manic-depressive insanity"—one of the two great arms of his nosology. This had the advantage of demarcating psychotic illness from psychoneurosis, which makes sense because each later acquired therapeutics of its own. Yet schizophrenia became the great beast that ate psychosis. Psychotic illness ceased to exist in any form outside of "schizophrenia."

In. those days, neither Kraepelin nor anyone else showed much interest in psychopharmacology. In 1913, in the last edition of his big textbook, of the over 200 pages dedicated to manic-depressive insanity, Kraepelin gave over three pages to "treatment"; he preferred lukewarm baths to drugs for mania and accepted, in a one-paragraph discussion, opium for depression.[43] (In his early days, Kraepelin did experiment with drugs as psychological probes, not for therapeutic purposes.)

By the 1970s, Kraepelin, the founder of modern psychiatric nosology, had been dead for half a century. But his influence lived on, and any effort to identify a medical dimension in psychiatry must be in some way labeled "Kraepelinian." Kraepelin saw the major diseases in psychiatry as "medical" in nature, meaning that they were distinctive illness entities—like tuberculosis and mumps—and they could be delineated on the basis of such clinical characteristics as course and outcome. He had little use for the study of brain anatomy in psychiatry, and he was silent on the role of the microscope, previously the field's primary research instrument for studying neural tissue. There have been quibbles about his exact importance—some writers emphasize the strong pushback his work initially encountered. Yet the quibbles were swept away by the majesty of his assertion that there were only two major disease entities in psychiatry. And this is what the field believes today, adding only anxiety. (Kraepelin refused to elevate symptoms of anxiety to the status of an independent disease entity.) The newborn psychopharmacology thus lay in a Kraepelinian cradle.

3

The Rise of Psychopharmacology

The utterly astonishing facts of the fifties were that terribly ill, hospitalized melancholics and schizophrenics often made startling improvements, including complete reversals to apparent normality, when given imipramine or chlorpromazine.—Donald Klein (2016)

The First World Congress of Psychiatry in Paris in 1950 was a vast meeting that brought together almost everybody who was anybody in the psychiatric world, including the Germans, who had previously been excluded in disgrace. At the end of a session on "biological therapies," Rudolf Karl Freudenberg, an émigré psychiatrist from Germany who had become an asylum head in England, said, "I should like to align myself with those who consider Psychiatry to be a psychophysiological science. . . . I hope that our deliberations have in fact proved that psychiatry is a psychobiological science."[1] In a psychiatry previously dominated by Freud's psychoanalysis, this was a new and refreshing perspective. (It is also interesting that Freudenberg was followed by Arthur Sackler, who with his brothers would shortly purchase the old Manhattan pharmaceutical company Purdue Pharma and turn to the manufacture of Oxycontin.) This congress was probably the founding event in the history of psychopharmacology.

These events took place against a background of psychiatry as a mature clinical discipline in Europe, with a hundred-year history, and as a fledgling sprout in the United States. The American Board of Psychiatry and Neurology was established only in 1936. In that year, the American Psychiatric Association numbered not more than 1,900 members and only six universities had residency programs based in psychiatric institutions (Johns Hopkins, Harvard, Yale, Columbia, Michigan, and Iowa).[2] Even though the number of psychoanalysts was small, psychoanalytic doctrines penetrated the teaching of the entire discipline.

Psychopharmacology itself flourished entirely outside of this academic carapace. There is no lineal connection between the early drugs, such as the barbiturates and the amphetamines—effective though they were—and the discipline of psychopharmacology. It was the new drugs like chlorpromazine that initiated the "era of psychopharmacology." Fritz Freyhan, a German émigré psychiatrist who became clinical director of the Delaware State Hospital in

Farnhurst—and a faculty member of the University of Pennsylvania—told a Senate subcommittee in 1960, "If we talk today about the era of psychopharmacology, we must remember that this is still a somewhat perplexing designation. There are people who would deny that we are in such an era. But I think that for all practical purposes we wouldn't be here today if something had not happened which had transcended all the usual delineations between clinical psychiatry and other areas of medicine. Here were drugs with such new effects that they could not be understood by anyone in terms of what had been known before."[3] Freyhan was right. It was an era, a true turning of the page.

What's in a Name?

It is probably an excess of pedantry to point out that the term "psychopharmacology," or "Psychopharmakon," first surfaced in 1548 from the pen of Reinhard Lorich, a professor of theology in Marburg, who used the term in the title of a collection of prayers for the dead.[4]

Nearly 400 years later, the first scientific use of the term "psychopharmacology" was in 1920 by Johns Hopkins pharmacologist David Macht.[5] Yet the term was not generally taken up. The first apparent use of "psychopharmacology" *in psychiatry* evidently stemmed from Melvin Wilfred Thorner, an assistant physician at Norristown State Hospital in Pennsylvania, who in 1935 dilated upon "The Psycho-pharmacology of Sodium Amytal"—he had mainly the treatment of catatonia in mind.[6]

Then the ball passed to Philadelphia—and to the argument that it was the drug industry that created psychopharmacology. In 1951, young Len Cook, at age 27 with his pharmacology PhD fresh in his pocket, had just gone to work for the Philadelphia drug house Smith Kline and French (SKF). The following year, 1952, SKF bought the license for chlorpromazine from Rhône-Poulenc, the French firm that had synthesized it. Two Smith Kline executives called Cook down to their office shortly thereafter. They said, "You know this looks like something interesting."

Cook replied, "I'm glad you said that, because from my limited experience I think we're into a whole new field. There's renal pharmacology, there's cardiovascular pharmacology etc. but I think we're into something totally new—I would call it psychopharmacology." Cook first used the term publicly in a seminar at Emory University in 1953.[7]

But not so fast, Dr. Cook! In December 1950, Jacques Gottlieb and colleagues at the University of Iowa submitted an article titled "Psychopharmacologic Study of Schizophrenia and Depressions" to the journal *Psychosomatic Medicine*. It was published in March 1952.[8] An academic priority for the University of Iowa?

THE RISE OF PSYCHOPHARMACOLOGY   29

Probably not. Probably there were dozens of other uses of the term "psychopharmacology" strewn about the literature. The point is not who has the priority—a tedious question at all events—but that in the early 1950s the concept of psychopharmacology was heavy in the air in the United States.

But how about Europe? It is a common belief among French scholars that they coined the term "psychopharmacologie." In 1950, Jean Thuillier, at the time an assistant in the psychiatry and pharmacology departments of the Paris medical school, told his examiners that his thesis, submitted to a professor of psychiatry and a professor of pharmacology, "must therefore be a psychopharmacology thesis." Thuillier said later that he knew of no previous use of the term.[9] Jean Delay was the psychiatry examiner. The usage may have clicked in his head because an article that Delay and Thuillier wrote in 1956 used the term.[10]

To be sure, in 1934, Henri Baruk, aided by funds from the Rockefeller Foundation, established what he subsequently called a "laboratoire de psychopharmacologie" at the mental hospital that he directed in the Paris suburb of Charenton.[11] Yet the lab seems to have been called at the time the "laboratoire de psychiatrie et de neurochirurgie expérimentales animals."[12] The title evidently didn't contain "psychopharmacology," because Thuillier later boasted that he had set up in 1960 at the Ste. Anne mental hospital branch of the National Institute of Health and Medical Research [INSERM], "the first institute in the world carrying the name of 'psychopharmacology.'"[13]

Word spread quickly from France to England. Willi Mayer-Gross, a Heidelberg psychiatrist who had fled to England in 1933, ended up finally at Joel Elkes' center in Birmingham. And in 1955 Mayer-Gross attended the conference on chlorpromazine that Jean Thuillier and Jean Delay had organized at Ste. Anne (see below). There, Mayer-Gross and Thuillier became friends, and Mayer-Gross invited Thuillier to come to Birmingham and lecture. Mayer-Gross introduced Thuillier: "From everything that will be said to you this evening, bear in mind this new word psychopharmacology. We already practice it here without realizing it, and everything we do tomorrow . . . everything we will want to do, will be gathered into this new discipline about which you are now going to hear."[14]

In Britain, the concept of "medical psychology" gained renewed currency, as psychiatry "moved back to its medical origins," as Anthony Clare at the Institute of Psychiatry in London, put it in 1982.[15]

"Chemical psychotherapy," "chemo-psychiatry," "behavioral pharmacology," and "experimental psychiatry" lingered briefly as rivals, then vanished. "A pharmacology preoccupied with tissues and organs is gradually giving way to a pharmacology of the behavior of total organisms," explained Elkes.[16] In 1957, Leo Hollister expressed a fondness for "pharmacotherapy" rather than "chemotherapy," "unless one truly believes in the existence of a 'schizococcus.'"[17] At a conference in Rome in 1958 that was the first formal meeting of the Collegium Internationale Neuro-Psychopharmacologicum (CINP), organized in Zurich the year previously, Delay ventured the expression "neuropsycho-chemie."[18]

The news spread even later to Canada. Heinz Lehmann, a German medical graduate at the time that he fled to Canada, was the chief of the Douglas Hospital in Montreal, and in 1957, at the time of the Second World Psychiatry Congress in Zurich, he was already a rising star. "What should the field be called?" he rhetorically asked the audience. He himself wasn't so thrilled with psychopharmacology. But even more, "What should the drugs that we are talking about be called?" There were various possibilities: "Ataractics? Tranquilizers? Neuroleptics? Happiness pills, or what?"[19]

Fifty years after Lehmann uttered these lines, we still are unclear about this. Such terms as "SSRIs" and "second-generation antipsychotics" evoke smiles from insiders.

Psychopharmacological Science

> As neurochemists tackling the problem of mental disease, we are scarcely beyond the stage of alchemy.—Alfred Pope, 1958, McLean Hospital[20]

Quite apart from drugs, in the first third of the twentieth century, neurochemistry attracted intense interest. In 1928, Nobel Laureate Richard Willstätter, emeritus professor of chemistry at the University of Munich, invited young Irvine Page to found at the nearby Psychiatric Research Institute what Page later called "the first department of neurochemistry in the world."[21] Page's *Chemistry of the Brain* (published in 1937) was a landmark volume.[22]

It would be difficult to overestimate the significance of chlorpromazine, probably the single most important drug in the history of psychiatry. Linford Rees, who pioneered clinical trials in England and was professor of psychiatry at St. Bartholomew's Hospital Medical School in London, said, "The main boost to the start of the whole science of psychopharmacology was the use of chlorpromazine in France."[23]

At Jean Delay's abovementioned conference in Paris in 1955 on chlorpromazine, Willi Mayer-Gross made it clear that there was such a thing as psychopharmacological science: "The only postulate I shall make at this juncture is that if a psychological symptom can be provoked by a drug, it will be reasonable to assume that it should also be possible to abort that symptom by pharmacological action." If one overlooks all the excited chatter about "neurotransmitters," this is as close to a general principle of drug discovery as we have, and Mayer-Gross gave examples of what the future might hold in store on the basis of this principle: depression. If reserpine can produce "a transient depressive picture," there must be drugs that can abolish it. Exactly. Two years later, imipramine was discovered. Anxiety: if hypertension can produce anxiety, drugs must be conceivable that can relieve it. Morphine, a sure reliever, was out of the question because of "the danger of addiction." Yet other agents might be conceivable? In 1955, meprobamate (Miltown) was introduced, and in 1960, Librium. How about the lack of feeling and "emotional blunting" that illness may produce? (Interestingly, he did not use the term "schizophrenia.") "Drugs are known which increase sensitivity and facilitate the irritability of nervous centers. It seems not over-optimistic to expect apparent blocking of emotions to become accessible to pharmacological therapy."[24] LSD and the hallucinogens were shortly to enter clinical medicine. Mayer-Gross, with his Heidelberg background in deep science, had made it clear that psychoanalysis was nonsense and psychiatry stood at the edge of immersion in real science.

Thus, the field began to follow science intently. Merton Sandler, then of Queen Charlotte's Hospital in London, spoke of his own early research in the late 1950s. When the latest edition of the massive *Federal Proceedings* came out, with its thousands of abstracts, Sandler would sit down and read through them carefully. "In 1957, there was a pearl in this particular oyster. It was an abstract by Armstrong and Shaw . . . that described, for the first time, the major metabolites of the catecholamines, noradrenaline and adrenaline, in the urine of patients with pheochromocytoma [a benign adrenal tumor that secretes these chemicals].[25] You wouldn't believe it, but up to 1957, we had no idea what happened to endogenous or administered noradrenaline and adrenaline." The description in this paper of various metabolites "broke the thing wide open. Julie Axelrod was immediately on to the enzyme mechanism involved, particularly catechol-O-methyltransferase (COMT). And it was partially for this reason that he won the Nobel Prize, and quite rightly." Then Sandler looked at tyramine (a product of the amino acid tyrosine) in the brain. It seemed linked to depression. "The metabolism of tyramine is largely carried out by monoamine oxidase (MAO). . . . We were able to show that in patients with unipolar depression, there was a significant deficit of tyramine conjugation with sulfate after an oral tyramine load."[26]

These were the intensely scientific origins of psychopharmacology. And the pioneers were militant about science. At the Second International Congress of Psychiatry in Zurich in 1957, Bernard Brodie, in whose lab at NIH the principle of neuronal reuptake had been discovered, deplored the readiness of many participants to jump directly to "schizophrenia" without first understanding "the normal functioning of the brain. I should feel more confident for the future of my car if it were fixed by a mechanic who knew how the normal engine worked."[27]

At the NIMH meeting on psychopharmacology in 1956, one participant said rather sarcastically, after a science-laden committee report, "I would like to ask the committee where they make allowance for the art of medicine in setting up their various scientific protocols." Jonathan Cole, the head of the NIMH's Psychopharmacology Service Center (PSC), immediately responded, "I think we have been talking here today about science. We are talking about the body of data which can be repeated, about which there is something repeatable, which can be communicated from one person to another. We have tried to get away from the art of medicine, which is very difficult to communicate. I, myself, would prefer to see a little more science and a little less art in this field."[28]

It is a measure of the alienation of the new field from psychoanalysis that, with the exception of Jon Cole, not one of the other organizers of the conference—Seymour Kety, Ralph Gerard, Joseph Brady, or Louis Lasagna—was a psychiatrist.[29]

Launch

There are sciences that are "theory driven," but, as David Healy pointed out, psychopharmacology is not one of them.[30] It is driven by events, and new drugs kept continually being discovered that challenged the old theories.

Two events directed the work of the budding psychopharmacologists, said neurochemist Theodore Sourkes. One was the synthesis of lysergic acid diethylamide (LSD) in the laboratories of Sandoz in Basel in 1938. LSD could produce a psychosis that seemed (to the eye of faith) a lot like schizophrenic psychosis. Here was "the possibility that schizophrenia was caused by a toxic substance." Second was the discovery in France in 1952 that chlorpromazine seemed to treat psychosis directly, tamping down the symptoms. This held out the possibility "of a chemical treatment of a mental disorder."[31] Both perspectives were startling.

On these two tracks, psychopharmacological investigation was launched.[32] Psychiatry does owe a profound debt to biology. As Ralph Gerard at the University of Michigan, one of the pioneers of biological thinking in psychiatry, put it in 1955, "When experience leaves an enduring trace, it must be some sort of material imprint. . . . There can be no twisted thought without a twisted molecule."[33] Biochemistry thus rushed into psychiatry's midfield. English psychiatrist Max Hamilton came to work in Elkes' service at St. Elizabeths Hospital in Washington DC, where he developed his famous depression scale. Hamilton later said, "Long ago, I came to the conclusion that ultimately the discoveries in psychiatry were going to be made by biochemists. . . . [But] the clinician is still critical. He is the man who leads the biochemist through the jungle."[34]

Simultaneously, interest in neurochemistry and in the neurosciences as a whole was blossoming. Investigators were pursuing such issues as whether acetylcholine plays a role in the transmission of the nerve impulse.[35] And from these sprouts emerged the enormous latter-day apparatus of neuroscience research. Yet these developments are not considered here, because at the practical level there is virtually no spillover from neuroscience and neurochemistry into psychopharmacology. It is hard to think of a single development in psychopharm that was triggered, or influenced, by a research advance in neuroscience. Advances in psychopharmacology took place either through serendipity, as apparent "side effects" from a molecule were actively pursued for independent therapeutic value on their own (e.g., the chlorpromazine story), or through the efforts of neurochemists who were working in industrial labs, as in the discovery of the benzodiazepines in the labs of Roche. There are examples of investigators who stood astride both camps, such as Joel Elkes, who organized the Oxford symposium on "The Biochemistry of the Developing Nervous System" in 1954 and who with his wife, Charmian, led the first chlorpromazine trials—but there are not many.[36] Of course, the initial discovery of neuronal reuptake occurred in a semi-academic, not an industrial, setting—namely, in Bernard Brody's lab in the National Heart Institute. But this trail grew indistinct as science (see below) and became fluorescent in the advertising copy of industry.

End of Psychoanalysis

> The danger of thinking of psychiatry as fundamentally a psychological field and not a medical specialty.—Michael Alan Taylor (2013)[37]

When Henry Brill introduced chlorpromazine to the huge mental hospital on Long Island, Pilgrim State, around 1954, he knew he was taking a big risk. In an environment dominated by psychotherapy, "pills" were viewed with hostility; Frank Ayd, a leading psychopharmacologist at Taylor Manor Hospital in Maryland, said, if Brill's patients had developed notable side effects, "the opponents would have gone for his head."[38]

Psychoanalysis turned out to be a terrible idea for psychiatry. But in trashing psychoanalysis, we are not trashing the mind. Psychiatry correctly treats the mind as an intervening link between brain and behavior. Paul McHugh, professor of psychiatry at Johns Hopkins and a foundational figure, said in 1998, "Psychiatrists cannot go directly from knowing the elements of brain (neurons and synapses) to explaining the conscious experiences that are the essence of mental life. . . . In other words, psychiatry cannot be replaced by neurology because brain facts cannot be substituted for mind facts." "The mind is an experience; the brain is a physical structure. They are *not* identical."[39] Too true. And in psychopharmacology one had the possibility of treating disorders that were *brain-generated*, such as melancholia and catatonia, and those that were *mind-generated*, such as PTSD and varieties of anxiety. The point, however, is that the study of mind-generated disorders was dominated at the beginning by the psychoanalysts, the adepts of Freud.

The analysts hated the new meds. One leading researcher on "tranquilizers" told a colleague around 1957 in a private note, "You are probably aware that there are a fairly well entrenched group of psychiatrists who have not written an Rx since they left medical school and whose entire way of life is threatened by the startling and sudden fact that psychiatry will no longer be limited to verbal persiflage."[40] Psychiatrists who had never written a prescription! Things were really about to change.

When Barney Carroll took over the adult inpatient psychiatry unit at the University of Michigan in 1973, he introduced a very different tone. The average length of stay in the 26-bed unit had been 18 months. (The average length of stay on the children's inpatient units was "over 4 years.") "In short order, George [Curtis] and I got the length of stay on our service down to around 6–7 weeks, which allowed us to get to know the patients, [and] to perform a supervised withdrawal of their previous, ineffective, drug treatments. . . . At the same time, we were able to conduct meaningful clinical research. [The psychoanalysts had done none.] By today's standards, however, even a 6-week length of stay would be considered scandalous [scandalously long]."[41]

It is hard now, in retrospect, to imagine the hold that psychoanalysis once exercised on psychiatry. Among insiders, it made the United States internationally a subject of curiosity. Michael Shepherd, a leading figure at the Maudsley Hospital in London, said in 1957 of psychoanalysis, "In the USA a remarkable attempt has been made in many centers to inject the whole system, python-like, into the body of academic opinion."[42] The psychoanalyst, or "my shrink," became the standard go-to figure for any mental issue. The parents of Jason, age 8, feared that he might be gay and took him to the "psychoanalyst," where he remained in treatment for his purported homosexuality for 4 years.[43]

Max Fink recalled that, around 1946, when he was just starting psychiatric training at Fort Sam Houston as an Army doctor, "One-third of the course was training in psychoanalysis," the rest on general psychiatry and neurology. "The reality was that everyone at that time thought psychoanalysis was the future of psychiatry."[44]

In the early 1960s, Don Klein went to work in psychoanalytically oriented Hillside Hospital on Long Island. He and Max Fink were the only two clinicians in the hospital allowed to write prescriptions; the rest of the staff administered psychotherapy. "At the time, everyone was called schizophrenic," Klein said. "Nobody was thinking diagnostically. To think in terms of systematic descriptive

diagnosis was [in the eyes of the analysts] a sure mark of a superficial mind because everybody knew that that was just the symptomatic manifestations of the
internal conflicts, which is where the real action was."[45] But, after 10 months of
psychotherapy, somebody would kick a nurse and Klein would be called in. He
was able to achieve remissions.

The infatuation with psychoanalysis put American psychiatry in an anoma-
lous international position. The United States was the only major country where
a contempt for diagnosis had become gospel. Carroll said, looking back, "Much
of the perceived unreliability in psychiatric diagnosis in the early 1970s was geographic. USA was the outlier. . . . In the rest of the world, there was generally good
reliability for differential diagnoses like melancholic/endogenomorphic depression versus reaction/neurotic depression or like schizophrenia versus mood disorder. The US side were the outliers. They were not just unreliable—they were
wrong."[46]

According to Harvard's Mandel Cohen, who was the godparent of biological psychiatry in the United States, "At one time in the early 1960s there
were . . . only two people with professorships in the whole country who were not
psychoanalysts: Eli Robins [at Washington University of St. Louis] and me. Most
departments wouldn't have anybody who wasn't a psychoanalyst. You can't prove
this, but it's true."[47] Robins was a student of Cohen's.

Jan Fawcett, later professor of psychiatry in Chicago, began his career at NIMH
in the early 1960s under the supervision of psychoanalytically oriented Dexter
Bullard from Chestnut Lodge in a suburb of Washington. "We were expected to
treat them with psychotherapy. I would see my patients every day, sometimes
seven days a week. They were extremely sick, psychotically depressed and highly
suicidal manic depressive patients. . . . To see the effects when we eventually put
them on medication was mind boggling."[48]

The psychoactive drugs were a body blow against psychoanalysis, because
with a few weeks of drug therapy you could make better patients who had spent
years "on the couch" and still had their depressive symptoms. At first, the analysts
pretended that the new drugs had no intrinsic efficacy, and if they seemed successful in state asylums, it was only because of the suggestive effects of the staff.
Psychoanalyst Mel Sabshin, later medical director of the APA and at the time
a staffer at the psychoanalytically oriented Institute for Psychosomatic and
Psychiatric Research and Training of the Michael Reese Hospital in Chicago, said
in 1956 that the staff were very oriented to "psychodynamic principles." The staff
found somatotherapy "distasteful." "One of the nurses said that she felt positive
toward insulin therapy [only because] the patient had eight hours of close contact with another person during the treatment." In his view, when chlorpromazine did (exceptionally) work on patients, it was because the prescribing doctor
gave the patients "a good deal of extra care."[49]

Then the analysts responded to the new discipline with a kind of generalized irritability. Psychoanalyst Roy Grinker, Sr., at the Michael Reese Hospital, said at a meeting in 1969 in Williamsburg, Virginia, "Now I will plead with you to drop the word phenomenology."[50] (He meant, stop talking about specific signs and symptoms.)

Jonathan Cole, director of the NIMH's PSC, said that drugs were sometimes given in "a very psychoanalytic setting. When a patient got a drug, the nurses would all go to the patient and say, 'Oh! You poor thing; you should be getting psychotherapy!' Patients who got drugs were pitied, babied, and made much of, and everyone thought it was a great shame whenever drugs were used."[51] Ralph Gerard had come from Michigan to Bethesda in 1956 to co-organize with Cole a conference at NIMH on psychopharmacology. Gerard addressed Chestnut Lodge psychoanalyst Frieda Fromm-Reichmann's theory that schizophrenia was caused by distant "refrigerator" mothers. Gerard told the conference, "To deal with a mother in terms of the conviction that schizophrenia in a child can only be due to maternal rejection can constitute a major trauma to her."[52]

Like two ends of a disciplinary teeter-totter, as psychopharmacology rose, psychoanalysis declined. Samuel Barondes, later chair of psychiatry at the University of California at San Francisco, who trained in psychiatry at McLean Hospital in Belmont, Massachusetts—an institution then much given over to psychotherapy—recalled, "[Drugs] were frowned upon at McLean at that time. I had two schizophrenic patients I treated during the whole three years I was a resident with psychotherapy but no medications. Both were adolescents with paranoid schizophrenia." He saw them three times a week for an hour of psychotherapy. His supervisor, Alfred Stanton, was the chief of psychiatry at McLean, and Barondes and Stanton would review tapes of the sessions. "But there was no discussion of medication." One of the patients couldn't walk in downtown Boston because he had the feeling the buildings were about to fall over on him. Barondes said, "I think this delusion would have dissolved if he were treated with Thorazine. I feel sad he wasn't treated properly because my teachers believed drugs didn't work very well. . . . It's ironic that over the years McLean became a major site for research on psychopharmaceuticals."[53]

The analysts fought back with the argument that psychopharmacology treated only "symptoms" without getting at the "root causes," which only psychoanalysis was able to discern. Fritz Freyhan, an émigré psychiatrist who had become research director of the Delaware State Hospital, gave that argument short shrift at the Second World Congress on Psychiatry in Zurich in 1957: "I always feel perplexed about the arbitrary division into symptomatic and curative therapies. In the absence of specific knowledge on the etiology of most mental disorders, one therapy is as symptomatic as the next. To advocate any therapy as directed at the illness process is at this stage of our knowledge pure conjecture."[54]

Psychoanalysis began to drift from the Main Street consulting rooms down to the psychiatric "street." Eric Strömgren, professor of psychiatry at Aarhus University in Denmark, said of psychoanalysis in the 1960s in Scandinavia, "One characteristic figure emerged: the bearded workers in the mental health field who detested genetics, preached psychoanalysis, and declared an allegiance to communism."[55]

With the launch of the first blockbuster drug in psychopharmacology in 1955, meprobamate, the field began choking on psychoanalysis. Finally, even at Chestnut Lodge, they surrendered. After Robert Cohen left NIMH in 1981, the administrators of the Lodge wanted him to come back (Cohen had been there much earlier). Cohen said, "They were running into problems, because the younger doctors who were engaged in psychoanalytic training didn't want to give medications to their patients at all, and [the administrators] thought that since I was a very senior person, I would be able to get them to use medication."[56]

Years on the couch replaced by . . . a pill. For Burton Angrist, a resident at Bellevue, the replacement happened rapidly. When he started his residency, he was, he said, "excited [by psychoanalysis] and couldn't wait to begin healing the sick with my clever psychotherapeutic insights. The only problem was that the sick were inconsiderate enough not to get better." How to sort this out? He consulted with Don Klein, the research psychopharmacologist. "Don generously reviewed my patients in detail and made suggestions about changes in dose, drug, etc. They all improved! I was *floored* and decided to get postdoctoral training in psychopharmacology."[57]

Thus, a page turned in the history of psychiatry. As Ralph Gerard said in 1957, "More than a billion meprobamate tablets alone have been ordered by their physicians for 160 million Americans in a little more than a year. . . . Psychiatrists of all schools . . . find their views shaken or supported by the emphatic re-entry of the brain into the mental arena." The piece was titled, "Drugs for the Soul: The Rise of Psychopharmacology."[58]

I cannot resist contrasting Ralph Gerard's piece with the words of the nameless physician of Mlle. Julie de Lespinasse, a popular Paris hostess, in the 1770s: Realizing that her problems were all emotional in nature, he told her, "We have no medicine for the soul."[59] Finally, Ralph Gerard proved him wrong!

A Culture of Psychopharmacology?

Robert Spitzer: "DSM has become a cultural event. No-one noticed the publication of DSM-II, but DSM-III and DSM-IV have actually become cultural events in that even the mainstream media take notice. It is amazing. I guess it defines things."[60]

Psychopharmacology became a kind of cultural reflex, a concept that made sense when all else failed. In the coronavirus lockdown of 2020, when everyone was going crazy staying at home, Gina Bellafante, a color writer for the *New York Times,* riffed in April on how the world had changed. "Had you told me at Thanksgiving that in six months we would all be confined to our homes and facing shortages of toilet paper, . . . I would have hugged you and smiled, and quietly called your psychopharmacologist to suggest adjustments."[61]

Psychiatry has always been up for adjustments. The field has functioned as society's moral gatekeeper, as evident in the diagnosis of "hysteria," in the traditional pathologizing of homosexuality, or in the rejection of sexual roleplaying as "sadism." Similarly, psychopharmacology has functioned as a means of throttling politically or socially undesirable trends. The early 1970s saw the beginning of female emancipation. Thus, an ad for Roche's Librium (chlordiazepoxide) told family docs: "Many women consider the roles of wife and mother to be inferior. A growing number deeply resent what they consider to be their 'second-class citizenship.' Indeed, in their resentment, some women may rebel not only against the feminine role in society but against femininity itself."[62] So, if you've got one of those malcontents in the chair in front of you, tranquilize her with Librium. Roche's message to budding feminists: Put a sock in it!

Psychopharmacology helped reorient attitudes to psychiatric disease. Illnesses untreatable for centuries had now suddenly become treatable. Thuillier said that psychiatry began to rejoin the rest of medicine "and definitively reintegrated itself in the 1950s with the discoveries of 'psychopharmacology' and with the new psychotropic medications (neuroleptics and tranquilizers). It was then that people started being less afraid of madness. Patients interned for long years returned to their family. . . . The madman was no longer insane, but a patient like all the others."[63] Under these circumstances, a culture of psychopharmacology started to develop for which there are few counterparts elsewhere in the sciences (there is no culture of optical crystallography).

But there were positive aspects, too, such as the impact of the new drugs on the mental-hospital environment. For the study of the hospital setting, a WHO working group proposed in 1958 the term "social pharmacology." They noted that the size and "atmosphere" of a psychiatric ward affected the amount of chlorpromazine or reserpine a patient could tolerate. The drug therapies changed the hospital culture by "mobilizing large chronic populations hitherto secluded in the continued-treatment units of the average mental hospital." This was bureaucratic speech for "back wards."

The new treatments abolished the hospital back wards, before, indeed, abolishing the mental hospitals themselves. The new drugs made possible the concept of "rehabilitation," which, the committee noted, "would have been very difficult to achieve in their absence." And, finally, the new drugs "have increased and made more urgent the contacts between the mental hospital and the community." This increased porousness of the hitherto tight barrier between hospital and community went under the name "social and community psychiatry."[64]

These were massive changes in the culture of the hospital. As Nate Kline apostrophized to a meeting of the ACNP in his presidential address in 1967, "We are probably only at the beginning of an era and still very much in the process of creating a new 'science' which may well alter the course of man's cultural and possibly his biological evolution."[65] Wow! For the early psychopharmacologists the sky was the limit: the drugs could create a new culture!

Kline was creating a legitimate drug culture as well as a science. A foundational creed of this culture was that people belonged on drugs and needed to *stay* on them. In the last years of his professional life, Mickey Nardo practiced in a charity medical clinic in the Appalachian hills of Georgia. There, everyone was on medications. "There's enormous pressure to medicate coming from the patients," he said. "It's not just that they expect medications, they want them— even the patients dissatisfied with the results. I think that must be why each new drug that comes along has a waiting following. I was taught [to] think of most depressions as time limited, but the patients in the clinic don't seem to think that way. A surprising number see them as an ongoing need."[66]

Then there were changes in the community culture. The uptake of the benzodiazepines in the 1960s and 1970s foreshadowed the massive success of the SSRIs in later decades. And, so popular were the benzos that the 1960s and 1970s were labeled by journalists the Age of Anxiety (and were so labeled in Librium ads as well), although the age was rather brief.

LSD became a recreational drug, and Harvard's Timothy Leary famously invited an entire generation to "turn on, tune in, and drop out." A number of other hallucinogens joined LSD on the street, and the drug culture of the 1960s was directly spawned by the success of psychopharmacology in producing hallucinogens.

But even off the street and in the living room, the belief arose that such elements of the human condition as tension and anxiety could be alleviated chemically. This would have been true of the barbiturates since 1903, but Luminal did not receive the same ferocious marketing as the new drugs. In March 1963, Fritz Freyhan told a Senate committee that drugs like meprobamate (Miltown) and Librium were "given, I believe, in a very liberal fashion in the hope that any sort of manifestation of anxiety, tension, or nervousness can be alleviated."

Hubert Humphrey, Senator from Minnesota (and former pharmacist), then observed, "In making a layman's tabulation of these so-called tranquilizers or drugs that deal with anxiety and relaxation of tension, we find that there are 39 so-called antidepressives, 100 sedative muscle relaxers, 17 phenothiazine derivatives [such as chlorpromazine], and 33 nonphenothiazine derivates, and many more." Freyhan then allowed that that was a lot. "There is, undoubtedly, overuse of tranquilizing drugs. . . . [Yet] I do not believe that there is a danger in the sense suggested by [Aldous] Huxley: That we may have kind of a tranquilized society which no longer is aware of political and other dangers, and that this may put us at a great disadvantage." So, in disclaiming Huxley's dystopian vision, Freyhan said, "I suspect that many people who take tranquilizers find out quickly enough that the medicine neither solves their personal problems nor absolves them from the experience of anxiety."[67] Here, the fear was that mass consumption of psychotropics might put us "at a disadvantage" vis-à-vis the Soviet Union. The Cold War was at its height. Was the country sinking into a culture of psychopharmacology?

(The term "tranquilizer," in use in the 1950s and early 1960s, embraced what we think of as quite disparate drug classes: all three of SmithKline's phenothiazines were marketed as tranquilizers, and in 1959 SKF had about one third of the total tranquilizer market[68]; but Wallace Labs' Miltown and Wyeth's Equanil, different brands of meprobamate, were also considered tranquilizers, although they had little antipsychotic value; and reserpine, Ciba's Serpasil, introduced in 1953 for hypertension, was the first real "tranquilizer," said to have a "calming effect."[69])

Part of the culture of psychopharmacology was the cultivation of diagnoses as a way of managing failed lives. Of course, not all patients with diagnoses have failed lives, but for some the diagnoses do provide cover. Max Fink, with decades of clinical experience, reflected in 2017 on, "The image of problems in adolescence, failure to successfully manage the transition to an independent, self-sustaining worker and family, ending with social failure, imagined thoughts and feelings, relief by alcohol, cannabis and opioids leading to social dysfunctions that the society labels either schizophrenia or bipolar disorder. As the subjects get older, the label changes to major depressive disorder." But then, Fink continued, some have real diseases. "Catatonia and melancholia take subjects out of this social failure world into a systemic medical world as these disorders are quite specific—identifiable, verifiable, and treatable—disorders that are ignored by the profession, happy in their delusions of schizophrenia, bipolar disorder, major depressive disorder, and substance abuse that mark the populations of psychiatric clinics."[70] Hence, the main psychiatric diagnoses served as rationalizations for failed lives—while the real diseases languished unrecognized by the profession. This is an interesting perspective and not necessarily unrealistic.

The Story Moves On

At a certain point, the baton passed from the United Kingdom and France to the United States. In the 1960s and 1970s, Americans were still enmeshed in psychoanalysis and the English had more or less free run internationally. Thereafter, this changed. Malcolm Lader, a pioneering investigator at the Institute of Psychiatry (attached to the Maudsley Hospital in London), was acutely aware of this. He said, "You have to remember that the United States was not interested in drugs. I was lucky, we had almost a 30-year clear run in the 1960s and 1970s when the Americans were not doing much psychopharmacology. It was only then that they finally gave up their flirtation with psychoanalysis and moved into psychopharmacology, and of course with their resources they've swamped the subject."[71]

In 1955, Albert Kurland at the Springfield State Hospital in Maryland helped begin the story. After an early chlorpromazine trial, he said, as Jon Cole recalled, "Gee, this stuff does something I've never seen before." He took out a second mortgage on his home, bought SmithKline stock, "and made a fair amount of money out of it."[72]

In 2017, Donald Klein at the New York State Psychiatric Institute wrapped up the story: "Chlorpromazine and imipramine had astounding unpredicted benefits on hospitalized patients with severe illnesses. Further, there was a rough correspondence with ancient phenotypes—psychosis and melancholia. Sounds like a good place to start." Glistening beginning! "Progress was terrific up to 1980s, when the salesmen took over."[73]

4

Things Get Rolling

In the dismal state hospitals, tiny little bells of hope began to ring. The take-off of psychopharmacology in the mental-hospital world began in the vast asylum system of New York State in the early 1950s. In 1953, Henry Brill, assistant state commissioner of mental hygiene, convened a conference on chlorpromazine. In 1955, he ordered the state system to introduce chlorpromazine, which led to the first decrease in the census of the state asylum system in peacetime. Under Brill's direction, some of the state hospitals began setting up psychopharmacology research units: In 1954, Sidney Merlis became director of research at the Central Islip Hospital. In 1955, Herman ("Hy") Denber set up a similar unit at the Manhattan State Hospital on Ward's Island. The new drugs were implemented in all these hospitals, and Brill, Denber, and Merlis—who count among the pioneers of psychopharmacology in the United States—began a series of publications on the drugs and their efficacy. In this way, psychopharmacology began its advance on the ground.

Ideas for a New Field

In December 1954, Nathan Kline at Rockland State Hospital in Orangeburg, New York, organized a symposium in Berkeley on "psychopharmacology." The symposium was jointly sponsored by the American Association for the Advancement of Science and the American Psychiatric Association. Kline said it was "the first major conference on the use of . . . new pharmaceuticals in the field of mental disease." Merlis and Denber were in attendance. The program was a roster of who was who in the budding science: Hollister and colleagues at the VA in Palo Alto reported their double-blinds trials of chlorpromazine and reserpine; Anthony Sainz from Syracuse talked about the cerebral action of reserpine; and Vernon Kinross-Wright from Baylor—famous for his ultra-high doses of chlorpromazine—discussed his clinical experiences.[1]

It was at such conferences that the young science jelled. In October 1956, the New York Academy of Sciences held a small session on the drug meprobamate. Gerald Sarwer-Foner, who came down from Montreal for the meeting, said later, "The psychiatrists in state hospitals believed that these drugs, reserpine and chlorpromazine, were antipsychotic drugs." Ignorant of the Paris World Congress, he wrote, "That was the beginning of psychopharmacology."[2]

In 1951 in England, pharmacologist and psychiatrist Joel Elkes established at the University of Birmingham the first department of experimental psychiatry in the world. It consisted of animal laboratories plus a 40-bed clinical unit. Also in Birmingham, in a local hospital, Charmian and Joel Elkes conducted the first blinded controlled trial of chlorpromazine (see Chapter 10). To give a sense of how fast things were moving, around 1953, Martin Roth, a biological psychiatrist in Newcastle, spent a sabbatical year at the Allan Memorial Institute in Montreal, the psychiatric department of McGill University. And Roth persuaded Theodore Sourkes, a biochemist in McGill's Department of Psychiatry, to collaborate. It was at Roth's initiative that, in the fall of 1955, Elkes invited Sourkes to come to Birmingham and give a series of lectures on "biochemical psychiatry."[3]

It is really the task of the academy to create science. But psychopharmacology was originated by hospital clinicians and industry; academics were Johnny Come Lately's. George Simpson told David Healy in an interview, "You had Heinz Lehmann in Montreal, Fritz Freyhan in Delaware, [Vernon] Kinross-Wright in Texas [Houston], Nate [Kline, in Rockland State hospital], [Herman] Denber, and Tony Sainz up in Syracuse. The drug companies also were here, so it was easier to go to your own back door than go elsewhere. But the early people were all hospital based. . . . Psychopharmacology began in the state hospitals and the VA and had to almost hammer the doors of academia down."[4]

Yet, even as the research institutes chanted "Science! Science!" uncertainty lingered that psychopharmacology was a real science of its own rather than a hybrid between two disciplines that otherwise didn't have that much to say to each other. Mogens Schou, the Danish clinician who conducted large-scale randomly controlled trials to show that lithium could prevent depressive relapses, said in 1959, "Psychopharmacology has been maliciously defined as 'the science in which psychiatrists try to be biochemists and biochemists to be psychiatrists.'"[5]

NIMH Misses an Opportunity

Yet, amidst this shower of initiatives, nothing matched the historical heft of the National Institute of Mental Health (NIMH), founded in 1949 in Bethesda, Maryland, as part of the National Institutes of Health. In-house research at NIMH was divided between "clinical," led by Robert Cohen, and "basic," led by Seymour Kety—a physiologist turned "psychiatrist" whose influence on psychiatry was so profound that he is sometimes referred to as "the father of biological psychiatry."[6] The "intramural" (in-house) research program at NIMH opened in 1953, and it was headed after 1957 by David Hamburg. From this intramural program flowed much of the research in psychopharmacology done in the United States. The clinical arms of the program were the beds at the Clinical Center, on campus at NIMH, and at St. Elizabeths Hospital, an asylum in Washington DC. In 1957, Joel Elkes opened the Clinical Neuropharmacological Research Center at St. Elizabeths. He had come over from Birmingham at the invitation of Cohen. (The name of the hospital is customarily written without an apostrophe.)

Following the conference, in 1956 NIMH also organized the Psychopharmacology Service Center (PSC) under Jon Cole, with the task of helping academic centers—often working jointly—to assess the new drugs.[7] This effort needed federal funding, because early investigators often found themselves overly dependent on Pharma for funding—and predisposed to favorable results.[8] In the late 1950s, the Center also granted research funds directly to several pharmaceutical houses.[9] Yet the PSC's ties to industry swiftly slackened under the influence of patent concerns (see Chapter 6), keeping Pharma's data secret, and a general fear that the PSC might turn into some kind of regulatory agency.

Under the PSC, the Early Clinical Drug Evaluation Unit (ECDEU) was established, which in 1960 began reviewing proposals for establishing local ECDEUs.[10] In the late 1950s, Congress had expressed interest in a program to evaluate the "tranquilizers," of which the antipsychotics were one component. And it was out of this program that, in 1957, Cole got an antipsychotic research program going at the VA hospitals, the first involving the VA facility at Downey, Illinois; chlorpromazine and promazine were the antipsychotics of choice.[11] Cole then organized a big nine-hospital trial of the phenothiazines in schizophrenia that in 1964 showed the effectiveness of these new drugs.[12]

The impact of the ECDEU on the field of psychopharmacology was huge: by the later 1960s, some 359 studies had been undertaken at 35 units; its impact on academic psychiatry, still enmeshed in the "unconscious," was, as Leo Hollister observed in 1970, close to zero.[13] In any event, in 1966, the PSC changed its name to the Psychopharmacology Research Branch; it got out of the business of funding external drug trials, and the ECDEU was dissolved in the mid-1970s. Therewith, the evaluation of pharmaceutical agents fell entirely into the hands of industry. One looks back with regret at the failure of the federal government to further involve itself in drug trials. A great turning point was missed.

NIMH and Depression

The NIMH spotlight turned on depression. In November 1964, Frances Kelsey, famed as the whistleblower on thalidomide and then an executive in the FDA's Bureau of Medicine, penned a note about colleague William (Biff) Bunney, Jr.'s "investigation of the possibility that depression may be related to specific catecholamine levels in the brain."[14] Bunney had wanted to study, among other agents, L-dopa. (Catecholamines, derived from the amino acid tyrosine, also include such neurotransmitters as norepinephrine.)

A new biological research agenda at NIMH was thus launched in 1965 when Biff Bunney and John Davis in the Adult Psychiatry Branch, in their project on the biochemistry of depression, proposed a research agenda about a link of the neurotransmitter norepinephrine to depression. They argued that, "Patients who are prone to depression may be sensitive to depletion of norepinephrine."[15] (Joseph Schildkraut at Harvard had just opened up a "norepinephrine hypothesis of depression"—see Chapter 8.) This was not work conducted at a high level of neurochemical theory. "We didn't know what a catechol was," said Davis later. "So my first question to Biff was, 'What's a catechol?' And, he didn't know either."[16]

"Experimental Psychiatry"

In August 1951, Joel Elkes, amid an American kind of scientific Cook's Tour, was chatting with Columbia biochemist Heinrich Waelsch, just before Elkes' return to Birmingham. Waelsch asked him "What is experimental psychiatry?" Elkes at that point did not have a good answer, and, to help the field jell, in 1954 Elkes arranged the first of a series of international symposia. At the first meeting, in Oxford in July 1954, the term "neurochemistry" was introduced, said Elkes, or at least it was used for the first time prominently at a conference. Waelsch edited the proceedings.[17]

The New York State Psychiatric Institute, jointly run by Columbia University and the New York State Mental Hospital system, and known as "PI," was a stout bastion of psychopharmacological research. Starting in 1948, Phillip Polatin, a 1929 graduate of New York Medical College, supervised at PI a large number of drug trials for different companies, including a trial of Ciba's *Rauwolfia serpentina* (reserpine) for "anxiety"; the trials were invariably small and uncontrolled. Yet it was pretty apparent whether a drug worked or not. Polatin had trained in psychoanalysis, and the purpose of the trials often seemed to be making the patients more accessible to psychotherapy.[18]

In the wake of the excitement caused by chlorpromazine (see Chapter 3), in 1955 the PI founded a Department of Experimental Psychiatry under the direction of Sidney Malitz. The department functioned in collaboration with the nearby Vanderbilt Clinic and was financed by a grant from NIMH. Malitz said at a conference at McGill University in 1959 that PI had set a special ward aside "for the evaluation of new psychopharmacologic agents." The agent that he and his colleagues were investigating at the moment was the first tricyclic antidepressant, imipramine (Tofranil).[19]

Thus, a number of new concepts, such as the PI's "experimental psychiatry," came into the mix that became psychopharmacology. In May 1954, the Josiah Macy Jr. Foundation sponsored a conference on "Neuropharmacology" in Princeton. Heavy-hitters like Kety from NIMH and Hudson Hoagland from the Worcester Foundation for Experimental Biology in Shrewsbury, Massachusetts, were in attendance. Four more conferences followed. The focus was drugs and the brain, not drugs and the mind.[20]

In 1959, Karl Rickels founded the Clinical Psychopharmacology Research Unit at the University of Pennsylvania, and in that year he received his first NIMH grant for drug study. From this base, in the early 1960s Rickels organized a whole family-practice trial network for outpatients. Known as the "Rickels group," the Unit at Penn specialized in what were then called the "minor tranquilizers" for anxiety disorders.[21]

Meanwhile, on the Continent

Meanwhile, on the Continent, events were also moving rapidly. In October 1955, Jean Delay held an "international colloquium on chlorpromazine and neuroleptic medications in psychiatric treatment."[22] It was this symposium that introduced the concept of "neuroleptic," which Delay understood, at a typically high level of abstraction, as "reducing psychological tension." Some have wanted to see this conference as the beginning of psychopharmacology, which it was not: Too many events preceded it to grant it priority. But, in fairness, the 1955 conference was the beginning of the *science* of psychopharmacology.

At the conference, some investigators, such as Fritz Flügel of Erlangen, called explicitly for pushing the dose of chlorpromazine to the point of producing frank Parkinsonian symptoms.[23] (Hans-Joachim Haase had initially described this "neuroleptic threshold" in 1954.[24]) "Neurolepsis" thus became a recipe for increasing the dosing until Parkinsonian rigidity and dyskinesia set in; these belonged to the so-called extrapyramidal symptoms of antipsychotic medication. As Hy Denber said in 1957, "Agents having very few physiologic or toxic effects are usually without action in the psychoses. The ability to induce an extrapyramidal action is a *sine qua non* of therapeutic effectiveness."[25] The amounts were often huge, and it was not unusual to find American psychiatrists dosing chlorpromazine at up to 2,000 milligrams a day.

In May 1957, Italian pharmacologist Silvio Garattini organized a large psychopharmacology meeting in Milan at which the idea for an important organization, the International College of Neuropharmacology, germinated (CINP are its Latin initials). David Healy viewed Garattini's 1957 book *Psychotropic Drugs* as "the first modern book on psychopharmacology."[26] (Yet another candidate for this could be Cologne professor Wolfgang de Boor's 1956 book—written in German and without much impact.[27]) A primal force in launching CINP was Sandoz's director of pharmacology, Ernst Rothlin. This was the first contact between industry and the new academic psychopharmacology. (There had previously been numerous contacts between psychiatry and industry—see Chapter 6.) Tom Ban pointed out, "It was very important to have someone of Rothlin's stature to bridge with industry because psychiatry was so slow to join."[28]

National psychopharmacology associations began to be founded. The first was the Czech association, established in 1959. The psychiatrist-director of the spa in Gräfenberg invited a research team from the Ministry of Health to spend a week there in the low season of early January. Said Oldrich Vinar, "When he invited us, I suggested that he also invite others who were interested in psychopharmacology because he had enough rooms to accommodate all of us and we could discuss the results openly. This was how the annual meetings started."[29]

As a kind of capstone to these events, in November 1960, Theodore Rothman, a Los Angeles psychiatrist, convoked at the Barbizon Plaza Hotel in New York a meeting designed to bring clinicians and basic scientists together. They decided that an American–Canadian organization was needed, and in October 1961, at the Woodner Hotel in Washington DC, the first meeting of the American College of Neuropsychopharmacology (ACNP) was held. ("Neuro" meant experimental research on animals; "psycho" meant investigations in patients.) Joel Elkes was elected the first president.[30]

There was a paradox here. All agreed that the proper classification of diseases, or nosology, became urgent with the new drug set, because you wouldn't prescribe the antimanic drug lithium for obsessive-compulsive disorder, and so forth. There had to be some differentiation. Yet the new psychopharmacology sounded the death knell of the old psychopathology, or careful individuation of diseases. The psychoanalysts were indifferent to psychopathology, yet not everyone else was. And in the pre-pharmaceutical era, a lot of ink was spilled in Europe over how many different ways there were to cut psychosis, for example. This interest now evaporated, because with only one drug class, "antipsychotics," you needed only one "psychosis." If there was only one nail, all you needed was one hammer.

Research Takes a Biological Turn

As these psychopharmacological shoots sprouted, at the same time research took a biological turn. Psychoanalysis yielded very little that could qualify as "research." It was mainly the recounting of clinical anecdotes. But as the science of the therapeutics of brain and mind started to be rediscovered, systematic research into the main diagnoses, such as depression and schizophrenia, revived. A landmark was the massive tome, *Psychopharmacology, A Review of Progress: 1957–1967*, cosponsored in 1968 by the ACNP and the Psychopharmacology Research Branch of NIMH. Here, Joseph Schildkraut at Harvard, John Davis at NIMH, and Gerald Klerman at Yale revived the subject of the "biochemistry of depressions" that had long slumbered.[31] They were all heavy hitters, and their work had a sentinel effect.

Led by Max Fink at New York Medical College and Charles Shagass at McGill University, a movement began to identify "neurophysiological response measures [as] objective measures to classify psychiatric populations," as Fink put it. Shagass' "sedation threshold" was seen as pioneering. (The sedation threshold was the point at which slurred speech developed in response to a barbiturate infusion, and it varied from diagnosis to diagnosis; see Chapter 8.) Fink used pharmaco-EEG to find distinctive electrophysiological profiles for the major illnesses and drug groups. This promising work—which Max Hamilton called "almost unique"—was soon overwhelmed by the vogue for neurotransmitters.[32] Pharmaco-EEG and the sedation threshold are now forgotten, and few younger psychiatrists are familiar with the terms.

But, in general, academic psychiatry did lag somewhat behind. In 1970, Thomas Ban became the founding director of the Division of Psychopharmacology of the Douglas Hospital in Montreal. This was WHO's first training center for teachers in psychopharmacology in developing countries.[33] As Bernard Carroll, who joined the Department of Psychiatry at the University of Michigan in 1973, wrote a colleague shortly thereafter, "More and more, our department is moving toward a biological approach to psychiatry."[34]

And the excitement in Chicago! Steve Paul, who later became head of neuroscience at Lilly, trained at Chicago in the early 1970s. He said, "We had a small class. Bob Freedman [later editor of the *American Journal of Psychiatry*] was in the class and a bunch of very good people. It was a very exciting department in those days. Herb Meltzer [unitary psychosis] was there and Heinz Kohut, the analyst, Bob Schuster [pioneered substance abuse research]. And many others. A tremendous department Danny [Freedman, editor of *Archives of General Psychiatry*] had pulled together, a small but extraordinarily fine department. Paul and Meltzer worked on deaminating enzymes that were responsive to LSD. Paul then went to NIMH where he worked with Julie Axelrod."[35]—This was the biological stratosphere of US psychopharmacology.

Thus, a glittering future lay before these young scientists and clinicians. To those who dismissed psychopharmacology as lacking the rigor of a real science, Joel Elkes said, at a dinner in 1961, "Psychopharmacology is for the first time, compelling the physical and chemical sciences to look behavior in the face, and thus enriching both these sciences and behavior. If there be discomfiture in this encounter, it is hardly surprising; for it is in this discomfiture that there may well lie the germ of a new science."[36]

Within the compass of a couple of years, these views had solidified. In 1965, Nathan Kline and Heinz Lehmann, two founding figures, said, "A new and tremendously exciting field has been opened in the past dozen years and the shape of the psychiatric universe will never again be the same."[37]

Drugs for a New Field

Drugs are brewed in the cup of science; they are drunk through a patient's lips, and "there's many a slip twixt the cup and the lip."[38]

In 1938, Albert Hofmann, a chemist at Sandoz in Basel, synthesized an ergot analogue that the company labeled lysergic acid diethylamide (LSD-25); 5 years later (1943), Hofmann discovered that the compound made him dizzy, that, in other words, it had psychoactive properties. It was then Max Rinkel at the Massachusetts Mental Health Center who, in collaboration with fellow staffer Harry Solomon, introduced LSD into psychiatric use in the United States, beginning in 1949.[39] Rinkel and Solomon conceived it "as a tool in experimental psychiatry." In 1954, John Gaddum and colleagues at the University of Edinburgh made the major discovery that LSD antagonized serotonin in animal preparations.[40] This set the stage for much research on serotonin as a neurotransmitter with a possible role in psychiatric illness. LSD enjoyed a brief therapeutic vogue in the 1950s for alcoholism and for the experimental induction of psychosis (it was a "psychotogen") before becoming a street drug. Some authorities mark LSD research as the real trigger of the revolution in psychopharmacology, although LSD's clinical diffusion was minimal.

Among the earliest labs for experimental psychiatry was the small room in the Department of Pharmacology at the University of Birmingham that Joel Elkes was accorded in 1942. With access to patients in the Winson Green Mental Hospital, Elkes and colleagues began work on the treatment of catatonic stupor and saw that Amytal relieved it, while amphetamine deepened it. It had already been well known that Amytal broke up catatonic stupor, and the observation was more part of Elkes' own scientific odyssey than a discovery for the literature. Elkes wrote later in his autobiography, "I felt instinctively that the drugs we were working with, and the drugs still to come, could be tools of great precision and power. . . . It is this kind of precision pharmacology of the central nervous system that made me hopeful, and made me take up my stances in the face of raised eyebrows . . . in psychiatric circles, where I was regarded as a maverick, a new-comer, and a curiosity."[41]

The 1950s were the golden years of psychopharmacology, as a rich cornucopia opened and a slew of powerful new agents poured forth. It was the very effectiveness of these new agents—and the research required to produce others—that nourished the field of psychopharmacology. The new drugs swept the old pharmacopoeia off the table. As Lee pointed out, "68.6 percent of all prescription drug products sold in 1951 were no longer available in 1960."[42]

The golden age opened with the discovery in 1949 that lithium was an effective treatment for mania, and the discoveries of Danish psychiatrist Mogens Schou, beginning in 1954, that lithium seemed an effective all-purpose agent in the treatment of mood disorders, including depression and mania. Yet the lithium research burned with a slow fuse, and not until 1970 was it accepted by the FDA (the United States was the fiftieth country to accept lithium therapy). So the psychopharmacology age did not really begin with lithium, but with chlorpromazine in 1952.

Before chlorpromazine, there was nothing specific for psychiatric symptoms. Thuillier said, "Aside from a few tablets of aspirin, antibiotics and even some cough syrups, the pharmacy of a psychiatric hospital in the past would include a supply of phenobarbital [Gardénal, Luminal], some sleeping medications, anti-epileptics and sedatives of every kind, but in a strict sense no specifically psychiatric medication. It was this way everywhere. The insane were a category of patients whose disorders knew no remedies."[43] This changed with the introduction of the first antipsychotic, chlorpromazine, and it was Delay who introduced chlorpromazine and coined the term "neuroleptic."[44] Thus, the vocabulary splayed across the table.

Jean Delay and his assistant Pierre Deniker began trials of chlorpromazine in 1952; by the following year, the drug was on markets in Europe as Largactil, and by 1954 it was marketed in the United States as Thorazine. Chlorpromazine really did change the frame. Freyhan recalled (writing for a German audience) the arrival of chlorpromazine:

In January 1954 a new epoch began. I could start my own studies with chlor-promazine that just had been introduced in the United States. The development of this psychoactive medication represented the beginning of a chain reaction that led to fundamental changes in clinical psychiatry. Within a short time there was a new science, psychopharmacology. . . . As far as clinical psychiatry goes, in the States it [had been] the stepchild of American psychiatry: pioneering work now originated from institutional [non-academic] psychiatry. It was the very few clinical research divisions of the state hospitals that occupied themselves systematically with investigation of the mechanisms of the new psychoactive drugs. At first, academic psychiatry was not just uninterested, but critical of therapy with medications as a shift from mechanical to chemical straitjackets.[45]

Chlorpromazine treated states of agitation without sedating the patients—unlike the barbiturates. So this specificity for agitation, and chlorpromazine's success in diminishing the symptoms of psychosis, made it the first real psychiatric drug. But it was also useful for a wide range of conditions, from pain in giving birth to serious depression. It was initially not confined to the treatment of psychosis, and only a rather arbitrary fiat of the FDA in 1970 mandated that it be marketed exclusively as an antipsychotic, or, alternatively, for schizophrenia. The 1960s saw the appearance of a whole row of other antipsychotics, such as Janssen's Haldol (haloperidol). Antipsychotics are powerful drugs, with many side effects, yet they are capable of normalizing the lives of patients with serious mental illnesses and constitute a key segment of the psychopharmacologic armamentarium.

Chlorpromazine was a sensation! A drug that could affect mental processes, diminish hallucinations and delusions, tranquilize the agitated, and pacify the furious. The food-stand owners outside the Ste. Anne mental hospital in Paris were astonished at how quiet it had become. Industry was far quicker than academics or clinicians to pick up this new lead. In 1953, Ciba in Basel brought out reserpine for hypertension, and the drug quickly became indicated in psychiatry. Art Prange, at the University of North Carolina, recalled, "People divided into two camps, the reserpine people and the chlorpromazine people. In our shop, they barely spoke to each other, at coffee breaks they sat at different tables."[46] (Chlorpromazine was a phenothiazine, reserpine an inhibitor of monoamine oxidase. Reserpine fell by the wayside in the, possibly erroneous, belief that it caused depression, and chlorpromazine won.)

In 1951, Roche in Basel marketed its hydrazine-derivative iproniazid for tuberculosis, then for depression (see Chapter 4). Geigy, also in Basel, hoping to get another chlorpromazine, fiddled the chlorpromazine molecule slightly and ended up in 1957 with imipramine, the first drug for vital (endogenous, or melancholic) depression. Carter Wallace in New Jersey floated meprobamate (Miltown, a propanediol)—the first blockbuster drug in psychiatry—in 1955 as a "tranquilizer." In 1959, Lundbeck in Sweden produced the first thioxanthene (chlorprothixene, Taractan). All of these drugs were first-in-class. By the end of the decade, psychiatry started to shift from Freud to biology.

Simultaneously with chlorpromazine, in 1951, a new class of drugs called monoamine oxidase inhibitors (MAOIs, as mentioned in Chapter 4) that inhibited a key brain enzyme was launched by Hoffmann-La Roche, initially for tuberculosis, and then, after images were seen of patients at a TB sanitarium dancing

about, in 1957 it was marketed for depression. The first MAOI was Roche's iproni-
azid (Marsilid), followed then by a slew of others. SmithKline's tranylcypromine
(Parnate) was launched in 1960 in the United Kingdom, and in 1961 in the
United States, and it remains the main MAOI on the market today.[47] None of the
MAOIs is in wide use today. This is a shame, because MAOIs, which are actually
quite effective in depression, constitute, alongside ECT, the remedy of choice for
"treatment-resistant depression."[48] In fact, in 2016, Jay Amsterdam, who led the
Depression Research Unit at the Hospital of the University of Pennsylvania and
was in the very top tier of academic investigators, called the MAOIs "among the
most 'potent' antidepressants on the planet." He deplored that "the marketplace
will not use them—even if they are as safe as mother's milk!"[49]

By 1960, a rough and ready classification of the available drugs had emerged.
There were, said Jon Cole and colleagues, three major groups[50]:

First were the *major tranquilizers*: Thorazine (chlorpromazine) and its phenothiazine cousins, among which Stelazine (trifluoperazine) and Mellaril
(thioridazine) played a prominent role.

Second came the *antidepressive drugs*: a mixture of agents later called the
"tricyclic" antidepressants, such as Tofranil (imipramine—the first antidepressant of them all), and the just-mentioned MAOIs, such as Marsilid
(iproniazid) and Nardil (phenelzine). Interestingly, Ritalin (methylphenidate), a drug famous today for its anti-ADHD properties, was included in
this group.

Third came the *minor tranquilizers* and *nonbarbiturate sedatives*. There were
no barbiturates on Cole's list. The best-selling of the minor tranquilizers
was Wallace Laboratory's Miltown (meprobamate): by 1971, the Danish
chemical company A/S Syntetic, the main global supplier of the drug, was
producing 500,000 kg a year.[51] None of the others on the list has survived
in memory, and their names, such as Ultran (Lilly's phenaglycodol), are
today foreign hieroglyphs. Nobody today has ever heard of the five "nonbarbiturate sedatives" on the list (try Noludar, Hoffmann-La Roche's
methyprylon).

The list is interesting because it shows how markedly the classification of
drugs can change over the years, and how swiftly drugs that are big in their day
can pass into oblivion (once the patents expire). The only enduring theme is
antidepressants: from the get-go, drugs against depression were prominently featured, either because depression has been widely recognized since the end of the
nineteenth century, or because it is such a winning commercial category.

The list is also interesting because it suggests that antipsychotics are an entirely different category from antidepressants. Yet, in 1958, Sidney Cohen at the

Los Angeles VA Hospital reported that the phenothiazine thioridazine (Sandoz's Mellaril) was effective in "severe depressive reactions."[52] And in 1962, Donald Klein and Max Fink at Hillside Hospital, in a much larger trial, determined that the phenothiazines were excellent antidepressants, and that a strict line between the two drug classes was unrealistic. "The depressive state was markedly alleviated," they reported.[53] (The finding had little impact on the theory that these very different diseases deserved very different drug classes. Klein said later, "Contradictory facts never sink a theory. It's a better theory that sinks a theory. These theories were obviously no good, but there weren't any better theories around."[54])

Then the great wheel rolled on. By 1972, the benzodiazepine Valium had become the nation's best-selling drug, up from #38 in 1966 (it was launched in 1963). Librium, the first of the benzos (launched in 1960) was #7 overall by 1972. Phenobarbital was at #14 in 1973, down from #3 in 1968. But the barbiturates were about to disappear from visibility. And by 1972, Ritalin and Dexamyl (SmithKline's popular barbiturate-amphetamine combo) were still up there in the money.[55] This is interesting because both drugs in Dexamyl, effective in conditions such as "nervous illness" and mixed anxiety-depression, were not unpleasant to take. They would, however, shortly be eclipsed by the torrent of benzodiazepines—for similar indications and also not unpleasant. (And then, as we shall see, the great wheel rolled still further and the SSRIs displaced the benzos.)

Psychopharmacology Goes Missing in the Trenches

Thus, in the 1950s, new drugs abounded in psychiatry. And the term "psychopharmacology" had certainly swept the deck in industry and hospital circles. Yet it is interesting that in the real world of pharmaceuticals, the concept of psychopharmacology was largely missing. In Paul de Haen's widely followed annual surveys of drug trends, from 1950 to 1959 psychopharmacology was not a concept. De Haen noted the introduction of "new ataractics" (antipsychotics), such as Sandoz's Mellaril. Front and center were "combination amphetamine-tranquilizer products to curb appetite" (a number of which contained methamphetamine). A shopping cart of MAOIs was included. De Haen listed Geigy's Tofranil "in the treatment of a variety of depressions." But de Haen was silent on the concept itself of "psychopharmacology."[56]

In the drug ads in the professional journals, there is an almost complete absence of the term "psychopharmacology." Librium, for example, was advertised as an "antianxiety" agent. The fine print of the ads did make use of such biological-sounding concepts as "pharmacotherapy," "psychotropic agents," and "CNS-acting drugs."[57] Merck branded Elavil (amitriptyline) as a form of "chemotherapy."[58] But the term "psychopharmacology," on everyone's lips in the halls of industry and academe, was almost completely lacking in ads aimed largely at family doctors. Nor was "psychopharmacology" used in ads in the psychiatry journals. (There were very occasional exceptions to this that prove the rule. For example, Merck said in 1968 of Triavil, its combo treatment of anxiety and depression—amitriptyline and perphenazine—that the agent was effective "during the early phases of psychopharmacologic therapy."[59])

Indications

The whole question of "indications" has also caused the leaves to tremble in the forest, because even today we have accepted the existence of such supposedly ironclad therapeutic categories as "antidepressant" and "antipsychotics," as though they were science-based classes of drugs as different as chalk and cheese. In an echo of Kraepelin's firewall between dementia praecox (psychosis) and manic-depressive insanity (mood), today we have insisted that these are separate diseases, and that they are treated by separate drug classes. They might have in common such symptoms as agitation or psychosis, but the mantra is that they are different diseases.

As any experienced psychopharmacologist knows, this is nonsense.[60] Therapeutic categories shift with the winds of commerce. As David Drachman of the University of Massachusetts told the Psychopharmacologic Drugs Advisory Committee in 1981, "The classes of drugs are introduced for theoretical reasons, usually the wrong ones. Then they are recognized to have some sort of beneficial effect, and then somebody looks for a rationale which is probably irrelevant." He said he had "absolutely no argument with the use of Ritalin [methylphenidate] to improve energy." Ciba had launched Ritalin in 1954 as an antidepressant. It then drifted into the fatigue market before ending up as a drug for troublemaking boys. Drachman thought it ideal for "improving energy in patients who had decreased cognition with dementia."[61] Thus, the larger categories, such as "antidepressant," were meaningless in the case of Ritalin. It worked for whatever it was marketed for.

Take the "antipsychotics," many of which have excellent histories as antidepressants. George Gardos, who trained at Boston State Hospital, said in 2003 that during his residency he had in fact "noticed that small doses of neuroleptics could be used for conditions other than psychosis, such as anxiety and depression. I did a study on [the antipsychotic] thiothixene and found that in low dose it had some antidepressant effect."[62] Indeed, at this writing, the so-called second-generation antipsychotics turn out to have all kinds of uses apart from psychosis! (See Chapter 18.) The fault here is not really that of the pharmaceutical industry, which is always happy to see markets expanded, but the Food and Drug Administration's insistence that drugs must be indicated for specific diseases, and that schizophrenia and depression are totally different.

Big Changes

In the background of these events, there were big changes going on. Contrast these two images.

It is 1958. The antipsychotics have just been introduced to the mental hospitals, and Nate Kline of Rockland State Hospital is testifying to the Committee on Government Operations of the House of Representatives. The antibiotics in medicine and asepsis in surgery were developments, he said, "so great that they revolutionized all subsequent therapy. The development and successful application of the psychopharmaceuticals was a thermonuclear-like explosion, which marked the end of one era and the beginning of another. . . . These drugs provide the long-awaited key which will unlock the mysteries of the relationship of man's chemical constitution to his psychological behavior." What practical difference, Dr. Kline? "No longer is the mental hospital racked with wild and meaningless shouting, nor do we see any longer the so-called disturbed wards of only a short five years ago." It was actually a problem that the patients now were "amenable to psychotherapy, occupational therapy, recreational therapy," which hospitals, alas, did not have the resources to provide. He went on to praise the pharmaceutical industry: Ciba for developing reserpine (which Kline had introduced clinically) and Squibb for supporting research at Rockland State. It was a "sunny uplands" view of psychopharmacology.[63]

Now fast-forward 15 years. The mental hospitals are emptying out, the patients are adrift on the streets. The center of gravity of institutional care has moved from the hospitals to the prisons. In the meantime, there has been much high-minded rhetoric about the now scorned asylums as sources of "institutionalism" and about the virtues of "care in the community." The rhetoric soon turned to gall. As the patients were turfed from the mental hospitals, they entered the welcoming arms, not of cozy halfway houses, but of predators. Mickey Nardo, who in the 1970s was director of training in psychiatry at Emory, recalled the uplifting rhetoric of the 1970s when he entered psychiatry. It was hostile to institutions: "Hospitals were for short term stabilization only. While the rhetoric was put in terms of a social reform movement, the motor driving it was the coming of the antipsychotics, which made change a possibility. By the time I arrived, the funding and the availability of even acute beds had fallen below the critical point. . . . The 'street people' (chronic mental patients) were beginning to appear in our cities on the streets and living under bridges."[64] With the help of antipsychotics, antidepressants, and ECT, these patients had done well in hospital. Nate Kline was right about that.

On the streets, they did less well. Nardo continued,

> Thomas Szasz was prominently mentioned. But there was a tragedy afoot. As services were cut, the patients that needed protective hospitalization lobbied to get in the front door and were quickly ushered out the back door. Social services that worked were overwhelmed and the dedicated people that worked in them burned out and ultimately bailed out. . . . Community outreach people with a reasonable case load suddenly found themselves with a telephone book full of people they had no time to call, much less visit. And worst of all, the cops and judges got fed up and started sending people to jails and prison—people who had been "manageable" before. It was sad to watch and that's all we could do. As a Training Director, I had to pull residents from various places because they wouldn't participate, and, to be honest, I didn't want them to.[65]

In the lives of these stranded and abandoned patients, there had once been a role for psychopharmacology. That role now came to an end for the street people.

The Benzos

It is only a slight exaggeration to claim that the productive phase of the Age of Psychopharmacology ended with the marketing of the benzodiazepines in the 1960s. Librium reached the market in 1960. (It is true that clozapine [Clozaril] is probably the most effective of the recently hyped second-generation antipsychotics. Yet clozapine is not a new drug: It was patented in 1963.) In 1963, Roche followed Librium with Valium (diazepam), among the best-selling drugs of all time. Wyeth marketed oxazepam (Serax) in 1965, and a number of other "benzos" followed in the late 1960s and 1970s. It is clear that the benzos are effective drugs, and their utility extends across a range of indications beyond anxiety. They were first advertised as "anxiolytics," to differentiate them from meprobamate (Miltown) and the barbiturates, which were considered "sedatives." So a lot of marketing went into "anxiolysis." In family practice and internal medicine, the benzos have been most useful for the mixed anxiety-depression once considered "nervousness." And they do relax tense muscles, smooth the furrowed brow, and function well as hypnotics.

Active minds saw some kind of a link—unofficial but real—between depression and anxiety. And in US psychopharmacology, Paul Leber, in 1983 the acting director at FDA of the Division of Neuropharmacologic Drug Products—let his own very active mind play a bit with this link. Are we going to grant the indication mixed depression-anxiety? At first he said No, then he reflected a bit: "The problem is with mixed states of depression and anxiety because what is first? Now, on the basis of some work that was done on outpatients, what do you think of the idea of outpatient dysphoria, the mixed state [of depression and anxiety], as being real? One that responds in the first week to benzodiazepines and in the third week to classic antidepressants? You would have to rework the nosology of the field."[66] So, he had thrown a hand grenade into the tidy DSM-III separation of depression and anxiety as separate *chapters* in the manual. But the hand grenade just lay there on the table and did not explode.

In sum, the benzodiazepines were a core component of the Age of Psychopharmacology and were knocked out of their market leadership by the SSRIs (for depression) in the late 1980s.

My God, We Hope . . .

New diagnoses, new drugs, astonishing increases in the rate of "mental illness." Robert Whitaker wrote, "In 2007, the disability rate [from mental illness] was 1 in every 76 Americans. That's more than double the rate in 1987, and six times the rate in 1955."[67] Six times more Americans disabled today than in the Eisenhower years! My God, we hope psychopharmacology didn't have anything to do with this.

5

Depression and Schizophrenia

There are few subjects on which information is more ardently desired, or more difficult to be communicated, than this of insanity.—John Ferriar, Physician to the Manchester Infirmary and Lunatic Asylum (1810)[1]

What dragged down psychiatry's scientific status in the twenty-first century was its inability to get beyond the two big diseases, depression, including bipolar disorder, and schizophrenia. Thoughtful observers found it increasingly incredible that the scientific method had not succeeded in disassembling these into their component disorders. Who could take seriously a discipline that preserved intact the vague, amorphous diseases of a hundred years ago?

Two Big Diseases

Depression and schizophrenia are really the backbone of psychiatry. Emil Kraepelin, the Heidelberg professor whose textbook has given us much of the structure of DSM nosology today, made them the core of the system of diagnosis that he enunciated in 1899, with "manic-depressive insanity" and "dementia praecox." And today, "major depression" and "schizophrenia" have chapters in the DSM that are miles distant from each other. The therapeutics are divided mainly into "antidepressants" and "antischizophrenics" (or antipsychotics). So these categories are as fundamental to psychiatry as are engines to automobiles.

In 1965, Max Fink and Don Klein reported a trial at Hillside Hospital of imipramine, chlorpromazine, and placebo in "depressive disorders." (They used a combo of chlorpromazine-procyclidine, the latter an antiparkinsonian anticholinergic agent.) Results? "Both drugs are effective in retarded depressive syndromes." The chlorpromazine combo was thought possibly more effective in agitated depressive states, imipramine more effective "in depressive patients with phobic anxiety features."[2] The trial established the efficacy of antipsychotics like chlorpromazine in the treatment of depression. There were several such trials in the literature; one could also see this as mocking the idea that depression and schizophrenia were really very separate illnesses.

All forms of depression were accompanied by anxiety, and most forms of anxiety (save the psychotic variety) by depression. There was, for the most part, a single illness—mixed depression-anxiety—and for years industry promoted agents for this indication. "Anxious depression has no geographic boundaries, neither does Ludiomil," shouted Ciba in 1982 on behalf of its new agent (in the US market) maprotiline.[3] Depression and anxiety were two sides of the same coin, and it was only by flipping the coin, as Alan Horwitz pointed out, that the "age of anxiety" becomes the "age of depression."[4]

Thus, one must be cautious about making dogmatic pronouncements about "depression" or "schizophrenia," because the terms don't actually mean that much. They are simply too heterogeneous. In 1959, at a meeting of the American Psychopathological Association, several participants expressed dissatisfaction with the state of diagnosis. Morton Kramer, a biostatistician at NIMH, said that, worldwide, "much of the knowledge that is used concerning the distribution of schizophrenia and other mental disorders . . . has come from the statistics of the New York State [asylum] system. If the diagnoses on which these data are based, and their reliability, is so very highly questionable . . . what knowledge do we really have about the distribution of these disorders in population groups right now?"[5]

At the same meeting, Benjamin Pasamanick from Ohio State University added that, at their university teaching hospital, they had been studying diagnoses at the ward level (the patients were randomly assigned to wards). "We found much to our shame, that the basis for diagnosis of psychoses, psychoneuroses, and personality disorders varied from ward to ward, and even within wards, when the ward administration changed. If this is true in a teaching hospital with a relatively small number of patients, what reliability can we expect in other institutions, even within a single hospital system?"[6] So, the formal diagnoses, what do they actually mean?

The above examples are from the world of DSM. But psychiatry has a diagnostic tradition of two centuries, 200 years of considering what is wrong with the patients and, once a diagnosis is in hand, of treating the patient on that basis. Over the course of those two centuries, much was learned about what can go wrong with the brain and mind. Part of the problem of psychopharmacology today is forgetting this precious store of wisdom and inventing new diagnoses that soon become profit centers for the pharmaceutical industry.

A great river of diagnosis flowed from nineteenth-century German psychiatry, dominating the global picture of diagnosis in the way that DSM does today. The nineteenth-century tradition was heavily biological, seeing mental illness essentially as brain disease. Wilhelm Griesinger, a professor of psychiatry in Berlin in the 1860s, was associated with the dictum that "mental diseases are brain diseases" (*Geisteskrankheiten sind Nervenkrankheiten*).

A new chapter began with Emil Kraepelin, who had little interest in biology. Kraepelin saw course and endpoint as the central diagnostic features, not brain tissue. One of his students, Karl Jaspers, who founded the modern study of psychopathology, turned the page on Griesinger and aspired to a much more patient-centered view of things. Jaspers was pleased that his own book, which debuted in 1912, was "free of the servitude" to the doctrine that "mental diseases are brain diseases" that had subordinated psychiatry to neurology and internal medicine.[7] Kraepelin and Jaspers oversaw the real birthing of modern psychiatric diagnosis, an infant who was almost drowned in the vast tide of Freudianism that engulfed the field in the first half of the twentieth century. But, driven by the success of the new drugs, psychiatry decided to make a new stab at diagnosis in order to individuate entities that were treatment-responsive.[8] This was a thoroughly admirable impulse.

Yet, there were problems with diagnosis. The main problem was that terms meant what their users wanted them to mean. As a result, there was chaos in communicating what it was patients actually had. The psychoanalytically oriented clinicians preferred "schizophrenia" for any disorder than seemed unamenable to psychotherapy. And terms like "hysteria" were freely bandied about in office practice, although exactly what the term meant was unclear, except that the female patient had somehow unsettled the diagnostician.

Why so much interest in diagnosis? Why does it really matter? The standard response would be, "No treatment without diagnosis, and some of the diagnoses require different treatments." But this is largely pious boilerplate: In reality, many patients meet the criteria for many different diagnoses, and the drugs have gathered so many indications that they qualify as panaceas.

Deeper Currents

But there is a better scientific reason, and that is to recognize the deeper currents that flow through the mind and brain with a view to matching them to your patient. In 1973, Richard Hunter at Queen's Square, at the time president of the Royal Society of Medicine, highlighted this problem: In psychiatry, he said, "Presenting symptoms are elevated to the status of a disease, like varieties of fever were in the eighteenth century."[9] Psychiatry's diagnoses were symptoms, in other words. As Bernard Carroll put it in 2014, "The essence of clinical work is to recognize underlying disease structures in the unstructured narratives of complex life situations."[10] Your patient has a complex life: What are the deeper currents steering it?

The current scientific understanding of diagnosis in the major diseases is that the symptom picture is genetically driven, but that the genes bear little relationship to DSM categories. One group of scholars—the "Brainstorm Consortium" led by Verneri Anttila at the Broad Institute of Harvard and MIT—argued in 2018 that in psychiatry, unlike neurology, genetic risk of major depressive disorder, schizophrenia, and ADHD is highly intercorrelated. It was not at all one gene, one illness. "Their current clinical boundaries do not reflect distinct underlying pathogenic processes, at least on the genetic level. This suggests a deeply interconnected nature for psychiatric disorders . . . and underscores the need to refine psychiatric diagnostics."[11] Thus, deeper currents.

This warning cry was largely drowned out in continuing ad hype about antidepressants and antipsychotics.

Schizophrenia

> I have known many in their childhood very sagacious, and extremely docile or apt to learn, that by their literature and discourse have caused admiration, who afterwards becoming young men, were dull and heavy.—Thomas Willis, *Soul of Brutes*, 1672[12]

One imagines the situation in the late 1950s and early 1960s. There had been a huge outpouring of drugs, such as Wyeth's Spartase and Upjohn's Monase, unclear in their indications. The medicinal chemists synthesized them, then they were put into monkeys in the animal lab, and the recipients were either tranquilized or stimulated. But what were the drugs good for in humans? As Frank Fish, then at Edinburgh, commented at a conference in 1959, "We have had so many drugs whose effects we do not properly understand, and we have sometimes very little idea of precisely what the condition is that we are trying to treat. This is a fantastic position and could be likened to what might have happened had somebody introduced simultaneously five powerful antibiotics in the middle of the eighteenth century [when there was no understanding of infectious illness]."[13] The drugs did something, but what were they good for?

Yet, amid all the confusion about diagnoses in little "p" psychiatry," in big "P" psychiatry, as we have seen, two huge diagnoses towered above all others: schizophrenia and depression. That is roughly the situation today, except that we have "bipolar disorder" as well. What did these terms mean?

Ever since 1896, when Emil Kraepelin popularized the term "dementia praecox," or literally "premature dementia," the authorities have argued about whether it was one disease or several.[14] Eugen Bleuler, the Zurich psychiatry professor who christened it "schizophrenia" in 1908, agreed with Kraepelin that it was just one disorder and that catatonia, paranoia, and hebephrenia were among its "subtypes"—not diseases of their own. Paul Janssen, the founder of Janssen Pharmaceutica, thought Bleuler was dead wrong about this. "It is very difficult to accept that this particular word [schizophrenia] invented by Bleuler can be one disease entity. This is important because we are constantly bombarded with the question: what is the etiology of schizophrenia. And my answer is that the etiology of schizophrenia is Dr. Bleuler."[15]

Schizophrenia managed to maintain itself intact for around a century, acquiring a kind of death grip on international psychiatry. But in the last several decades, voices have become louder in proclaiming that there are in fact several distinct diseases sheltering within this omnibus label. Catatonia has been definitively withdrawn from it, becoming a disease of its own.[16]

When Kraepelin launched dementia praecox (schizophrenia) as a single disease of its own, there was much dissent. In the day, many observers challenged the view that Kraepelin's creation was a valid entity. "Schizophrenia is probably not a unitary disease at all," said Kraepelin's successor in the Chair of Psychiatry in Munich, Oswald Bumke, in 1919.[17] The two men heartily detested each other, but Bumke spoke for many. Yet the dissenting voices were drowned out. By the 1930s, schizophrenia had become one of the two great disease entities in psychiatry. Kraepelin's manic-depressive insanity was the other.

The great dilemma plaguing psychiatry for a century was what to call, as Paul Leber put it, "an acutely exacerbated, somewhat threatening, very excited patient . . . who basically is out of control." Schizophrenia or psychosis? "Schizophrenia" rather than "psychosis" was on everybody's lips because in 1998 the FDA shifted its focus from antipsychotic to antischizophrenic.[18] This public shift was the more ironic because in private—in supposedly confidential remarks to the Psychopharmacologic Drugs Advisory Committee—Leber challenged the idea of a unitary psychosis or schizophrenia. He queried the Advisory Committee in 1995, is psychosis like dropsy [a general term for edema]? Are we saying "I have an anti-dropsy effect, an anti-Bright's Disease effect? . . . Maybe we shouldn't be giving such claims [as "antipsychotic phenomena"] anymore and it is time to start breaking it out from the stage of dropsy into the individual components. That is sort of what I think the diagnostic question has to be."[19]

Purely on the basis of clinical course, there were four wildly different outcomes in schizophrenia: one episode ever and no following impairment (20 percent); sporadic acute episodes with no disability in between (35 percent); residual symptoms after the first episode, which then do not subside between following episodes (10 percent); a chronic disease with disability worsening after each episode (35 percent).[20] These cannot possibly all be the same disease.

Thus, it is true that schizophrenia was—and remains today—one of the great diagnostic disasters of psychiatry. It has the disadvantage of not actually existing as a single disease, despite the fact that psychiatry has embraced it as such for over a century. Many authorities, voices lost in the wind, have asserted this. Thomas P. Rees, an experienced hospital superintendent, said in 1951, "As for schizophrenia, I think that the term has little meaning. It often signifies no more than that the patient is mad; it carries no clinical picture, no prognosis, and unclear indications for treatment."[21]

There was a long European tradition of throwing doubt on the unitary nature of Emil Kraepelin's "dementia praecox" and Bleuler's "schizophrenia." Leo Alexander, the director of the Neurobiological Unit of Boston State Hospital, was born in Vienna, Austria, in 1905 and read German. In 1958, he ginned up early doubts about schizophrenia as a disease. He called the diagnosis useless. "Patients with schizophrenia show markedly different clinical courses with or without treatment. Hence the term 'schizophrenia' has very little to offer." Schizophrenia, he said, was "too amorphous . . . where we are dealing with a mosaic of disturbances rather than a single disturbance."[22]

But most of the literature on which Alexander relied, written in an unfamiliar language, failed to cross the Atlantic.

Great confusion about symptoms, prognosis, and treatment resulted. What constitutes schizophrenia has remained unclear. In the 1920s, when English psychiatrist Eliot Slater was taking the qualifying exams for his diploma in psychiatry, he was quizzed in the written examination about dementia praecox. "I looked at it aghast," he later said. "I had never heard of this disease." So, he gave it his best shot. "I sat down and wrote. I threw in everything I had ever heard of. The disease was commonly insidious and progressive but could be interrupted with acute attacks." The examiners gave him a pass. Anything he might have said had an equal chance of being right.[23]

Hans Hoff, professor of psychiatry in Vienna, is said to have shouted, "I define what schizophrenia is!"[24] This is not the soundest of scientific bases.

So, how many different diseases are entombed in the vast sarcophagus of schizophrenia? Catatonia has already been extracted. Oneirophrenia, or dreamlike psychosis, may be just around the corner. Laszlo Meduna, who in the 1930s had moved from Budapest to Chicago and was among the most thoughtful of disease-classifiers, revived this older diagnosis in 1950 to mean "sensory deceptions."[25] Note that Emmanuel Régis, who taught psychiatry in Bordeaux, described in 1899 an "état de rêve" (dream) as one of the délirs toxiques. He cited others who had written on an "état de confusion en forme de rêve."[26]

The first notable US attempt to systematically dismantle schizophrenia as a unitary disease came in 1963 from Warren Gerard, a noted clinical neuroscientist at the University of Michigan, who wrote, "Our hypothesis was that schizophrenia is a nosological mixture and that its separate components could be disentangled by giving a wide variety of tests to a sufficient number of subjects." In fact, only two subgroups were found, "paranoid" and "others." Yet Gerrard cherished the hope that in further research—which, alas, time denied him owing to his death in 1974—"We will indeed have split schizophrenia into the schizophrenias . . . groups identifiable biologically as well as behaviorally."[27]

In the 1980s, George Brooks at the University of Vermont and Courtenay Harding at Yale undertook a series of retrospective studies of schizophrenic patients admitted in the mid-1950s to Vermont State Hospital. In 1987 they found that, contrary to Emil Kraepelin's view of dementia praecox as a deteriorating condition, a majority of patients studied at follow-up had not gone downhill at all but were leading normal lives: "68% of the 82 subjects who met the DSM-III criteria [retrospectively] for schizophrenia at index hospitalization did not display any further signs or symptoms (either positive or negative) of schizophrenia at follow-up."[28] The authors didn't attempt to disaggregate their patient pool into separate illnesses, but evidently there were two clinical populations: Those who went downhill and those who recovered.

Then there was "amentia." Was this schizophrenia? Willy Mayer-Gross, with his background in Heidelberg psychiatry, described it as a "subacute delirious state," in which the clouding of consciousness is less deep than in delirium. "The leading symptom is incoherence of thinking, and this fragmentation extends to all mental processes, including perception and action. In more lucid moments the patient seems to realize the disturbance. He asks questions expressing his helplessness and perplexity—'Where am I?' 'What is going on here?'" But the patients uniformly recovered.[29]

There clearly is a distinct illness where young people develop a kind of anxious, withdrawn prodrome, then move into a full-scale incapacitating illness. As early as 1928, German investigators discovered that schizophrenics had larger cerebral ventricles than did non-schizophrenics.[30] (Half a century later, Daniel Weinberger and colleagues at NIMH reproduced these findings, completely unaware that they'd been scooped.[31])

Some of these "schizophrenics" recover, at least to the point of being able to lead a life marked by social "deficits." Others do not really recover.[32] Much has been made of "good outcome" versus "bad outcome" schizophrenia, which may or may not be two separate illnesses.

Childhood "autism" was once considered a form of schizophrenia, but it no longer is.[33]

It is likely that, in the years ahead, the "schizophrenia" concept will dissolve entirely as its components are extracted, and the great whale will flop on the beach breathing its last.

The aim here is not to list all the many disease fragments that, at one time or another, have been lumped into the schizophrenic pot, but to demonstrate that the schizophrenia monster has more or less eaten the study of psychosis in a way that is absolutely incompatible with science but thoroughly congenial to commerce: maintaining a single "psychosis" concept for the sale of "antipsychotics." Tom Ban told David Healy in an interview,

> Psychopharmacology focused attention on the biologic heterogeneity of schizophrenia but this was obviously contrary to the interest of the drug firms. In trying to prevent the falling apart of the neuroleptic market, industry is lavishly supporting and propagating neuropharmacologic research on receptor changes in schizophrenic brains or linkages through the D4 receptor to genetics. This kind of research is based on the assumption that schizophrenia, a concept, is one disease, whereas psychopharmcologic research should be trying to disentangle the biologic heterogeneity of schizophrenia found in clinical investigations. There is no support from industry for this kind of work . . . and it is rather unfortunate that there is no appreciation for psychopharmacologic research in schizophrenia at the American universities.[34]

Underbrush

Some underbrush has grown up around the massive schizophrenia tree.

One patch of underbrush insists that there are "positive" symptoms, such as psychosis with its hallucinations and delusions, and "negative" symptoms involving social withdrawal, mutism, and negativism. This distinction was reintroduced by John Strauss and William Carpenter in 1974, updating Hughlings Jackson's nineteenth-century discussion[35]; but it seems unhelpful. Many of the negative symptoms are in fact catatonia, a separate illness that responds very well to treatment. Some of the negative symptoms do in fact respond readily to treatment (but some do not). Leo Hollister said to a colleague at the Veterans Administration Hospital in Palo Alto, "Roy, how would you like to have all the patients on the ward on chlorpromazine?"

The colleague responded, "Oh, my God, I've got too many patients now talking to me, who never said a word before, it's all I can do to keep up with them."

Hollister continued, "If that isn't treating a negative symptom, I don't know what is."

Hollister had some data on treating negative schizophrenia, but his long-time collaborator, psychologist John Overall in Texas, had thrown away a lot of the file, so it was never published. "So, we never did that, but there's no question this is a myth and it's all the more developed now because of the atypicals [second-generation antipsychotics, supposedly treating negative symptoms], which are another myth."[36] These anecdotes are not, of course a substitute for good data, which do not include catatonia and do include only the core illness. But when respected senior figures like Hollister, with decades of experience with very sick patients, express such thoughts, they must be listened to.

Another patch of underbrush places psychosis at the core of schizophrenia. But several authors, including René Kahn in Utrecht and Richard Keefe at Duke, have questioned making psychosis the central experience in schizophrenia. "Schizophrenia is a cognitive illness," they argue. Declines in cognitive function usually precede the onset of a psychotic break by as much as a decade. Further, "It is clear that cognitive function in schizophrenia is related to outcome and little influenced by antipsychotic treatment. Thus, our focus on defining . . . the disorder on the basis of psychotic symptoms may be too narrow."[37]

These authors are not alone. Veteran clinicians recognize that many of their chronic patients do not necessarily have "the noisy things," the delusions or hallucinations of core psychotic experience. To be sure, they may have a thought disorder that makes them sound crazy, and they are very ill, which is another sense of the term "psychotic." But what the core patients may evidence is a slow and subtle deterioration of function. This may involve several things, including "emotional blunting," meaning that they themselves do not express emotions or respond to them in others. Nor, if untreated, can they hold any but the most menial jobs; and they are, as mentioned above, often "thought-disordered," meaning that they have cognitive disturbances.[38]

Furthermore, their capacity for executive function is often obliterated, meaning they are unable to get anything done. As Daniel Weinberger, a premier schizophrenia researcher at NIMH, told an interviewer in 2007 about the schizophrenic patients he had seen as a resident at the Massachusetts Mental Health Center, "One of the things I found to my amazement was that the hallucinations and delusions which were the most obvious florid characteristics, was not what was wrong with them. . . . What was wrong was they could not function."[39]

It is these deficits—emotional blunting, executive dysfunction, and thought disorder—that are the problem in core schizophrenia, which some authorities believe should be called "hebephrenia," going back to a term that Ewald Hecker introduced in 1871, in an article that initiated Kraepelin's interest in dementia praecox.[40] More recently, Michael Alan Taylor has argued for "hebephrenia [as] the original notion of schizophrenia."[41]

Various classifications have been proposed. Can we classify schizophrenia on the basis of good or poor premorbid state, as Sam Guze and Eli Robins at Washington University of St. Louis proposed in 1970? They concluded that, "good-prognosis 'schizophrenia' is not mild schizophrenia but a different illness."[42] The contribution created waves and remained an article of faith among Wash U graduates. As the DSM drafters wrestled in 1978 with the problem of schizophrenia, Donald Goodwin, then chair of psychiatry at the University of Kansas and a Wash U graduate, wrote Harrison Pope at the McLean Hospital, telling him of the Wash U views: "A good-prognosis schizophrenic was a person who <u>look</u>ed schizophrenic and whom practically everybody in the U.S. would call schizophrenic but had certain good prognosis features: abrupt onset; affective symptoms, usually depressive but sometimes manic; an air of bewilderment, confusion, or perplexity; and a good 'premorbid' personality." These good-prognosis patients, he said, "were likely to experience a complete recovery (regardless of treatment), while schizophrenics without these features were likely to remain ill."[43] Then, in 1978, Goodwin backpedaled a bit from these views, yet they represent an influential effort to dismantle the diagnosis. (Seymour Kety, who was drawn into the discussions in 1977, thought it very interesting that "the so-called acute schizophrenic [good prognosis] responds well to lithium."[44])

Another patch of underbrush in schizophrenia concerns medication.

Some patients needed to be on medications long term, indeed forever, others did not. A 20-year follow-up study of 70 schizophrenic patients found that at each follow-up, 30 to 40 percent of the patients were no longer on antipsychotics. A recipe for disaster? No. The investigators found that, "Schizophrenic patients not on antipsychotics for prolonged periods were significantly less likely to be psychotic and experienced more periods of recovery; they also had more favorable risk and protective factors. Schizophrenic patients off antipsychotics for prolonged periods did not relapse more frequently."[45]

Benjamin Wiesel, a staff psychiatrist at the Hartford Hospital in Hartford, Connecticut, found plenty of schizophrenic patients in the outpatient service who didn't need medication: Many of them were stumbling around with their "brown bags" full of medicines. "They were dopey, half-sedated, a little toxic. We took away the medication completely and gave them nothing. We'd say, 'Just taper it off and come back in a month.'"

They'd come back in a month and we'll say, 'How do you feel?'"

"They'd say, 'Gee, I feel alive again.' Absolutely amazing, like the walking dead who suddenly come to life."[46]

So, here were two groups, those who needed medication and those who didn't. These are surely different diseases, if one definition of a "disease" is distinctive response to treatment. Louis Gottschalk, who graduated in medicine in 1943 and was the first research psychiatrist at NIMH, said of his experiences at Longview Hospital in Cincinnati, "Our findings . . . demonstrated that not all chronic schizophrenic patients had to be kept for the rest of their lives on a major tranquilizer. So, we discontinued the old practice, and a fair number of patients who were off medication for a while could be discharged."[47]

There are forms of schizophrenia that seem to be lifelong afflictions, others that have an onset suddenly in previously normal late adolescents and early adults. Robert M. Kessler, a neuroradiologist at NIMH, nailed this in an interview: "There are people who fell out of the womb as awkward kids; they may have been a little bit funny looking, didn't do well in school, are socially isolated, and then, as teenagers begin to hallucinate, and now they're suddenly called schizophrenics." Kessler juxtaposed these individuals with, "people who are very social, do extremely well, who have high achievement, go to Ivy League schools, have very high IQ's, have lots of friends . . . and then in their mid to late twenties or late thirties have a psychotic break and become schizophrenic. The one who was never right from the first may have a very different disease from the one who was a philosophy major."[48]

The Science Wavers

This issue is not going to be sorted out in the present volume, but the point is that dubiety grew. The science wavered.

In theory, the gap between mood disorders and madness is filled by "schizoaffective" disorder. Yet this is fictive. It pretends that schizoaffective disorder is a separate class of illness. But the reality is that almost all schizophrenia is interpenetrated by depression.[49] At the extremes, schizophrenia may be differentiated from depression, but in the vast middle, depression may initiate an episode of schizophrenia, be present throughout, and persist even after the schizophrenia has subsided. Yet the firewall in DSM is just as strong as Kraepelin's initial firewall in separating dementia praecox from manic-depressive insanity. The firewall is, moreover, very profitable for industry because it means that two medications should be prescribed rather than just one.

In an attempt to dismantle the firewall, in 1975 Joseph Schildkraut and Don Klein proposed "schizophrenia-related depressive disorders" as a separate class. (The three additional classes of their nosology were manic-depressive disorders, endogenous unipolar depressive disorders, and a "residual group" that included "nonspecific syndromes," such as "most situational depressions" and "nonspecific depressive syndromes occurring in the context of other psychiatric disorders.")[50] Klein, of course, was on the DSM-III Task Force. When asked why none of this made it into the 1980 third edition of the DSM, he replied simply, "I was outvoted."[51]

Rival classification systems sprang up. In 1957, in a distinctive system, German psychiatrist Karl Leonhard asserted that there are some kinds of psychotic illness, which he called "affect-laden paraphrenia" (part of the "unsystematic schizophrenias") that respond beautifully to neuroleptic medication; others, which he called the "systematic schizophrenias," do not.[52]

It's not just that these types of schizophrenia are clinically different. They are also biologically different, to the point of reinforcing our confidence about dealing with separate diseases. The dexamethasone suppression test (DST) measures biological dysfunction in one of the body's main endocrine axes: the axis from hypothalamus in the brain, to the anterior pituitary gland at the base of the brain, to the adrenal gland, atop the kidneys (the HPA axis). If you give a normal person an injection of the artificial steroid dexamethasone, hours later their serum cortisol will be lower: the HPA axis has suppressed the secretion of cortisol because it recognizes that the body already has enough steroid hormone on board. But in serious illnesses, the level of cortisol remains high: The patients ("nonsuppressors") do not reduce their cortisol. In one study of "schizophrenia," nine of ten patients with the catatonia subtype showed nonsuppression, four of six in the hebephrenia subtype were nonsuppressors, and zero in eighteen patients with the paranoid subtype were nonsuppressors.[53] This is a huge biological difference! These cannot be the same disease.

There was so much difficulty about schizophrenia that it became a byword for the diagnostic difficulties of US psychiatry. The Americans, ensnared in psychoanalysis, diagnosed schizophrenia much more often than anyone else, because they needed a term for patients inappropriate for "the couch." Charles Bowden, who trained in psychiatry at the psychoanalytically oriented New York State Psychiatric Institute (PI), recalled that the diagnosis of schizophrenia was so frequent that there was a special category of patients known as " 'PI Schizophrenics'. . . Patients with any psychotic features, even if transient and related to drug taking, or to stressors, or bipolar disorder or addictive disorders, tended to have their psychosis equated to schizophrenia."[54] This was an obvious scientific travesty.

Despite these qualms, US psychiatry persisted in treating schizophrenia as being real as mumps. A review in 2019 in *JAMA Psychiatry,* a leading journal, said flatly, "Schizophrenia is a common, severe mental illness that most clinicians will encounter regularly during their practice."[55] The ongoing attachment to schizophrenia is, in other words, further evidence of the disqualification of psychopharmacology as a scientific field.

Many Different "Depressions"

Given that "depression" is by far the commonest diagnosis in psychiatry, the misadventures that have befallen mood disorders have also shaken the scientific status of the field. If "major depression" is an artifact, then what else is artifactual as well?

In London in the mid-1960s, Barry Blackwell, who had trained in psychiatry at the Maudsley, unaccountably decided to try family medicine for a bit. He noticed that the "depressed" patients he saw in the office were very different from those he had seen in the hospital:

> At the Maudsley, I had been used to seeing people with severe depression who had "classical" symptoms: hopelessness, lack of energy, poor concentration, severe sleep disturbances, early-morning ruminations (the ceaseless round of painful thought), suicidal ideas, and complete lack of pleasure.
>
> In family practice, I saw a different picture. Like a thirty-year-old mother of two young children burdened with household chores and an unhelpful husband. Reluctantly, she complained to me of being irritable, easily angry at the kids but quickly guilty afterward. She had difficulty falling asleep, woke feeling tired, and reluctantly admitted she had lost all interest in sex.[56]

These clearly were two different kinds of illness, not differences in severity but qualitative differences in kind, one melancholia, the other, let's say, neurasthenia. In 1959, W. Furness Thompson, the research vice-president of Smith, Kline & French, said, "There seem to be several kinds of depression and they don't all respond to the same therapeutic agents." SmithKline had on offer Compazine (prochlorperazine), introduced in 1956 as a moderate phenothiazine "tranquilizer" for "mild conditions," such as neurasthenic depression; Thorazine (chlorpromazine), the first member of the phenothiazine class and intended for severe depression and psychosis; and Stelazine (trifluoperazine), a phenothiazine for "severely psychotic cases," which would include psychotic depression.[57] This kind of differentiation seemed self-understood.

But surely this has always been recognized?

Actually, not. The typing of depression has a long history, except that it was not called depression. Melancholia is more than very serious depression. It is a separate illness involving not just mood but mentation and the entire body. The diagnosis goes back to the ancients and represents what one might think of as "settled clinical opinion." Even today, if you say "melancholia," people immediately know what you mean.

Melancholia disappeared from psychiatry early in the twentieth century, because both Kraepelin and Freud found it old-fashioned. It was replaced by other terms, such as "involutional psychosis" and "endogenous depression." In 1965 Herman van Praag, then in Amsterdam, reactivated Kurt Schneider's 1920 phrase "vital depression" for the melancholic form of depression,[58] and it enjoyed currency in Europe. Psychiatrist Gordon Parker at the University of

Sydney then rehabilitated "melancholia" in an influential 1996 book.[59] In 2006, Michael Alan Taylor at the University of Michigan and Max Fink at Stony Brook wrote a practical guide to the diagnosis and treatment of melancholia.[60] Parker, Taylor, and Fink thus revived the concept scientifically but their work made little impact on US psychiatry.

There were other types of depressive illness, too, given how rich a theme low mood, low energy, and slow thought are. Clinically, melancholia differs sharply from the lesser depressions: 98 percent of patients with "severe" depression have a stooped posture, while only 32 percent of those with "mild" illness show this. Ninety-four percent of the severe cases have suicidal ideas or wishes, but only 47 percent of the mild. Feelings of inadequacy are found in 90 percent of the severe cases, and 56 percent of the mild. Loss of gratification (anhedonia) is present in 92 percent of the severe cases, and 65 percent of the mild. The originators of these data assumed there was only one "depression," with different degrees of severity.[61] Yet the numbers make the case that melancholics stand out in clinical practice. It is a truism that you can recognize a melancholic patient the moment that he or she walks through the door.

There was biochemical evidence of different depressive subgroups. Starting in 1975, Merton Sandler, professor of chemical pathology at the University of London's Royal Postgraduate Medical School, and colleagues tried giving depressed patients an extra dose of tyramine. They had found that in these patients urinary levels of tyramine (in the form conjugated with sulfate) were low in depression. By 1986, they were proposing "tyramine-conjugation deficit" as a trait marker in endogenous depression. And in 1989 they reported that this subgroup responded well to tricyclic antidepressants.[62] The subgroup should have become the object of intensive investigation: a biologically homogeneous group of patients in the otherwise terribly heterogeneous group of patients with "major depression." It should have, but it didn't. (A Columbia group did, however, confirm the validity of "the tyramine challenge test as a marker for melancholia."[63]) Sandler concluded the neglect arose because the urinalyses required for the test were too difficult to perform.[64] It may also have been because the field had become blinded to anything not having to do with neurotransmitters.

In 1947, New York psychiatrist and founder of Hillside Hospital Israel Strauss articulated the unfocused sense of ill-ease—which Barry Blackwell found in his office general practice—when he told a psychiatric meeting: "I would venture to say that in 75 percent of [a young doctor's] practice he will be dealing with patients in whom, in one form or another, the emotional state is a dominating factor."[65] The problem is that, after 1980, many of these patients were diagnosed as "depressed."

Psychiatry's grip on the different depressions began to slacken with the closure of the asylums in the 1970s and 1980s. The asylums had been a boon for the understanding of serious illnesses because the inpatients could be followed closely and the evolution of their conditions could be understood. Mark Kramer called them "the secret sauce of discovery." Then there occurred, he said, "the increasing separation of researchers from their ring-side inpatient clinical seats." Instead, the understanding of illness passed to outpatient physicians, in the academy and the community. Kramer said, "Outpatient general physicians could not make subtle nosological distinctions but could be swayed by the stream of increasingly sexy amitriptyline ads in major medical journals. . . . It was deinstitutionalization . . . by which we lost our best benchmark of potentially big clinical outcomes."[66]

So that was the situation before DSM-III: many different depressions, some representing what were probably different illnesses. I say "probably" because modern research on types of depression slowed greatly after DSM-III was published in 1980.

A lot of this story turns around a single putative disease: major depression. Major depressive disorder was conceived in 1980 by Robert Spitzer during the drafting of DSM-III. Industry had no role in its making but gladly accepted it as a billion-dollar gift. There was to be only one depression, major depression, and one class of antidepressants would be indicated for its relief: Prozac and its SSRI cousins.

The Previous Consensus

The scientific consensus that had evolved before 1980 about the structure of depressive illness was thus rubbished. That consensus said that there were, essentially, three depressions, and so unlike one another were they that it made little sense to refer to the whole illness basin as "depression." The three were:

Neurasthenic depression, or what used to be called nerves, later termed "psychoneurosis." (The analysts did not originate the term but they popularized it for forms of illness that presumably responded to psychotherapy.) Psychoneurosis was not necessarily even a mood disorder, given that many patients were not sad, but tired, anxious, phobic, sleepless, obsessed with details, and feeling poorly in their skins. Neurasthenic depression responded in a hit-and-miss way to many different drug classes, including amphetamines, benzodiazepines, and the SSRIs.

Atypical depression. This is a diagnosis that went back to around the Second World War and that had been revived by Donald Klein. A paradoxical kind of depression, atypical depression meant overeating, oversleeping, and an exceptional sensitivity to the environment (being dumped by one's boyfriend, for example). Studies found that atypical depression was different from melancholia and major depression, although nonetheless somewhat heterogeneous in composition.[67] There was some indication that the treatment for it was the now seldom prescribed drug class monoamine oxidase inhibitors (MAOIs), such as Parnate.

Melancholia (endogenous depression). This was core serious depression in which the mood was either deeply sad or emotions were lacking entirely, the patients feeling deadened in spirit. Patients were also slowed in thought and movement and experienced anhedonia, meaning a complete lack of joy in their lives or of any future horizons. In 1980, in the depression outpatient program at the University of Michigan, 53 percent of the major depressions, as defined in the Research Diagnostic Criteria, were judged melancholic.[68] Patients referred to the program would already have been seriously depressed to begin with, so among patients in the community with major depression, the percent who were melancholic would have been lower. In another study of patients diagnosed as having major depression, only 37.6 percent met the criteria for Kraepelin's manic-depressive insanity, and only 13.6 percent for Kurt Schneider's vital depression.[69] Both of the latter diagnoses would qualify as "melancholia."

Harder to pinpoint but nonetheless real was the patient's notion of "distinct quality of depressed mood," an almost undefinable sense that something was very wrong and that it was different from mourning. In 1980 DSM-III allowed, under the "fifth-digit code" for melancholia: "distinct quality of depressed mood."[70] In 2013, DSM-5 watered this down, making melancholia into a "specifier" without a code (and not mentioned in the index): "a distinct quality of depressed mood characterized by profound despondency, despair and/or moroseness or by so-called empty mood."[71]

And there was biology. As Bernard Carroll pointed out in the *Lancet* in 1980, "We now have biological evidence [a positive dexamethasone suppression test] to support the isolation of endogenous depression as a separate disorder apart from the undifferentiated, heterogeneous group of conditions termed major depressive disorder"[72] (see Chapter 5). William Styron left a moving memoir, *Darkness Revisited*, of his own experiences with melancholia. Melancholia was also distinctive as the only illness in the mood basin that responded well to treatment: it responded adequately to the tricyclic antidepressants and exquisitely to electroconvulsive therapy.

This emphasis on depression was relatively new. Henri Ellenberger, the Swiss psychiatrist who settled in Montreal (and wrote one of the great works in the history of psychiatry), described in 1955 "the consternation of a German psychiatrist hearing that certain American colleagues regarded manic-depressive psychosis as a form of schizophrenia; for him this was about as fantastic as the assumption that a camel is a subspecies of the elephant."[73] But with DSM-III, depression became the disorder that ate American psychiatry.

Disaster

The two narratives of depression and schizophrenia are especially important for understanding the end of the Age of Psychopharmacology because both turned out to be artifacts that dragged the field into disaster. Both had begun well. As noted, serious depression was the old melancholia, a diagnosis of such power that it can be traced back to antiquity. And when Kraepelin conceived dementia praecox in 1893 it came as a revelation to a field that had classified the psychotic illnesses in terms of current disease picture rather than as disease processes.[74] Thus, Kraepelin had said there were basically two great disease processes in psychiatry: the process that led to manic-depressive insanity, a serious mood disorder; and the process that led to dementia praecox, a relentless disintegration of the personality leading to dementia. Not every line of Kraepelin's analysis was correct. He vastly exaggerated the gravity of the prognosis in dementia praecox. Yet it was a grand diagnostic coup de main that transformed the field's diagnoses.

By the beginning of the new millennium, both diagnoses had become smoking garbage dumpsters: DSM-III had split Kraepelin's manic-depressive illness into "bipolar disorder" and "major depression." There is no convincing evidence that the depression of the former is different from that of the latter, or that the occasional eruption of mania into a depressive picture is so significant as to represent a disease of its own. Both "bipolar disorder" and "major depression" are within themselves vastly disparate and have become pretexts for the sale of drugs.

In 2016, Mickey Nardo asked, What constitutes depression? "Would it be people who say they're depressed? Which is what unhappy people nowadays say to describe how they feel—bad marriages, no marriages, the burden of a difficult biography, personality disorders, situational crises, grief, loneliness, etc. The formal diagnosis of depression has become corrupted in the recent era—simplified to mean almost any constellation of discrete symptoms and causes."[75] But all members of this vast population were candidates for drug treatment.

Furthermore, Kraepelin's dementia praecox, a century later now called schizophrenia, was ripe for dismantling and disaggregation. Yet that has not happened. Schizophrenia has remained in the middle of the diagnostic field, exactly as it had at Bleuler's Zurich Cantonal Psychiatric Hospital in 1910. Entire libraries have filled up with literature analyzing a disease that basically did not exist.

These were the main diagnoses of psychopharmacology, and they were, for scientific integrity, a poisoned chalice.

6

Industry

Early Days

There is an innate tension between science and commerce, between what is proven true and what is possibly profitable.—Barry
Blackwell (2012)[1]

Industry efforts to woo physicians did not begin in the 1950s. At a meeting
in 1933 of the Sections of Therapeutics and Psychiatry of the Royal Society of
Medicine, one veteran practitioner said that medical men who were still newbies
"often entered upon a somewhat indiscriminate use of hypnotics, stimulated by
a constant supply of free samples and desk blotters from the manufacturers.' "[2]
From free desk blotters to the free ballpoints of recent memory: Twas thus
ever so.

Of interest to us is not penny-ante bribery by the detail men but the big
bribery story by the head office. It is simultaneously a story of science and a story
of commerce.

It was in 1858 that the pharmaceutical industry began, with the discovery by
August Kekulé, then at Ghent, that carbon atoms can link to themselves to form
long chains. Kekulé, who became a professor in Bonn, further learned in 1865 that
a ring of six carbon atoms can be closed into a benzene ring. This formed the basis
of the dye industry, an industry that then—with such firms as the predecessors of
Geigy, Ciba, Sandoz, and Bayer—turned into the pharmaceutical industry.

Before the Second World War, in the United States such "full-line" firms as
Merck and Pfizer bought medicinal chemicals in bulk and processed them into
pharmaceuticals for sale to pharmacies or directly to physicians, who dispensed
them to patients.[3] (The idea was to displace the compounding pharmacist as the
manufacturer of pharmaceuticals.) As one report noted, "These segments of the
industry gave the industry many of the aspects of an exclusive gentleman's club."[4]
All this activity was vastly accelerated by the introduction before the First World
War of a new pill-making technology that Colonel Eli Lilly and W. E. Upjohn
were quick to adopt. In 1900, with aspirin, Bayer in Leverkusen became the first
drug company to market a major product in tablet form.[5]

In the 1920s, the transition of drug manufacture into an industry rather than a profession was already in full swing. Robert Fischelis, who was secretary of the state board of pharmacy in New Jersey in the 1920s, recalled that in the old days the average pharmacy filled "around thirty prescriptions a day. Well, now thirty prescriptions a day would keep one pharmacist fairly busy. In the days when there was a good deal of compounding, it was a full day's work, but when ready-made products came on and the pharmacist didn't have to pack capsules anymore, or mix liquids, he could fill these prescriptions in a very short time."[6] Castoria, a laxative for infants, sold nearly 20 million bottles in 1929. The retail sales of the Emerson Drug Company's sole product—Bromo-Seltzer—totaled at least $20 million a year. The Lambert Pharmaceutical Company spent at least $5 million for the advertising alone of Listerine.[7] The days of the corner druggist as a compounder of medication were over.

A hundred years later, these developments eventuated in psychopharma-cology. And it was industry-driven psychopharmacology that triggered, as Thomas Ban put it, "the ongoing transformation of psychiatry into a medical discipline. This is happening because the industry has rendered pharmaco-therapy accessible in the treatment of mental illness." Ban pointed out that, ini-tially, academics, namely psychoanalysts, were opposed to this transformation. Thus, "the teaching of the treatment of mental illness has slipped out of their hands."[8]

The preliminary meeting to organize the International College of Neuropsychopharmacology (CINP) was held in Milan in 1957. Ciba was the sponsor, although Ernst Rothlin, the founding figure, worked for Sandoz. Today, that might spell undue influence on the part of the donor's products but, as Frank Ayd recalled, in 1957 there was none of that. "Ciba did not try to control the or-ganization in any way." "Ciba's major function was to contribute the money to fund the travel expenses for the people who participated."[9]

Ayd, extensively involved in drug trials at his private psychiatric hospital, Taylor Manor in Ellicott City, Maryland, was among the earliest to use chlor-promazine. "I reported the first case of severe dystonia with chlorpromazine," he said. "In fact, I filmed this patient and I took it to Smith, Kline & French and showed it to them. They had never seen or heard of this and they arranged for me to show the film at the annual meeting of the American Neurological Association in Atlantic City."[10] Readers accustomed to industry behavior today will read these lines with disbelief. Rather than trying to cover up or prettify the side ef-fect, Smith Kline asked him to show a movie of it to doctors!

Industry employs scientists who have no manifest interest in propagating untruths—whatever agitprop the marketing people put out. Why shouldn't in-dustry have a big role in deciding what agents to pursue? The problem is that industry is interested only in remedies that can be patented. It is the exclusivity of patent protection that drives profits. As Max Fink put it in 2002, "The commercialization of academia limits the opportunities to develop a robust science of psychopharmacology. The few interventions that hold promise, lithium, ECT, and hormones, do not have the patent protection that would encourage industrial entrepreneurs to invest in their study, leaving their development to a few independent researchers. The promise for meaningful advances in psychopharmacology in the next decades is not very strong."[11]

The Industry Story Begins

Until the 1930s, the "pharmaceutical industry" in the United States existed mainly in the shadow of the chemical industry. As pointed out above, many big firms started out as "long-line" houses, with long lists of chemicals supplied to drug stores, who then compounded remedies. But the First World War created a demand for more sophisticated medicines, and the budding pharmaceutical industry began setting up its own labs. Merck led with the Merck Institute for Therapeutic Research in 1933, then came the Lilly Research Laboratories (1934), the Squibb Institute for Medical Research (1938), and the Abbott Research Laboratories (also 1938). Many early drugs emerged from these labs. As Thomas Ban put it, "Modern psychopharmacology was created by the drug companies and people from the drug companies have played an important role in moving psychopharmacology ahead during the past 40 years."[12]

Here, we need a certain sense of realism. The research labs of firms like Lilly and Merck did real research and constituted a culture of their own. But, referring to much of the rest of industry, Haskell Weinstein, the former medical director of Pfizer's division Roerig, debunked for the Kefauver Committee in 1961 the scientific value of in-house drug company "research." "Much that is called research in the pharmaceutical industry has little relationship to what most people engaged in academic and research activities would consider to be scientific research. . . . Mostly, . . . [it aims] to modify the original drugs just enough to get a patentable derivative, but not to change it enough to lose the original effect."[13]

Yet there was real research. The 1950s were the great decade of innovation. For "big science" as a whole, the 1960s were then "the go-go years," as Roy Vagelos, CEO of Merck, put it: Government funding, the expanding universities, industry recruiting, and a ton of new posts at NIH made the decade a kind of scientific apogee.[14]

After the 1962 Kefauver-Harris amendments to the drug act of 1938, a process of retraction began: There were mergers and bankruptcies as FDA regulations greatly increased the costs of registration and only large firms could afford to satisfy the requirements. In 1968, there were 111 drug companies in the United States, plus 25 associated subsidiaries, usually with their headquarters in Europe. By 2019, the number had dropped to 35. But, of the latter number, there were really only about nine big companies oriented toward research.[15] The process of concentration had been immense. Pfizer, one of the nine, had acquired over the years American Cyanamid, American Home Products, Pharmacia, Upjohn, Warner-Lambert, and Wyeth, as well as the pharmaceutical branch of Monsanto.[16]

Europe was the actual center of gravity of psychopharmacology in the early days, and, as we have seen, it was the pharmacologist Ernst Rothlin, the former research director of Sandoz, who was instrumental in founding CINP in Zurich in 1957. Rothlin was the first president of CINP, and the first meeting in 1958 in Rome was financed by Ciba and other members of a consortium of heavily Swiss-based drug companies with branch operations in Italy. At that meeting, Rothlin asked the question that was on everyone's mind—certainly on industry's mind: "If we admit that some psychotropic drugs influence psychic and emotional processes, the logical question which follows is 'How do they produce their effects?'"[17] (This is the question that 60 years later, and after billions of dollars of research, still has not been answered.) The members of the new organization were absolutely immersed in industry. Yet was there any question of KOLs selling out their principles for industry coin? Not at all.

Right up to the 1980s, the American pharmaceutical industry remained a tail wagged by a big European dog. Of 148 "medicinal innovations" identified between 1800 and 1930, 44 percent came from Germany, 16 percent from France, and 14 percent from the United States.[18] Of all the New Clinical Entities (new drugs) introduced between 1961 and 1973, 23.6 percent came from France—and from that country's traditionally vibrant pharmaceutical industry; 15.1 percent from Germany, a country that before 1933 had been the world leader in drug research; and only 9.0 percent from the United States.[19]

But in one area the Americans were ahead: sales of psychopharmaceuticals. In the United States in 1994, 17 percent of total drug sales were psychiatric in nature; in Europe, 11 percent; in Japan, 5 percent.[20]

"Science-Based Competition"

A quick look at the major players shows how, in the early days, they engaged in behavior that was very different later.

Merck

Merck and Company, originally a German firm, founded a US branch in 1891 that became fully independent in 1919. The US company grew steadily, acquiring Sharp and Dohme in 1953, to become MSD.

The Merck Institute embodied the new badge of scientific respect. Alfred N. Richards, who joined the pharmacology staff of the University of Pennsylvania in 1910, was arguably the godparent of American pharmacology. In 1922 he developed the first course in clinical pharmacology in the United States. He became a Merck "consultant" in 1930, on the condition, as historian Nicolas Rasmussen explained, "that Merck never use his name publicly without his explicit approval, and that the firm impose no constraints on what he might publish in the scientific literature."[21] An oil portrait of a distinguished-looking Richards, with a cigarette in his hand, hangs in the lobby of Merck's head office in Rahway, New Jersey. And on Richards' recommendation, the Merck Labs hired Viennese pharmacologist Hans Molitor as the director. The company provided ample material support, and the scholarly output of the Merck Labs was considerable, "nearly fifty papers from 1939 to 1941," as Lesch stated.[22]

When Edward Scolnick came to Merck from NIH in 1982 (to become chief of research 3 years later), he landed in the middle of Merck's "science-based culture." How did Merck decide which drug to develop among the profusion from the laboratory benches? "Merck's winnowing process has evolved over three decades into committees of scientists who discuss one another's work with brutal frankness. It's a system of peer review modeled on one used at the NIH," and, said Scolnick, it "allows a really good debate about what we should be doing."[23]

There was at Merck a kind of corporate "caste" system, the scientists being the highest caste, the marketers the lowest. At the Merck Research Labs, said Roy Vagelos, chief executive officer of Merck, "The MRL scientists looked down on marketing as an inferior, low-status activity. Marketing was at best a necessary evil. . . . At Merck, the scientists were industry royalty and the marketing folks were commoners."[24]

Vagelos, as chief executive officer of Merck, was one of the towering giants among industry leaders—a man who radiated integrity, competence, and leadership. The industry was, and is, highly competitive, and Vagelos saw the competition as honorable and ultimately in the public interest as the companies sought to best one another with ever superior products. It was he who used the phrase "science-based competition."[25] This was the way it was supposed to be.

And "Mother Merck" inspired a lot of confidence among the loyalists. William Potter, who had gone from NIH to work for Merck, told fellow members on the Psychopharmacologic Drugs Advisory Committee in 2008, "I know this may not sound believable, but sometimes companies actually do studies and introduce drugs way beyond what the finances would dictate. So companies are not always making money when they introduce drugs."[26] Potter had a big scientific reputation and was not an industry flack.

The literature has shown a tendency to demonize the industry. But it would be hard to demonize someone like Merck's Vagelos, who valued his coworkers and thought well of their common work. He wrote, "In the university and in business, a few people were reasonable candidates for sainthood, and some were fundamentally immoral. But most were someplace in between, trying hard to do the right thing, to lead productive lives, and to make positive contributions to society."[27] Yet this sunny statement should be slightly redacted: instead of "to make positive contributions to society," we should write "to uphold shareholder value." Because at the end of the day, Merck was a business—not a mini-NIH—and companies had to make money or face a takeover (and massive job losses). So it is not necessarily bad that the story is driven by money—that is how things work—but this reality is with us on every page.

Vagelos hired Mark Kramer, who would head Merck's psychopharmacology division. Kramer later said, "I knew that I would be entering a company that in psychobiology only had Elavil [amitriptyline]. But I was recruited to help develop the first atypical antipsychotic—remoxipride. [On remoxipride, see Chapter 18.] That sounded awfully good to me, as that is what the field needed. I'd researched and treated thousands of schizophrenics. It also seemed to me that with the right serendipity this was the place I might be able to acquire massive funding to translate my 'jazz style creativity' [Kramer played jazz in a band] into a new science for my beloved field of Psychopharmacology."[28]

A landmark in the early collaboration of academics and industry was the publication in 1961 of Frank Ayd's *Recognizing the Depressed Patient*. Ayd was a prominent figure in early drug trials. Merck's amitriptyline was said to be "his drug." According to Mark Kramer, Merck distributed 50,000 copies of Ayd's book to local medical docs, "and this practice likely began to dilute diagnosis [blurring the line between melancholia and non-melancholia]. This distribution of literature may have happily contributed to the de-stigmatization of depression. It certainly increased sales of amitriptyline. If it had not been for Frank, as the story goes, Merck would not have developed amitriptyline for depression. Buried in an old file cabinet at Merck, I found the monograph to be accurate for the times, and laudably lacking all signs of gloss. So, via Dr. Ayd's book one can already discern a faint distant image of 'Mount Science and Sales.' "[29] Thus, both sides come out looking good: Merck is moved by academic input to develop what turned out to be an important antidepressant, and Frank Ayd legitimated for many colleagues the idea of working productively together with industry.

The company's Neuroscience Research Centre was in Harlow in the United Kingdom. But Merck began to disengage from Central Nervous System (CNS)

drugs in 2001 when it sold to GlaxoSmithKline the rights to a potential antidepressant it had decided not to develop. "Merck did not consider the CNS to be a
core area," said *Scrip*, an industry newsletter, "and would seek to license out all
CNS products that required a large US sales force."[30]

Lilly

In 1926, the Eli Lilly Company in Indianapolis, feeling a need for in-house
physicians to clinically evaluate its new products, created a clinical research program that became the Lilly Laboratory for Clinical Research. Beds were in the
Indianapolis General Hospital. In 1931, Paul Fouts of the Thorndike Laboratory
in Boston joined the staff, and in 1937, together with O. M. Helmer of the
Rockefeller Institute and others, he became the first to use nicotinic acid in pellagra.[31] In 1937, Irvine Page came from the Psychiatric Research Institute in
Munich to Indianapolis as the lab's new director and turned the lab's attention in
the direction of hypertension.[32] Years later, the lab became involved in research
with psychiatric drugs.

By the 1980s, the Lilly Laboratory had a lot of top-flight academic talent on
board. Psychiatrist Alan Breier had come from NIMH and Charles Beasley, who
had interned at Yale, had trained in psychiatry in Cincinnati. Jay Amsterdam,
who ran the Depression Research Unit at Penn, had worked with Lilly staff in
the 1980s and 1990s. "Many of their registration RCTs [for FDA] had a clear
academic and clinical aspect to them that separated them from the rest of the
Pharma lot." Amsterdam had participated in several Prozac studies, which "were
really fun to do—as it was real applied clinical science on Lilly's dime without
the need to write a NIIMH grant. I 'grew up' professionally with some of the internal and extramural Lilly folks, and quite a few I knew as good researchers at
the NIMH and other institutions before they went to Lilly."[33]

In terms of psychopharmaceuticals, Lilly's famous Prozac is discussed in
Chapter 16. Lilly's other main product, olanzapine (Zyprexa), approved in 1996,
became in 1998 the first "schizophrenia" drug to join the billion-dollar club[34]
(and it represented one-third of Lilly's sales for 2001[35]). The company seems to
have had no compunction about flogging the drug's off-label use. In 2000, one
of their physician-consultants wrote to the head office about Zyprexa: "Once the
ground is extensively plowed with good credible clinical information, not limited by the GPP [Good Promotional Practice] guidelines that restrict information to schizophrenia and acute mania, then (perhaps) turning the sales force
loose may be appropriate."[36] Of course, this was not necessarily company policy,
merely one consultant's opinion. But he must have thought his words would land
on fertile ground—Turn the sales force loose!

Janssen/Johnson & Johnson

Today, Johnson & Johnson, with a market value of over $350 billion, is the most valuable pharmaceutical company in the world.[37] It was founded in 1886 to make first-aid kits for railway workers. It launched its first pharmaceutical product in 1931. The company had always had a big public-service ethic, as Steven Brill pointed out, and when Robert Wood Johnson II took over in 1947, he created the "credo," a statement of principles based on responsibilities to doctors, nurses, and patients. Shareholders came last in the credo. Johnson stepped down in 1963, 2 years after acquiring the highly innovative Belgian firm Janssen Pharmaceutica.

Paul Janssen said that the Beerse firm did not start out as a pharmaceutical company. He told David Healy, "In 1953, my objective was not to create an international pharmaceutical company but to create an independent research company. Marketing did not even enter the field."[38] They sold licenses for their products, such as haloperidol (Haldol) and fentanyl, to firms like McNeil. Janssen Pharmaceutica, the drug company, was created in 1956.

Janssen Pharmaceutica, which Johnson & Johnson bought for a few million dollars in 1961, was said to be "the richest prize [ever] acquired by any American firm."[39] Leo Hollister called it "the most productive pharmaceutical company in history." Hollister likened Paul Janssen to "the Henry Ford of psychotherapeutic drug development," and nominated Janssen, unsuccessfully, for a Nobel Prize.[40]

Did Janssen have to pay clinicians large amounts of money to conduct trials? No. "In those days, it was relatively simple," Janssen said, "to find clinicians who were willing to do whatever was required simply for the sake of their patients and because they were interested. Jean Delay [professor of psychiatry in Paris] and Jean Bobon [professor of psychiatry in Liège] never asked me for a dime." Janssen said he might later do them a favor. "To discuss money was simply not done, it was even considered very impolite. Jean Delay I am sure would have been angry if somebody had raised the subject with him. Today I am not exaggerating when I say that it is simply impossible to do clinical research without discussing money first. . . . The world has completely changed."[41]

In 1986, a crisis began as Haldol—the money-spinning antipsychotic that Paul Janssen had created—came off patent. Risperdal was its successor, and there was huge pressure to expand the Risperdal market to make up for the shortfall[42] (see "Sally," Chapter 17).

Sandoz-Ciba-Geigy-Novartis

Today, Novartis is the third most valuable pharmaceutical company in the world (following Roche at second place and J&J, of course, at first).

The royal road of modern psychopharmaceuticals was laid down in Basel by several firms that started out as dye traders and manufacturers: In the heyday of the Industrial Revolution, dyes for all the new woven cotton and wool cloth were urgently needed. Thus it was dye chemistry that laid the basis of modern organic chemistry and of pharmaceuticals. It began with the Geigy company, founded in Basel in 1758 as a dye works. Ciba was founded in Basel in 1859, also as a dye works (in 1884 it became a proper chemical company). Sandoz was established in Basel in 1886, in the dye area as well (the company is known for synthesizing LSD in 1943). Ciba, Geigy, and Sandoz did not complete fiercely against one another, and after the First World War they formed a cartel.

As well, these companies all worked smoothly with the academy. Swiss professors of pharmacology often had industry appointments. Hanns Hippius and his academic group of psychopharmacologists in Berlin began working with the Wander company in Berne—Wander and Sandoz would merge in 1967—on the antipsychotic clozapine, and they published a brief note in 1966 at a CINP Congress in Washington DC.[43] In 1971, Hippius and pharmacologist Günther Stille, a consultant at Wander, explored the possibility of having an antipsychotic without neuroleptic (disordered movement) properties.[44] And after clozapine ran into trouble in the mid-1970s and Sandoz wanted to withdraw it, Hippius came down to Berne to plead with them not to do so (see Chapter 18).

Sandoz's first big psychiatry drug was the sedative Calcibronat, a calcium-bromine salt that reached the market around 1936. As noted, after the merger, Sandoz acquired Wander's exceptional drug Clozaril (clozapine), which went on to become one of the best antipsychotics in history (see Chapter18).

Ciba's first big psychopharmaceutic success was reserpine, a rauwolfia alkaloid, marketed as Serpasil in 1953 for hypertension and shortly thereafter for psychosis.

In 1970, Ciba and Geigy merged, forming Ciba-Geigy. And in 1996 Ciba-Geigy merged with Sandoz, giving rise to Novartis. The psychopharm pipeline ran dry early at Ciba-Geigy, which failed to have a psychiatry drug after Ciba's tricyclic antidepressant maprotiline (Ludiomil), marketed in Europe in 1975, in the United States in 1980.

Hoffmann La Roche, the former Basel dyemaker (founded in 1893), remained independent of this merger. Roche began producing narcotics in 1909, barbiturates in 1922, and nonbarbiturate hypnotics in 1943. It became best known in the psychopharmaceutical area for the benzodiazepines, the first of which, Librium (chlordiazepoxide), launched in 1960.

Astra and AstraZeneca

Astra, founded in 1913 and headquartered in Södertälje, Sweden, got into the export market for its drugs only in 1934. Imperial Chemical Industries (ICI) was founded in England in 1926; in 1993, it demerged three of its businesses, including pharmaceuticals, to form a separate company Zeneca. Astra and Zeneca merged in 1999 to form AstraZeneca, with its head offices in London. Research offices remained in Södertälje, Sweden.

Astra and its subsidiary Hässle had a towering scientific reputation. It had collaborated with Nobel Laureate pharmacologist Arvid Carlsson and English investigator Alec Coppen to research serotonin, producing the first drug that blocked its reuptake, zimelidine (Zelmid). Ivan Östholm, a pharmacist with Hässle from the early days and later head of research, recalled, "I am convinced that the foremost reasons for Hässle's success, despite our small resources, were the new directions indicated by our university consultants and our early employment of highly qualified people in our own research and development department."[45] Note that there is no reference to "marketing plans."

Yet it must not be thought that Astra was indifferent to marketing. Its 1994 annual report said, "A powerful marketing organization and efficient production are essential if pharmaceutical companies are to compete successfully in the international marketplace." An "R&D pipeline" must be backed by "effective marketing."[46] By 1996, AstraZeneca's Losec (omeprazole), a stomach-acid inhibitor, had become the best-selling drug in the world.[47] In 2005, AstraZeneca's antipsychotic Seroquel (quetiapine), approved in 1997, reached the $2 billion club in annual sales.[48]

Sam Gershon, a key Australia-born player in psychopharmacology, had extensive dealings with Astra in the 1960s. "At that time," Gershon said later, "the head of research at Astra was a very remarkable person and did honestly use consultants to examine their material for the truth and they also quickly killed Zimelidine at the hint of side effects. Then after the takeover of the company [by Zeneca] the company quickly swung in the other direction. But there were in many companies people looking for the truth, and with the changes, the picture followed the compass, in the OPPOSITE DIRECTION."[49]

Bernard Carroll, who also consulted a good deal for industry, said that Astra Pharmaceuticals in Sweden was known for doing the right thing. "The Astra Sweden model that I knew in the mid-1980s–early 1990s seems quaint today. They were indeed . . . principled people. I didn't need to twist any elbows at Astra over remoxipride [Roxiam]—they themselves took the initiative to close it down, just as they had done 10 years earlier with zimelidine [Zelmid] over cases of Guillain-Barré disease. Their thinking was that they didn't want unclean hands from unacceptable harm to patients, considering that neither zimelidine nor remoxipride was a major breakthrough."[50] (Remoxipride was withdrawn worldwide by 1994 and Merck, the American licensee, requested that its NDA be cancelled.)

Carroll said that he "sat in on some of those discussions—nobody seriously suggested trying to finesse the problem. Paul Leber at the FDA later commented that they could have winged it with a black box warning but that was not the company's ethos."[51]

I'm going to quote Bernard Carroll again on the subject of disinterestedness of research because he later became a fierce foe of Key Opinion Leaders, clinicians acting as shills for pharmaceutical companies. In his view, the science was altruistic, not opportunistic. "Back then the whole point of experimental therapeutics . . . was to give us a point of leverage into the proximate mechanisms of these successful new drugs. The follow-on goal was to advance our understanding of the mechanisms of clinical depression. The 'business of psychiatry' was never a consideration in the construction of the catecholamine hypothesis or the serotonin theory of depression in the 1950s–60s."[52]

Smith, Kline & French

Smith, Kline & French (SKF) played a pivotal role in psychopharmacology, introducing Benzedrine in 1932, acquiring the American license for chlorpromazine (Thorazine, Largactil), launched in 1954, and bringing out paroxetine (Paxil) in 1993 in the United States. In 1950, the company issued what was one of the most successful drugs in the history of psychiatry, a barbiturate-amphetamine combo that it called Dexamyl. The compound was later withdrawn after the FDA declared both of its components to be addictive.[53]

SKF was founded in 1841 for the production of patent medicines, and only in the 1920s did it begin to go over to "druggists' specialties." But it was under Francis Boyer, who joined the firm in 1936 as executive vice-president (later becoming president and chairman until his resignation as director in 1970), that SKF experienced its explosive growth from a small supplier for drugstores to one of the US 500 corporations, with psychoactive products accounting for about two thirds of its sales. The company was not unfamiliar with CNS products, given its successful line from 1901 of Eskay Neuro Phosphates.

SKF employed a long list of significant scientists, such as Leonhard Cook, the virtual founder of CNS chemistry (see Chapter 8). Among its later presidents was Henry Wendt, who majored in history at Princeton before joining industry. (I, of course, have a PhD in history, and when, in an interview for a book I was writing, I asked Wendt if he had ever taken a course from Eric Goldman, a distinguished Princeton historian, he looked at me in astonishment, thinking I was a physician.)

On changes in the SKF company name: in 1982, Smith, Kline & French became SmithKline Beckman, its headquarters moving from Philadelphia to a London suburb; in 1989, SmithKline Beckman became SmithKline Beecham (SKB), again moving its headquarters, this time from London to Brentford, England; in 2000, SKB became GlaxoSmithKline—GSK. The company was known as SB in England.)

Executives Who Aren't Marketers

Many of the big figures in the early days were leaders in industry and at the same time held important university positions. Alfred Pletscher was director of biological research at Roche and simultaneously professor of pathophysiology in Basel (and also a key member of. Bernard Brodie's lab at NIH in the mid-1950s, as neuronal reuptake was being plumbed).[54] Ernst Rothlin, a former director of Sandoz and professor at the University of Basel, was, as we have seen, instrumental in founding CINP in 1957–58.[55] And Robert Domenjoz, director of pharmacology at Geigy, was also professor of pharmacology at the universities of Homburg/Saar and Bonn (Roland Kuhn addressed him as "Herr Professor."—see Chapter 4).

Who is at the top of a pharmaceutical firm makes a crucial difference. The CEO, who is usually not a scientist, provides guidance in drug development and promotion. Competition among companies has always been fierce, but for many years there was a feeling that working in the industry was an honorable pursuit and did not involve selling one's soul to mammon.

FDA executive Gerald Meyer (who headed liaison with the pharmaceutical industry and Congress) was interviewed in 1995 about his contacts in the industry. Meyer was not a creampuff, and the interview is filled with acerbic opinions about the often-brutal internal politics of the FDA. The subject was the extent to which the industry needed the FDA:

> There is a large number of people—Doug Watson from Ciba Geigy, and Fred Lyons from Marion Merrell Dow, Bob Black from Zeneca . . . Pat Zenner from Roche, and on—who would say, "Wait a minute now. We need FDA. It is important for us that the hurdle you have to pass through to get your new drug approved is a high hurdle, or we'll have a bunch of schlock competitors out here killing people, and that isn't going to help our business a bit."[56]

So, these were, in Meyer's view, the good guys. All were at some point CEOs of the US branch of their international companies. And none of them had come up through marketing.

Douglas G. Watson was a Scot with an MA in pure mathematics from Cambridge University who, from 1971 onward, had risen through the executive track at Ciba Geigy, becoming CEO of the US branch in 1996 just as it merged with Sandoz to form Novartis; he stepped down in 1999.

Fred W. Lyons, Jr., graduated from the University of Michigan College of Pharmacy and earned a master's degree from the Harvard Business School. He became president of Marion Laboratories in Kansas City in 1980 and stayed on in the top job after Marion merged in 1989 with Merrell Dow Pharmaceuticals. Far from being a marketer, he had served for 3 years as chairman of the board of directors of the Federal Reserve Bank of Kansas City.

Bob Black had earned a BA in biology from San Francisco State University, joined the US branch of the UK Pharma giant Zeneca in 1965, and became CEO, stepping down as Zeneca merged with Astra in December 1998.

Patrick Zenner received a BSc from Creighton University and an MBA from Fairleigh Dickinson University. He began work for Hoffmann-LaRoche's US branch in 1969, spent several years in Basel learning the ropes, and then in 1988 was elected to Roche's executive committee and board of directors—he has been CEO since 1993.

All these men were, essentially, "lifers" with their various companies and may well have identified with their companies' reputations as important and dignified American institutions.

Yet there was change in the wind. Alex Gorsky, the CEO of Johnson & Johnson, had started out at its subsidiary Janssen as a Risperdal marketer.[57] After Roy Vagelos retired as CEO of Merck in 1994, Raymond Gilmartin, who had no background in science, took over the helm. He created a new bureaucracy that, according to one news account, "included marketing people, who sat in on the earliest stages of drug development."[58] The research culture that Vagelos and Mark Kramer described began to dissolve.[59] Speaking of the late 1990s, Kramer recalled, "Marketing presence at high-level meetings was increasingly felt by me as intrusive. . . . By the late 90s marketer-salesmen had a strong presence at high-level meetings." Around 2000, Merck formed, Kramer said, "worldwide business strategy teams (WBSTs). . . . Looking back, I now regard these as nodes of growing authority in which the really knowledgeable scientists in therapeutic areas could be insidiously brainwashed into taking a low road."[60] A new era was dawning in pharmaceuticals.

"A Gentleman's Game"

Drug-making was once a gentleman's game. Relations among executives were courtly, not cut-throat, more like a gentleman's club than a Go-Kart race. Klaus Bogeso, Lundbeck's drug-hunter in Copenhagen, said in an interview, "There was a gentleman's agreement that you didn't interfere with other people's invention areas." So companies didn't file for a patent until they were ready to market the drug. "But nowadays you know that everything can be stolen so you simply cannot wait to file a patent."

His colleague Vagn Pedersen at Lundbeck added, "We promoted our products, but we never mentioned the products of other companies. Now today you can find some nasty things being said about a competitor's products. That was unheard of 25 years ago."[61]

In England, Burroughs Wellcome was the big player, and as it contemplated merger with Glaxo, its chief executive, Richard Sykes, "made it clear that he still regarded the company as a serious research company that would have nothing to do with lifestyle drugs like Prozac." After the merger in 1995, as David Healy pointed out, Sykes was gone.[62]

Relations among the American Bigs may be described as a kind of chummy confidentiality. Wallace Janssen (no relation to Paul), who was director of public information for the FDA in the 1950s and early 1960s, said, "Once a firm got a license they belonged to 'the club' and any problems had to be settled inside, in private rather than in public It wasn't good to settle things in public. All the people who belonged to the club were good people and they would do the right thing if and when any problems arose."[63] Of course, later the clubbiness completely dissolved.

To be sure, the 1961 report of the Kefauver Committee to the Senate on drug prices tut-tutted about the gentleman's club as "oligopoly." As an alternative to letting the Patent Office decide about priority, "The companies may themselves decide which should receive the patent. The others thereupon withdraw their applications, in exchange for which they are licensed by the company receiving the award. This process of intercompany agreement on priority is quaintly referred to in the trade as 'arbitration' "[64] (This "gentlemanly" aspect of the industry is one of the last residues of the view that science could be trusted because its creators were gentlemen. As Stephen Shapin put it, "Veracity was understood to be underwritten by virtue. Gentlemen insisted upon the truthfulness of their relations as a mark of their condition and their honor."[65])

Thus, a real sea change took place in the climate of industry as the story approached its denouement in the 1980s and 1990s, and the gentlemen fell upon one another with knives.

"Two Worlds"

It was not that ties between industry and academics were unknown. As mentioned, before the Second World War the scientists working for companies that were members of the big trade associations—the American Drug Manufacturers Association and the American Pharmaceutical Manufacturers Association—formed a joint committee called the Combined Contact Committee to "deal with problems of drug testing and drug standards," as Janssen later said. He added that the FDA scientists also participated in those meetings.[66]

Working *with* industry was different from working *for* industry. In 1950, a grant from Smith, Kline & French plus a Fulbright Award enabled Joel Elkes to travel from his newly founded Department of Experimental Psychiatry in Birmingham to the United States for an academic tour. And SKF introduced Elkes to Seymour Kety, director of basic science research at NIMH, where they talked intensely through a "four-hour lunch." It was doubtless this encounter that led to Elkes' being invited in 1957 by Kety and Robert Cohen, chief of clinical research at NIMH, to found a Clinical Neuropharmacology Research Center for NIMH at St. Elizabeths Hospital in Washington DC.[67]

If an academic wanted to study a drug, they would make application and the company would send the drug and maybe reimburse the academic's expenses. In the early 1980s, James Kocsis at the Payne Whitney Clinic in New York wanted to run a trial with Lederle Labs' new norepinephrine reuptake inhibitor Asendin (amoxapine). Kocsis was interested in comparing it to the older tricyclic antidepressant Elavil (amtriptyline). Against expectations, Elavil beat Asendin. Kocsis said, "This study was funded by the company that manufactured Asendin. I was a little worried, number one, that they wouldn't let me publish it and two, if I did publish it, I'd never be welcomed or have another collaboration with any pharmaceutical company for the rest of my life. I was worried I'd be blackballed. And guess what, neither happened. They did allow me to publish it."[68] Thirty years later, such a narrative would have been unlikely.

But accepting money from industry could be contaminating. Tom Ban, who then was at the Douglas Hospital in Montreal with Heinz Lehmann, said, "I practically had to stop Heinz from paying for our lunch with a medical director of one of the Swiss companies. In the late 1960s, the only way he accepted it was with the understanding that we pay the next time."[69]

Even though industry scientists and practicing physicians worked closely together, they inhabited, in a sense, two worlds. Owen Wade, professor of clinical pharmacology at the University of Birmingham medical school, crossed the Atlantic to point this out at a conference organized in May 1970 at the Smithsonian Institution's center in Elkridge, Maryland: "The industry needs good clinical pharmacologists. I would like to see . . . many more of the men who work in industry, especially the scientists, working with doctors. The scientists at present don't think the way doctors do. They believe in drugs in a way that no doctor actually believes in them."[70] So, in Wade's view, industry science and medical science represented two separate cultures, but the one didn't dominate the other. The industry culture didn't give millions of dollars to the doctors' culture to be subservient.

But working for industry had a different coloration. Len Cook, who went to work for SmithKline in 1952, became arguably the most distinguished scientist in industry employ. Yet what awaited him at the beginning was a cold-water bath. When he told his pharmacology professor at Yale he was accepting a job at SmithKline, the prof said, ""Okay, if you want to be a whore, if you want to prostitute yourself, go ahead."[71]

Tom Ban said, "In the late 1950s and through the 60s people in close contact with industry were kind of looked down on in academic departments. It was pretty stupid but this is how it was."[72] When internist-pharmacologist Donald S. Robinson left Marshall University to head CNS Research for Bristol-Myers Squibb around 1984, his move met with frowns. "A career in industry had a negative connotation for many academicians," said Robinson in an interview. "Industry was considered a cut below in terms of the quality of research. The cutting edge resided in academia."[73] Robinson ended up shepherding the development of Squibb's antidepressant BuSpar (buspirone), which was generally regarded as an effective drug until its eclipse by the SSRIs.

Thirty years later, the situation had changed. Leslie Iversen, who had been born in England of Danish parents—and who had a PhD in biochemistry—went to work for Merck in the early 1980s. There, lots of science was done on "rainy afternoons." "When you finish your week's work on a Friday afternoon, particularly if it's raining, and do an experiment because you have a good idea, that is what I call a 'rainy afternoon experiment.'" His colleague Nadia Rupniak had a bright idea: "She did a substance P antagonist study using an animal model predictive of anxiolytic-antidepressant activity. In the model the infant pup is separated from the guinea pig mother and the pup emits distress by vocalization." Could a drug like substance P diminish the mother's or the pup's distress? Apparently so. Merck immediately put substance P into clinical trials, but with disappointing results. "Merck management learned some of the rules about antidepressant drugs, namely, that they don't always work in clinical trials." "The probable explanation is that the patients included in the study were suffering from mild depression, and the placebo effect, which is well known to be greatest in mild depression, killed the outcome." Iversen left Merck in 1995, "privileged to work in world-class lab in the US and to work for a world-class company."[74] There is nothing negative about any of this.

Industry was glad to get patients from clinicians, but the companies weren't always so thrilled when outside investigators brought in compounds. Arvid Carlsson described this as the "NIH problem: Not Invented Here." Company chemists prized their own compounds and were unenthusiastic about giving priority to outsiders. Carlsson said in an interview with David Healy and the present author in 2007, "We [outsiders] had the NIH problem. That's a very serious problem. We have suffered a lot from that, because we always had to compete with their own drugs, and all the time we lost, of course, and the other drugs that they prioritized are forgotten. Our molecules are still around. They did the wrong thing, by giving priority to their compounds."[75] So, here, relations between industry and academics were competitive rather than collaborative.

The waters swirling around mood disorders were treacherous, and industry needed academics to help them navigate—but the academics themselves had trouble navigating. In March 1977, Ives Laboratories appeared yet again before the Psychopharmacologic Drugs Advisory Committee seeking approval for a new tricyclic antidepressant, trimipramine (Surmontil). (They had struck out in an earlier submission in June 1968.) Two trials were necessary. So the company commissioned Karl Rickels at the University of Pennsylvania, a noted specialist in the treatment of small-d depression and anxiety disorders, to conduct one trial, and Don Klein and Arthur Rifkin at the New York State Psychiatric Institute to do the other. The decision was almost fatal. Rickels ended up studying "neurotic depressive outpatients," and Klein and Rifkin treated "psychotic depressive inpatients." These were vastly different clinical populations. How the Ives executives could not have seen disaster looming is unclear. Members of the committee asked, Are these not separate diseases? And if so, one trial for each won't be enough. Trimipramine hung by a hair's breadth as the committee puzzled over whether there was one depression or two. But then the resistance crumbled. One member said maybe the differences weren't so dramatic. Klein used his powerful reputation to assert that the evidence was "very supportive." Trimipramine passed the committee, six votes to one.[76] So there were real stakes for industry in lining up academics who could plot a straight course on depression. Note that at this point the company made no effort to centralize the analysis of all data under lock and key at its headquarters.

Mark Kramer, fresh medical and pharmacology degrees from Temple University in hand, recalled going to work for Merck in 1989. He told friends, "I think you would have loved the scientific and ethical atmosphere at Merck (known affectionately in 1989 as Mother Merck). I kid you not: for me it was not a job—it was a calling and a monthly 'defense of thesis.' " He said of his colleagues, "These were the best scientists in the world, not because of their Harvard or MIT pedigrees . . . but because they were truly effective top-shelf wunderkinder." Later, came more sober reflections: "I said, we in industry had all been duped by biological psychiatry, and nobody knew why. Circa 1989 I'd not appreciated that the founding fathers of biological psychiatry, APA etc. had only survived psychoanalytic hegemony via selling their souls to industry. Duped. That we were developing medicines for concocted disorders, not yet diseases, was pretty much off my radar."[77]

Looking back, Kramer said there had indeed been a kind of golden era of industry–academy collaboration. "Until financial engineering overwhelmed science in big Pharma, 'real' innovation (drugs that worked and were as safe as possible) in psychopharmaceuticals had invariably been the primary goal of industry when working closely with academia." Then Prozac and its cousins took over and the industry became blinded by profit. This was a major mechanism driving the transition from science to marketing. Said Kramer, "In the wake of the mega-profits generated by SSRIs, with shareholders pressuring for more of the same, [innovation] had been stalled."[78]

Jay Amsterdam distinguished rigorously between KOLs and industry scientists. "The problem is that Pharma discoveries and science ultimately appear in fictitious ghost-written medical literature"; "the nameless, industry-hired scientists who made the discovery" are crowded off stage.[79]

Thus did the two cultures collaborate. Michael Alan Taylor, at the University of Michigan, said, "When the first generation of psychotropic agents was being developed, the pharmaceutical industry scientists worked with academic psychopharmacologists to produce drugs that were effective. The goal was useful and safe agents. New drugs were tested by the academics who designed and ran the studies and analyzed and published the data. Industry provided the drugs and supported the research but was minimally intrusive."[80]

This began to change in the 1980s, Taylor continued, with the introduction of drugs that were "weakly effective."[81] To demonstrate statistically that they worked at all, large numbers of "patients" (newspaper-ad recruits) were needed, so that the p-values would be beneath 0.05—a number that is clinically meaningless because it doesn't measure effectiveness but tells us that the result, however feeble, is unlikely to have been obtained by chance. To get these large numbers, patients from a number of different centers were lumped together and the results compiled at the drug company's headquarters, not by the individual clinicians.

Don Klein recalled how helpful Geigy had been to him and Max Fink when in 1962 they undertook the first trials of imipramine (Tofranil) in depression at Hillside Hospital. "We assumed it would be some sort of supercocaine, blasting the patients out of their rut. Remarkably, these anhedonic, anorexic, insomniac patients began to sleep better, eat better, and after several weeks often underwent a normalizing transformation, saying 'the veil has been lifted.'" Klein and Max Fink then spent the next 2 years figuring out which dose was optimal. "The company provided us with imipramine, assuming that whatever we did with it would contribute to psychopharmacological knowledge and that in the long run that would be helpful to them. This pattern of support has disappeared."[82]

So, collaboration there should be, but as Marcia Angell, former editor-in-chief of the *New England Journal of Medicine,* pointed out, it should not be an embrace, but "cooperation should be at arm's length, with both sides maintaining their own standards and ethical norms."[83] And indeed, before 1980, it was largely at arm's length. As we know, there was collaboration between industry and the academy going back to the 1920s. Yet, as Angell pointed out, there is a difference between working together and selling out. Nardo said in 2014, "It seems far, far away from now. It was the 1960s, and the notion that someone on a medical faculty might have financial ties to a pharmaceutical company was *unheard of*." Then, suddenly, it was 1983. Nardo continued, "There was a new chairman [at Emory], and it was a new day (post 1980 DSM-III). The new chairman wanted me to start a Grand Rounds series with outside speakers. We had no funds for such a thing, but he said not-to-worry, he'd take care of it." At the end of that year, Nardo left Emory.[84]

Industry can produce new drugs, but it can't test them on humans. Therein lies the basis of the intrinsic collaboration between the Academy and Pharma. Leo Hollister remembered that, as SmithKline launched chlorpromazine in 1954, the company searched for academics to put the drug into patients. "When we were starting off, Smith, Kline & French said, 'We'll give you all the chlorpromazine free. You can treat every patient in the hospital.' They wanted to see what the impact was if we saturated the hospital with it. In those days we didn't get six figure grants for doing fourteen patients. We got nothing. Everybody was clamoring for the drug, but there was no money involved. I thought that was a pretty good deal."[85]

The One Culture Invades the Other Culture

Nardo: "Medicine is replete with stories where [the] system broke down" (e.g., thalidomide). "But this story in psychiatry has something unique. The system didn't 'break down.' It was invaded."[86]

The filigree of ties uniting academic researchers and industry began to unravel in 1962, when the Department of Health, Education and Welfare (DHEW) modified the patent arrangements for drugs developed with the aid of NIH grants: Previously, the understanding had been that if industry evaluated in its animal labs drugs devised by academic researchers, the company would have first dibs on the patent. In 1962, DHEW stipulated that the government would determine who had patent rights, the government itself, industry, or the academics. This introduced into the patent issue unacceptable uncertainty for industry, and industry stopped evaluating compounds that came in from outside. In 1963–65, for example, one academic researcher in mental health tried to get two pharmaceutical firms to evaluate his compounds. "Both firms declined to sign the patent agreement required by PHS [Public Health Service]," said a government report. (NIH was still part of the Public Health Service at this point.) Arrangements for testing were finally made with the Psychopharmacology Service Center of the NIMH (see Chapter 10). Then the Center told the researcher that, because of budget cuts, it could accept no more new compounds.[87] Jon Cole, head of the Psychopharmacology Service Center, later said that trying to get drug companies onside was a waste of time.[88] In the big scope, none of this was of overwhelming importance, but it was a straw in the wind.

On January 18, 2012, Joseph Glenmullen, a Harvard psychiatrist, was sworn in as an expert witness in the *Texas v. Janssen* trial over a treatment algorithm that Janssen had sponsored that absurdly favored their antipsychotic drug Risperdal—and made them an enormous amount of money[89] (see Chapter 19). (One of Glenmullen's previous reports in another trial had come to the attention of Senator Charles Grassley of Iowa, leading to a Senate investigation of academic reimbursements by industry.) In this trial, it was Glenmullen's testimony that finally broke Janssen's will to fight. Glenmullen's assessment of Janssen's behavior is of interest and gives an insight into the scope of the invasion by industry into science. (It is also interesting that Glenmullen said he had spent "over 3,000 hours on this case," and at a rate of $550 per hour had apparently billed the State of Texas almost $2 million![90])

What were some of the fibs Janssen had told? "The company's business plans, marketing plans made it very clear that the company was taking the position that Risperdal caused very little or no diabetes."

"I concluded that the science did not support that claim," said Glenmullen.[91]

In a "Dear Doctor" letter that Janssen had sent out in 2003 denying a link between Risperdal and diabetes, there were eight references.

Q: "Do these eight references support Janssen's claims that Risperdal is not associated with diabetes?"

Glenmullen: "No, two of the eight do not." He gave details. They showed just the opposite.[92]

Q: "Is that good medical science to cite a study for a proposition that's just the opposite?"

Glenmullen. "Bad medical science."

In another of the studies, it emerged on the basis of company documents that Janssen had "manipulated" the results before publishing them. The original results said that Risperdal and Zyprexa caused an equally high risk of diabetes.

So what did Janssen do? "They took all the female patients out. They took all the Asian patients out. And when these patients were taken out, that changed the result in favor of Risperdal."

Q: "Do you know of any accepted scientific standards that would permit that kind of manipulation of data?"

Glenmullen: "No, I do not."[93]

Now, it turned out that Janssen had done three additional studies of this question. None were mentioned in the "Dear Doctor" letter or shared with FDA. One was a high-quality prospective and blinded study of Risperdal versus Zyprexa that Janssen had denied existed. Patients on both drugs gained lots of weight, and 2.8 percent of the Risperdal patients developed diabetes. This was three times the threshold for concern. Janssen completed the study in 1999. In 2000, the FDA wrote the industry asking for studies that looked at the diabetes question. Janssen remained silent about this study.

For the second study, a week before the submission to the FDA was due, a Janssen executive instructed, "Do not include." A third similarly high-standard study found Zyprexa and Risperdal comparable, and it was hushed up.

The "label," or instructions for use, that Janssen had devised in 1994 said there could be "weight increase and weight decrease." The sentence was buried in a section of the extensive label that dealt not with serious health concerns but was "a laundry list of side effects." "And it's difficult for a doctor to know how much weight increase, what the significance of that is, and especially when right after it, it says weight decrease. The doctor doesn't know what to make of that. That's very different from a warning saying this class of drugs is associated with serious weight gain and diabetes."[94]

The prosecutor had much more, but time was up for the day, and the court adjourned. Janssen settled the next day.

PART II
WORSENING

7

DSM

When I am sitting in clinic at 4 pm on a Tuesday afternoon, trying to make decisions on whether to medicate, what to prescribe, and what else to do, I would like a DSM that makes sense of what I am actually seeing in the clinic. When I look at drug studies, I don't see my patients.—Audrey Newell, University of Michigan (2008)[1]

A capital reason for the decline of psychopharmacology was the growing view that many of the diagnoses in the official *Diagnostic and Statistical Manual of Mental Disorders* (DSM) didn't really exist. That they were fictions, not diagnostic science. The pivot here was the third edition of the DSM in 1980.

This revolutionary new edition began in the late 1960s in the office of Eli Robins, head of psychiatry at Washington University of St. Louis. But Robins, ill at the time with the multiple sclerosis that ultimately killed him, wasn't there. Instead, he loaned his office to a small discussion group of residents led by fellow resident John Feighner. Lots of drug research was going on in the department at the time, and there was intense interest in diagnosis. Paula Clayton, then a resident but not part of the group, later said, "They met in Eli's office every Wednesday for months. . . . It was John who said, 'We really have to get this into writing.' So they met every Wednesday and wrote the paper."[2] Fritz Henn, also a resident at the time, said, "We all sat around a table and made these criteria up from old Kraepelin stuff."[3]

The paper that began the revolution in diagnosis in psychiatry was written, in other words, by a group of residents—with some input from staff. (The whole concept of "operational criteria" had been initiated by Mandel Cohen at Harvard, and his student Eli Robins brought it to St Louis.[4]) Distinctive about the paper, in addition to their efforts to get a handle on the real diagnoses, was the drawing up "diagnostic criteria" for each diagnosis. You couldn't make a diagnosis of depression, for example, unless the patient had all of the criteria A through C, which included dysphoric mood, at least five of the eight additional criteria (poor appetite, sleep difficulty, etc.), and the illness had lasted for at least a month. The paper, officially authored—in outrageous unfairness—by the staff of the department, with the exception of Feighner, appeared in 1972.[5] The criteria became known as the "Feighner criteria," and the paper became, according to historian Hannah Decker, "the most cited paper ever published in a psychiatric journal."[6]

Sam Guze was, along with Eli Robins, a main figure in the Wash U school of psychiatry, and increasingly he became its voice as Robins lay ill. Washington University became a biological beachhead. As Feighner's teacher, Guze remarked, "There is no such thing as psychiatry that is too biological."[7] Guze and Donald Goodwin later wrote, "In the sixties and seventies, Washington University's Department of Psychiatry gained the reputation of having a strong alliance with biology taking a medical view of psychiatric illness and placing heavy reliance on reproducible data. It believed in diagnosis, and the belief caught on."[8]

Guze and Robins had famously advocated what came to be called the medical model in 1970 as a means of describing diseases.[9] (They didn't use the term "medical model" in 1970, but Guze and collaborators did in 1973.[10]) Guze was bemused by the success of the Feighner article but explained it thus: "It met an important scientific need at a time when American psychiatry was slowly and imperfectly groping its way back to medicine. . . . Our article was a proposal for a new beginning in a discipline that for a generation had rejected our premise [that a reliable classification system is essential for scientific psychiatry]."[11]

The residents gathered at Eli Robins' office table, and the clinicians who moved on the periphery around them, constituted a kind of "college." Gerald Klerman called the informal coalition of scientists and investigators who had started to form around Washington University in St. Louis, the New York State Psychiatric Institute, and several West Coast institutions, the "neo-Kraepelinians." It was psychologist Roger Blashfield at Auburn University in Alabama who described them as a "college," and said that the college followed "principles latent in Kraepelin's approach . . . strongly advocated a scientific approach, supported the medical model, engaged in biological research, and eschewed the psychoanalytic perspective."[12]

That is the micro-picture. The big picture is that Emil Kraepelin, in the various editions of his textbook around 1900, had lumped all the mood disorders into one big basin: manic-depressive insanity. My own view is that this makes sense.[13] But the ideas of Karl Leonhard, the East Berlin psychiatrist who in 1957 penned a revolutionary recasting of the major illnesses, did not like the big Kraepelinian illness pool and implemented a strict division on the basis of polarity: unipolar depression versus bipolar disorder.[14] The Leonhard acolytes soon ensured that this dichotomy became gospel. (One blogger cited "the belief of many people . . . that if they have more than one emotion, they're bipolar."[15]) In the meantime, the Freudians had conceived "neurotic depression," or "depressive neurosis." As Nassir Ghaemi observed, "Thus, the pre-1978 version of proto-DSM-III already was a mishmash of ideas on a sometimes-weak scientific basis.

This led to the radical rejection of Kraepelin's broad unitary manic-depressive illness [in favor of a division] into bipolar versus major depressive disorder; much more data since then pointing in the opposite direction has been rejected."[16]

Thus, the St. Louis–New York axis attempted to rethink some of this "proto-DSM-III" ideology with "major depression" and, in later editions, "bipolar disorder." But the axis was not solely responsible for ushering in new diagnostic thinking. Edinburgh psychiatrist R. E. Kendell later said, "Things rapidly gathered momentum [after Feighner in 1972] for a variety of reasons, of which a convergence of interests between Spitzer's group in New York and Eli Robins' protégés was only one. [Gerald] Klerman at ADAMHA [the Alcohol, Drug Abuse, and Mental Health Administration, est. 1973 as a super-agency over NIMH] must have had a considerable influence on the direction and scale of government research funding in the 1970s, and his lineage was Yale and Harvard rather than St Louis or New York. Other workers like [Joseph] Mendels in Philadelphia and [Richard] Abrams and [Michael] Taylor at Stony Brook were also part of the movement."[17] In their various incarnations, these individuals were the senior leadership in biological psychiatry. They united in scorning the previous psychoanalytic direction of US psychiatry and wishing something different.

DSM-III Begins

We are the guardians of nosology!—Robert Spitzer (1984)[18]

Industry had virtually no role in the deliberations of the Task Force leading to DSM-III. Yet, in the area of depression, industry was not entirely indifferent, and the FDA was prepared to be accommodating. At a meeting of the Psychopharmacologic Agents Advisory Committee. (as it then was) in March 1977, the committee got around to how many trials you needed for depression. Two seemed to be the right number. Thomas Hayes, the leader of the Neuropharmacology Unit, said, "The point . . . is one which I bring up with some reluctance, but I am even more reluctant to fail to face it now and have to face it later. To my recollection, demonstration [of efficacy] in various categories of depressed patients had been held up as a requirement for other proposed antidepressant drugs, such categories being inpatient and outpatient, but not exclusively, and that there be substantial evidence in any group." The discussion was then adjourned for the day with this hot potato still on the table: Do we double the number of trials we require or not?

On the following day, the Committee again returned to the subject: How many trials in which kinds of depression? Hayes said, "I will give you odds that I know what you are going to say, and that is that the data in regard to either the psychot-ically depressed group or the outpatient group is not sufficient, that one part of it is complete but the other is not."

John Overall, the VA psychopharmacologist, seemed to be leaning toward two studies for each depressed group.

Hayes then showed his hand: "I suppose you do not necessarily have to have two of this and two of that." In other words, two studies of "depression" in general would suffice.[19]

The discussion is interesting because in 3 brief years, the DSM Task Force would erase the distinction between depressed inpatients and outpatients, and say there was only one depression, "major depression." Industry clearly had a strong interest in this outcome, although the transmission belt of their interest is unclear.

Why is DSM-III important, as opposed to being just another piece of academic litter destined to slumber forever in the libraries? Here is the frame: Around 1980, the old psychoanalytic paradigm had become exhausted, and psychiatry itself was on the back foot from antipsychiatry and the competing psychotherapies. Yet psychiatry broke out of the crisis with the discovery of new diagnoses that seemed eminently suitable for drug treatment and with the financial support of the pharmaceutical industry. The way into the future seemed secure: industry money together with drug-friendly academics would safeguard the medica-tion side of psychiatric care. The document that cemented this alliance of in-dustry and willing academics was DSM-III. The argument was that it "provided a common language for psychiatry." Michael Alan Taylor judged this as "baloney." "Gibberish spoken by all is still gibberish."[20]

But there was a commercial angle, too. Nardo said of DSM-III: "It opened the door for an unholy merger between industry and academic psychiatry that led to levels of scientific corruption unequaled in the medical profession in its history."[21]

This story really began in 1965, when Joseph Schildkraut at Harvard published an influential article suggesting that depression was a disorder of norepineph-rine metabolism.[22] Schildkraut later said, "I very much knew the potential in this paper. And I had known I was writing about more than catecholamines in de-pression. I was really writing about the place of biochemical studies in psychi-atry." He decided to stop his psychoanalytic training.[23]

Schildkraut's proposal was such a staggering departure from the conventional wisdom that it really set the leaves in the forest to rustling, including at NIMH, where Martin Katz was the chief of "extramural research."

Along with Don Klein and other influential figures, Robert Spitzer, too, was at the New York State Psychiatric Institute (PI), and since at least 1969 Spitzer had been in contact with the chiefs at Wash U. At a NIMH-sponsored meeting on the "psychobiology of depression" at Williamsburg in 1969, Katz evidently corralled Eli Robins, wishing to use Robins' knowledge of depression; Katz encouraged a grant application from Robins and Spitzer on depression.

Spitzer was not at Williamsburg, but Gerald Klerman, then at Yale and the éminence grise of American psychiatry, was. Klerman had evidently been very impressed with drafts of the Guze-Robins article, published in 1970, on diagnostic criteria for schizophrenia, and he thought that the same might be done for depression. So, at Williamsburg, and later in Bethesda and St. Louis, Klerman was somewhere in the mix, wheeling, dealing, and bringing people together. (Bernard Carroll considered Klerman, rather than Spitzer, the true architect of the disaster of DSM.[24]) The NIMH grant was awarded, and the work began in 1972.[25]

The idea was that Robins, Spitzer, and Spitzer's coworker at PI, the psychologist Jean Endicott, would take on the St. Louis Research Diagnostic Criteria (RDC) and "generate a system for diagnosing and classifying disorders that was generalizable."[26] These efforts reached fruition in 1978 (see Chapter 18), but in the meantime Spitzer became involved in the DSM revision. The DSM revision did not arise directly from the "psychobiology of depression" work.

Here is the chronology: In 1973 the American Psychiatric Association (APA) decided to revise the DSM. The APA offered the job of heading the Task Force to Henry Brill, a veteran psychiatrist at Columbia and a sometime official in the vast mental hygiene system of New York State. Brill turned them down, so they acceded in 1974 to Bob Spitzer's request to head the Task Force. Don Klein said later, "Spitzer got the job because it was unimportant. The whole notion of diagnosis was just a nuisance and not central to anybody's concern. . . . It was all psychoanalytic, all mental illness was thought of as a defense against anxiety."[27]

It was Spitzer's job to come up with a new statistical classification for psychiatric illness. For the APA, the distinction between a "statistical classification" and a "nosology" was probably not foremost in their minds. A nosology, as Julius Hoenig pointed out, uses science to arrive at disorders that are valid. A statistical classification uses group consensus to arrive at disorders that are negotiated. It is more like a checklist, functioning like a filing cabinet, than an intellectual construct with an "inner theoretical consistency."[28] The APA brass didn't really need a nosology. They had psychoanalysis. DSM was a classification.

Almost as a footnote, the NIMH project of reclassifying illness was realized in 1978, when Spitzer, Endicott, and Robins—exactly as NIMH had wished—published the RDC. This was really a separate project from the DSM revision, although they have often been conflated. Observers have tended to see the 1978 RDC as anticipating the 1980 DSM. Yet that is not correct. Eli Robins, for one thing, was not on the DSM Task Force. The classification of depression in the RDC was a finely articulated, subtle instrument: There was Major Depressive

Disorder, with eleven different varieties; there was also Minor Depressive Disorder, and Intermittent Depressive Disorder.[29] By contrast, DSM-III, 2 years later, contained none of these refinements: It hit depressive illness with a single great mallet called Major Depression.

The APA Board, which commissioned the Task Force in March 1973, was unclear about theoretical marching orders, but they did specify they wanted "national concerns [to be] overriding" in the revised DSM, which would have meant preserving psychoanalysis—a classification in other words as it had taken form in DSM-II.[30]

As a draft of DSM-III was circulating in 1979, a tremor went through the world of psychoanalysis. In 1979, Boyd Burris, president of the Baltimore–District of Columbia Society for Psychoanalysis, wrote to analyst Jules Masserman, who at the time was president of the APA, "Unfortunately for us all, DSM-III in its present version would seem to have all the earmarks for causing an upheaval in American psychiatry which will not soon be put down."[31] In retrospect, among the few virtues of the revised DSM in 1980, chief is that it broke with psychoanalysis. The Task Force verified that "psychiatry is not psychoanalysis," as Nardo put it.[32] There was a desire, in the words of Joe Zubin at Columbia (Spitzer's mentor) to "cut nature at the joints."[33] Well, they really failed at that. The main diagnoses were chaos.

There was an anticlassification tradition in the psychoanalytic dominance of American psychiatry. The analysts knew why everything happened in the mind, owing to the unifying theory of unconscious conflict. The PI school had to struggle against this tradition. The anticlassifiers insisted there were no psychiatric diseases, only problems in adjusting to life. Donald Klein at Columbia, who was on the DSM-III Task Force, and John Davis of the University of Illinois at Chicago mocked this tradition in their influential psychopharmacology manual published in 1969. "One might even take the stand that defecation is part of life. Since diarrhea is simply excessive defecation, it should not be considered a disease at all, but rather a style of life." Their approach was the opposite: "We believe that there is a variety of discrete etiologies causing specific diseases among some psychiatric patients."[34]

Spitzer was appointed at the PI and some of the meetings took place there. In addition, members of PI who were not on the Task Force nonetheless had a powerful voice in the discussions. Spitzer himself appointed all the members of the Task Force, although there was, he later said, some restlessness about the large contingent from Washington University—a point that lost some of its force when Robert Woodruff of Wash U committed suicide.[35]

Spitzer said that he wanted something quite different from the Freudian nosology, and when the Task Force convened in September 1974, he insisted on "a classification of mental disorders that would rest on "etiology . . . only when it is clearly known," which ruled out all the speculative psychoanalytic musing about unconscious causation.[36] Indeed, the DSM Task Force ended up with a document that was very much a classification, the product of a good deal of horse-trading around the Task Force table.

The dynamic tension in this story is between the psychoanalytic establishment at APA, uncertain about how psychopharmacology was shifting the ground beneath their feet, and the anti-analysis workers at St. Louis and PI, themselves not really psychopharmacologists but, let us say, brain-and-genetics-oriented. Sam Guze recalled an encounter he had at APA with Karl Menninger, one of the gods of psychoanalysis. Menninger had expressed unhappiness that psychiatry seemed to be moving toward a new classification of illnesses and he thought a descriptive paragraph was much better. Guze raised his hand and said, "Dr. Menninger, you know those of us who are interested in the importance of diagnosis want a label that could substitute for that paragraph. What we want that paragraph to include are the key items that research will have shown us are important for classifying that person." Guze said he had tried to make the point in a nice way. "Menninger smiled and took another question."[37] But after DSM-III was published in 1980, the analysts stopped smiling.

What Menninger didn't realize was that, unlike in the rest of medicine, in psychiatry things can change very rapidly and often in a not highly rational way. Look at how swiftly the hysteria diagnosis, once on the tongue of every clinician, was ended in 1980 with a stroke of the pen by DSM-III. This was rational. Look at how swiftly electroconvulsive therapy (ECT) was consigned to a kind of outer darkness by a movie, *One Flew Over the Cuckoo's Nest*, in 1975. This was irrational, given that ECT is the most powerful treatment that psychiatry has on offer. Look at how rapidly effective drug classes, such as the tricyclic antidepressants (TCAs), were replaced by ineffective treatments, such as the SSRIs. From the viewpoint of industry, this was rational, given that the SSRIs had patent protection for a decade or so and the TCAs didn't. From the viewpoint of offering patients a benefit, it was irrational.

Thus, psychiatry moves in jerks. The swing to psychoanalysis in the 1920s was a swing away from the biologism of the nineteenth century. The swing to psychopharmacology in the 1950s and after was a swing away from Freud's doctrines. These swings may be built into the beast. In 2011, Nardo said, "Psychiatry has moved in monotonous cycles where new approaches are widely embraced, over-utilized, then become the new problem rather than stay in their former role as solution." There were the old "snakepit" mental hospitals that were overturned by the new model of community care, which, in its turn was overturned by the problem of the "homeless." "Now psychopharmacology and neuroscience," Nardo continued, are waning "as their limitations and ill effects are more apparent. It's in the nature of medicine to move through paradigm shifts and cycles like this, but psychiatry has less access to an anchoring basic science, and so it swings wildly compared to the rest of medicine."[38]

But in none of these previous swings was *commerce* the driving force. It was science that gave birth to the Age of Psychopharmacology, as the spectrophotofluorometer at the National Institutes of Health made it possible to track the activity of the amine neurotransmitters. But it was commerce, in league with venal academics, that put an end to the psychopharmacologic era, as industry corrupted the trial and marketing of drugs. Commerce, to be sure, was not responsible for the catastrophe of the DSM that created heterogeneous entities for which effective treatments could not possibly be conceived—because the entities themselves, such as Major Depression, were fictive. As the mantra goes, you can't develop drugs for diseases that don't exist.

Who Called It Science?

The Task Force that guided the revised edition of the DSM met on a number of occasions and corresponded extensively. But their mode of resolving the disputes that inevitably arise among a group of colleagues around the table was unnerving: They decided issues by voting rather than by appeals to science. It was as though the speed of light had been decided by vote.

The work of the Task Force consisted of listing "operational criteria" for each diagnosis, symptoms the patient needed to have before the diagnosis could be conferred. This sounds pretty rigorous. There were five symptoms for major depression. Psychiatrist James O'Brien, based in Mira Loma, California, interviewed Spitzer. "How exactly did you decide on five criteria as being your minimum for depression?"

Spitzer took a sip of orange juice and thought for a second. "It was just a consensus. We would ask clinicians and researchers: 'How many symptoms do you think patients ought to have before you would give the diagnosis of depression?' And we came up with the arbitrary number of five."

O'Brien: "But why did you choose five and not four. Or why didn't you choose six?"

"Spitzer smiled impishly, looking me directly in the eyes. 'Because four just seemed like not enough. And six seemed like too much.'"

O'Brien commented later, "Thanks. Pick a number, any number! SCIENCE!"

Carroll: "Science? Who called it science?"[39]

In 1979 the Task Force was close to a final draft. Spitzer had argued throughout for schizophrenia as a unitary diagnosis, rather than "the schizophrenic psychoses."[40] Yet Nancy Andreasen, a major schizophrenia expert at the University of Iowa, was unhappy with some of the draft. She said on March 14 that in chronic schizophrenia, "poverty of content of speech combined with affective blunting and an avolitional state" were much commoner that delusions or hallucinations. She said of the proposed text, "It is a patchwork, due to repeated attempts to rewrite it quickly. I would like to overhaul it completely." She then went on to make specific suggestions, such as the failure to use the classical term "derailment" instead of "loosening of associations." (In fact, "derailment" comes from the powerful German term *Entgleisung* [train wreck] and captures better the speech catastrophe of being unable to stay on subject.)

How to resolve these disputes? A vote, of course. On March 20, a ballot went out with five questions, on which Task Force members were required to pass judgment. One question: "Nancy wishes to include the concept of poverty of speech and tangentiality." Do you agree or not?

Robert Spitzer, head of the Task Force, had a tendency to behave in a rather dictatorial manner and somehow came out on top of almost all of the disagreements. The tabulation of the vote has not been preserved, although Spitzer's views seem to have been endorsed, because his follow-up note has a triumphalist ring. He argued on March 28, 1979, "We agree with Nancy that poverty of speech . . . is very common in schizophrenia. We do not believe that it is a characteristic symptom of the disorder." ("We" meant himself and his coworker Jean Endicott, although it is unclear to what extent she participated in the drafting of his memos sent on "their" behalf.) He disliked derailment: "When trains leave railroad tracks, they rarely get right back onto them, whereas schizophrenic speech frequently veers off but returns back to a central theme."

Yet, not all were happy with this mode of conducting business. On April 4, Donald Klein, the director of research at PI, challenged Spitzer: "Your use of the questionnaire technique seems somewhat erratic. . . . I'm sorry to have to raise these issues publicly, but, again the issue of arbitrary judgment without proper consultation raises its ugly head."[41]

I have reproduced this exchange in some detail, not because of its intrinsic importance—there were dozens of such exchanges in the course of drafting DSM-III from 1974 to 1979—but to make the point that opinion and arbitrary fiat guided the entire DSM process, not science. Nardo said, "They preached evidence-based medicine but they practiced expert opinion."[42] What emerged in 1980 could not possibly be viewed as a scientific document—but only as a political one.

DSM-III was a "consensus-based" document. While consensus is wonderful in committee dynamics, it has a major intellectual handicap: real differences may disappear in the bland pudding of agreement. As Tom Ban, who led psychopharmacology at Vanderbilt University, pointed out, "Consensus-based diagnoses . . . are detrimental for progress in nosological research. They cover up the component diagnoses that might be selectively affected by psychotropic drugs.

The use of consensus-based diagnoses has not provided the necessary feedback for developing clinically more selective and thereby more effective psychotropic drugs."[43] This pithy statement nails exactly why DSM has been fatal for progress in psychopharmacology.

It was DSM-III that guided the subsequent Age of Psychopharmacology. DSM-III's major depression became psychiatry's favorite diagnosis, and the scads of Prozac look-alikes to relieve major depression became psychiatry's favorite treatment. The Age of Psychopharmacology collapsed in the end because of the scientific inadequacy of the diagnostic classification and the therapeutic inadequacy of the SSRIs, which, as they went off patent early in the new century, seemed little better than placebos in the treatment of real depression.

The Birth of Major Depression

> If you are stupid and put people with TB into your angina study, you are not going to show that your antianginal drug works.—Robert Temple (then director of the Cardiorenal Division of FDA, 1981)[44]

In 1981, Bob Temple was not thinking of antidepressant trials, but he could have been. The great obstacle to the discovery of new, effective drugs in mood disorders has been the hodge-podge of major depression that DSM-III created in 1980. DSM-III was received with incredulity in many circles, especially the part of it collapsing all the previous depressions into major depression. In all the controversy since surrounding DSM, this has probably been the most acute issue.

Of the various defects of the third edition of DSM, the greatest was the creation of the diagnosis of major depression, conceived as a political move to drive the analysts and their "depressive neurosis" out of psychiatry. It became a dambuster for the flood of "antidepressants" that sluiced over American society in the following decades.[45]

The term "major" had been floating around the depression basin for some years. At a conference at McGill University in 1959, Michael Shepherd from the Maudsley Hospital in London used the phrase "major depressive illnesses."[46] DSM-II in 1968 had a category called "major affective disorders."[47] The diagnosis "major depressive disorder" was originated in 1975 by Spitzer in an early draft of the RDC, with numerous subtypes.[48] By the final draft of the RDC in 1978 there were eleven subtypes of major depression, which made the diagnosis flexible.[49] Then, at the very end of the DSM process in 1979, as the Task Force was unable to agree on how to classify depressive illness, the disease designers again returned to "major depression." But this time there was really only one major depression, with no subtypes. (You could "specify" if melancholia or psychosis was present, but these were not subtypes.) For Spitzer, major depression was now a single disease.

Spitzer conceived rejigging the depression section as part of his agenda to drive psychoanalysis out of psychiatry. A favorite analytic diagnosis, depressive neurosis, could be destroyed under the pretext that there was only one depression, major depression. The scientific consensus that had evolved before 1980 about the structure of depressive illness was thus rubbished in DSM-III. Henceforth, there would be only one depression—major depression." The analysts were so stunned by this sophistry that they never organized a major counterattack, and DSM-III sailed through the Assembly of the APA with only a few feeble squeaks against it.

The "scientific" justification for folding the two depressions into one was a single research study that said severe depression and reactive depression had the same number of stressful events.[50] So they must be the same disease!

Mickey Nardo commented in 2015, "Robert Spitzer was so worried that the psychoanalysts and psychotherapists would reframe any equivalent of the former 'depressive neurosis' to fit their own model, that he left it out altogether. By lumping together widely diverse groups of patients into his Major Depressive Disorder (MDD), he created a category exploited to the tune of billions by industry, got many people overmedicated . . . and created a thirty-five year fiction."[51] Elsewhere, I have discussed in detail the meanderings of the Task Force that ultimately eventuated in this portmanteau diagnosis.[52]

To be sure, melancholia made it into DSM-III as a "fifth-digit code for the subclassification of major depressive episode," but even this afterthought was watered down. Around 1980, Paula Clayton, a former St. Louis trainee and colleague, now head of psychiatry at the University of Minnesota, said in an audio cassette introducing the new DSM, "Melancholia has such a severe ring to it that patients won't like it when they see it on their insurance forms." She recommended writing on the face sheet of the chart just "3," which stood for melancholia in the fifth-digit column of the major depression code. "It doesn't have to be written on the front sheet. It could be just major depression, recurrent, or something."[53] Or something! The psychiatric world was about to say goodbye to melancholia.

Mickey Nardo said of these events, "One of the enduring flaws in the DSM-III system—the lumping of the Major Depressive syndromes with the much more common reaction depressions—was driven by the zeal to remove depressive neurosis from the diagnostic system. The net result was to shut down productive research on those major syndromes (by dilution) and to open the door (by inclusion) to industry and their minions . . . for a decades-long antidepressant marketing spree. We were not led from 'atheoretical with regard to etiology' [Spitzer's initial rationale] to 'a highly prevalent, chronic, recurrent, and disabling biological disorder' by scientific discovery—it was by rhetoric, extrapolation, and the persistent vilification of defeated enemies."[54] (Nardo, a sometime psychoanalyst, was sensitive to DSM's anti-analytic slant.)

Senior figures, who had long treated inpatient depression as an entity very different from the outpatient sort, found infuriating the creation of just a single depression called major depression. Said Mickey Nardo, "I just couldn't get my mind to put people who became depressed after some life event in the same category as people who just got depressed out of the blue."[55]

In February 1979, as drafts were circulating, Bernard Carroll at the University of Michigan wrote Spitzer, "It is a serious mistake to have only one basic depressive typology or category. . . . I believe that there should be two categories of depression. These should be endogenomorphic and non-endogenomorphic depression. . . . I am sincerely suggesting these changes to you with the greatest possible sense of urgency. I honestly believe that you will be buying yourself (and the rest of us) a lot of grief if you allow the unitary category of major depressive disorder to remain."[56] (By endogenormorphic, Carroll meant the illness that Donald Klein had described in 1974: "All depressions with similar symptomatology regardless of precipitation, are labeled endogenomorphic."[57] For Carroll, non-endogenomorphic—a term that was not taken up—meant more subjective psychological or characterological sensations of depression. This usage did not survive.)

Carroll was considered one of psychiatry's most trenchant critics, and it is of interest that he later said, "The essential strategic blunder of DSM-III . . . was the decision to walk away from hard-won clinical insights concerning melancholic and nonmelancholic depression. This problem was compounded by two more blunders: the characterization of generic major depression as melancholia lite, and the lack of syndromal depth in the DSM-III-IV definitions of generic major depression as well as the melancholia specifier." What is syndromal depth? You have two very different mood-disordered patients in front of you. It would be wonderful to give them differential diagnoses other than major depression. Carroll defined this kind of depth as "the texture one gets when salient information like your patient's past episodes and family history are considered in addition to the list of allowable symptoms." He wrote this in 2011. "As best I can tell, DSM-5 will continue with the crippling heterogeneity of generic major depression."[58] He was not wrong.

Industry had no role in the making of major depression but gladly accepted it as a billion-dollar gift. There was to be only one depression, major depression, and one class of antidepressants would be indicated for its relief: Prozac and its SSRI cousins. There were other antidepressant drugs available, but how to choose among them? Carroll said, "Clinical diagnosis became a quagmire of undifferentiated depressive complaints, with no guidelines for selecting treatment approaches."[59] The rival drug classes were quickly forgotten, and today, what young psychiatrist prescribes MAOIs (monoamine oxidase inhibitors) or tricyclics?

There was, in fact, a second depression in DSM-III, although news of it was largely drowned out amid all the industry noise about major depression: "dysthymic disorder" replaced what the drafters had been calling "chronic minor depressive disorders."[60] In 1979, shortly before the launch, Spitzer promised to put "neurotic depression" in parentheses after it, thus giving the psychoanalysts a short-lived victory (In fact, "depressive neurosis" was the term used, a neurosis, not a mood disorder. Depressive neurosis vanished from later editions; there was, unsurprisingly, no industry interest in "adjustment disorder with depressed mood," which might not have required medication.) Spitzer said that he had to go to a psychiatric dictionary to look up exactly what dysthymia meant, so it was not a great victory for science.[61] Don Klein, in a furious blast at Spitzer for having ceded to the political pressure of the psychoanalysts on depressive neurosis, made this very point: "To respond to this sort of unscientific and illogical . . . pressure in the fashion that Dr. Spitzer suggests is unworthy of scientists who are attempting to advance our field via clarification and reliable definition."[62]

Blundering into a Swamp

Untutored by history and incurious about the physical side of psychiatric illness, the designers of DSM-III blundered into a swamp.

There was the swamp of micro-diagnoses when macro would have served perfectly well. DSM-III contained 265 diagnoses. According to Henry Pinsker, a staffer at the Beth Israel Medical Center in New York, that would be about 259 too many. He told Spitzer in 1982, "Most of our residents get by with just five diagnoses: Major Depressive Disorder, Manic Disorder, Bipolar Disorder, Adjustment Disorder, and Borderline Personality . . . Schizophrenia is rare."[63]

Another problem was privileging the current clinical picture ("phenomenology") over other such nosological principles as lab tests, family history, and response to treatment. As news of the proposed new edition started to filter out, observers were appalled. At a meeting of the American Psychopathological Association in 1978, Max Fink called attention to electroencephalography (EEG) as a diagnostic aid (countering the mantra that "There are no diagnostic signs in psychiatry"). Fink then said, "I came to this meeting to introduce response measures and laboratory test procedures for classification of populations. I think the APA Task Force has ignored these data and selected phenomenological aspects primarily. Phenomenology marked the many earlier classification systems, and the fact that the system is revised again is evidence enough that such a strategy is expedient but inherently of limited value." He said the next classification should be based on other criteria, "such as treatment response or drug response, which may reflect the pathologic processes in the brain which seem to be the basis for most mental disorders."[64]

Fink and Spitzer then clashed over this. Spitzer asked doubtfully, "Let's say we recommended that an EEG be performed when one is considering schizophrenia. What help would that be?"

Fink: "It would be of great help." Fink said the EEG would rule out epilepsy, also that there was a subgroup of schizophrenic patients with a biologically distinctive EEG pattern ("B-mitten pattern").[65] This would be of considerable interest in dismantling the giant "schizophrenia" diagnosis. But the leads were never followed up.

DSM-III-style major depression was a blow to psychiatric research. At one swoop, psychiatry lost one its main research diagnoses, a decision that, as Bernard (Barney) Carroll put it, created "melancholia lite" and "compromised the past 37 years of clinical research into depressive disorders. The loss has been incalculable."[66]

Barney Carroll, by this time chair at Duke, was counted as one of psychiatry's éminences grises: he had enormous clinical experience combined with an interest in basic neuroscience coming from a PhD in endocrinology. He was asked: How could such a blunder have happened? Carroll: "The revisions of DSM-III were never based on evidence from studies but on ad hoc group expert opinion replacing magisterial expert opinion." The well-considered opinions of senior figures with huge experience would have been considered "magisterial," but no one on the Task Force, with the possible exception of Don Klein—certainly not Spitzer!—had that kind of clinical judgment. Carroll continued, "The entire DSM-III exercise was a confidence trick, engineered by the APA following the principles of pragmatism, palatability and payoff for administrative needs. Clinical science took a back seat."[67]

Major Depression Careens Down the Road

It quickly became apparent that there was a major problem with major depression: The category was simply too disparate. Max Fink commented on psychiatry's shift in depression from Kraepelin's manic-depressive illness to major depression. For manic-depressive illness, there were only "a small number of people. When it became major depression, fifty percent of the people are depressed. That's absurd. That's not reality. That means there's something wrong with the label."[68]

In 1983, one European psychiatrist told Spitzer, "Major depression, as it is described in DSM-III, is unacceptable for European psychiatry. The old distinction between endogenous and neurotic depression was more useful for us."[69] In September 1984, Spitzer wrote Don Klein, "There is a general concern with the heterogeneity of the clinical pictures that now are given the DSM-III diagnosis of Major Depressive Episode." He and Klein danced around the question whether the depression responded to good news or not. The question of quite different kinds of depression came up only when Klein proposed "atypical depression," a type of mood disorder that responded to MAOIs. Spitzer had no time for this.[70] (Atypical depression has since been judged as one of Klein's great contributions to psychopathology.)

In the mid-1980s, it was time to prepare for the next edition of DSM, which was launched in 1987 and was called DSM-III-R, the R meaning revised. The disease designers wrestled more with depression than any other issue. What should we do about melancholia, the oldest diagnosis in psychiatry and the mainstay of the European diagnostic tradition? By August 1984, Klein, who had always been a burr under Spitzer's saddle, finally lost patience. "One of the more irritating consequences of DSM-III has been the plague of affective disorders that have descended upon us."[71]

At APA, there was a "melancholia" committee. Votes were held. In March 1986, Spitzer decided arbitrarily to simply abolish melancholia![72] But in the published version the following year, melancholia was merely downgraded from the fifth-digit code status it had enjoyed in DSM-III (having a code number) to a "specifier" (without a code). It is interesting to see how unhitched the disease designers had become at this point from all of the field's diagnostic traditions.

In 2011, "Tom," a veteran psychiatrist, told the *1 Boring Old Man* blog, "Diagnoses such as neurotic depression and neurotic anxiety seemed to work well. They were distinct conditions from the involutional melancholia and endogenous depression that seemed to signify severe major depression with likely heavy biological bases. The pharmaceutical revolution has brought madness to the field and dumbed it down, with horrible consequences."[73]

Much of the deplored "recent increase in mental illness" was in fact the work of DSM-III: The threshold for defining people as ill declined considerably. In 2012, Allen Frances, chair of Psychiatry at Duke University, and Laura Batstra at the University of Groningen in the Netherlands, noted an increase in the lifetime risk of mental illness from 32 percent in the early 1980s to 48 percent a decade later, "a whopping 50 percent increase." Mental disease is spreading? "It is extremely unlikely that we are witnessing any true increase in morbidity. Human nature changes slowly, if at all. In contrast, diagnostic labels and ways of assessing them are extremely elastic and malleable to current fashion. Clearly there has been a massive relabeling, expanding the concept of mental illness to include symptoms and behaviors that previously were considered an unpleasant, but expectable, part of everyday life."[74]

The triumphal on march of depression did not happen spontaneously, as a result of the power of the concept. It happened because the pharmaceutical industry systematically marketed depression to the medical profession and the public. A diagnostic guide should call people's attention to conditions they can actually make better. It seems almost perverse that such a readily treatable disease as melancholia should be downplayed in both diagnostics and therapeutics. Mark Kramer was well aware why industry wasn't interested: "Nobody in-house wanted to study severe patients. That would have restricted labelling to severe."[75]

DSM Conquers the World But, Alas, Without Melancholia

[The] DSM is the primary source of American domination of world psychiatry.—Nassir Ghaemi, Tufts University (2013)[76]

DSM conquered the world like Atilla sweeping across the steppes. Previously, psychiatry was alight with rival diagnostic systems and fine psychopathological labels for conditions, such as "mythomania" (chronic lying). After DSM-III, in 1980 only three or four big disease entities were left standing: major depression, bipolar disorder, schizophrenia, and the childhood diagnoses, such as ADHD. All the rest of the historical psychopathology had been eliminated, one has the feeling, because the widely unread DSM team were unfamiliar with much of it.[77] Thomas Ban wrote scathingly of these developments, "By the end of the 1980s, psychopathology and psychiatric nosology, the disciplines which enabled psychiatry to detect the differences in the pathologies of the processing of signals in the brain and in the organization of these pathologies in time, were forgotten languages in psychiatry."[78]

A diagnostic guide should call doctors' attention to conditions that are treatable. Melancholia, as we have seen, is one. Catatonia, which only recently has come into its own, is another very treatment-responsive syndrome. The first-line treatment is a benzodiazepine, such as lorazepam; the second-line approach is convulsive therapy: It's only a slight exaggeration to say that if ECT doesn't work in catatonia, you've got the wrong diagnosis.

Less familiar yet highly drug-responsive, is the "phobic anxiety depersonalization syndrome" that Newcastle psychiatrist Martin Roth described in 1959.[79] Clinicians need first to recognize it and then realize that it is highly treatable with the MAOI phenelzine (Nardil).[80] In 1976, shortly after Tom Ban arrived at Vanderbilt, the chair of the department, Marc Hollender, referred to Ban for consultation one of his long-term psychoanalytic patients. Ban at once diagnosed "a phobic anxiety-depersonalization syndrome," and recommended that Hollender prescribe phenelzine. For Ban, this was self-evident. The patient "promptly responded."[81] Other highly treatment-responsive entities go back in psychiatry's past: Karl Schneider's "vital depression" (1920),[82] and Karl Leonhard's "affect-laden paraphrenia" (1957).[83] One looks in vain in the DSM for these diagnoses, and it is fair to say that psychiatrists trained with DSM as their bible will misdiagnose many of these distinctive syndromes as depression and prescribe Prozac.

In the 30 years since DSM-III's appearance in 1980, melancholia disappeared almost completely from view, submerged in the swamp of major depression. (This was comparable to submerging catatonia in the swamp of schizophrenia.) Spitzer wanted to ban melancholia entirely from DSM-III-R, published in 1987.[84]

Fink and Australian psychiatrist Gordon Parker mounted a sustained campaign on behalf of melancholia.[85] To no avail. The next classifications—DSM-III-R (1987), DSM-IV (1994), and DSM-5 (2013)—ignored completely Fink's and Gordon Parker's advice. "Thanks to DSM-5," said one psychiatrist, "clinical depression is being dumbed down to a bad hair day."[86]

In February 2012, Mickey Nardo said of melancholia, "Back in December . . . I had recently seen a case and it was fresh on my mind. Although it's a term from antiquity, the disease is still with us just like it has always been. It got removed from the DSM-III for reasons that still make little sense to me. It makes little sense because the condition hasn't gone away. Of all the failings of the DSM-III, DSM-IV, and the coming DSM-5, none seems so absurd as removing this unique clinical syndrome. It is as distinctive as an acute schizophrenic decompensation—once seen, it's never forgotten."[87]

But the DSM-5 Task Force had no interest at all in melancholia. Fink's group wanted to place the melancholia/non-melancholia distinction above the unipolar/bipolar distinction. William Coryell of the University of Iowa, a member of the Task Force, said there was not a chance of that happening! Indeed, the Task Force turned their back on Coryell himself for even daring to suggest it. Coryell told Fink in April 2010, "The interest I have shown in modifying the criteria for melancholia has not been shared by any of the other workgroup members and, given Gordon [Parker's] firm belief that a modification entails a fundamental change in the boundaries for major depression, there would be no point in my pursuing it further."[88]

The significance of DSM for psychopharmacology is that major depression opened the door to what are now routinely called antidepressants, meaning Prozac and its cousins. This has been a historic defeat for psychopharmacology because the SSRI antidepressants drove effective drug classes out of business. The MAOIs, for example, were effective drugs for serious depression. One experienced hand had this to say in 2015, "I'm firmly convinced MAOIs are better than SSRIs, especially for resistant depression. I think the caveat that there is a difference in efficacy between the old and new antidepressants was the influence of DSM-III and not real science."[89] This theme occurs time and again in discussions of DSM and especially the depression chapter (chapters, plural: by the time of DSM-5 "bipolar disorder" got its own chapter). The DSM series departed from the pathways of psychiatric science and was kept on life support by the needs of the pharmaceutical industry for marketable indications.

Huge Numbers of Ill People

The extraordinary enlargement of the concept of "mental illness" that DSM permitted made it possible to assert that huge numbers of people were mentally ill. A survey by SAMSHA (the Substance Abuse and Mental Health Services Administration, the federal mental-health body) in 2014 found that 4.3 percent of adults over 18 had serious, disabling depression. Among youth 12 to 17 years old, the figure for major depression with severe impairment was 8.2 percent. That is almost one in ten.[90] It gets worse: The Mental Health Surveillance Survey by SAMHSA found that in 2017, 20.7 percent of all women had a mental illness of some kind, and 15.1 percent of all men were similarly afflicted.[91]

Various official estimates of the *lifetime* prevalence of major depression around 2012 vary from 13.2 percent to 22.3 percent. So, one in every five Americans will have serious depression (which, in theory, major depression is) in the course of his or her lifetime.[92] Some current estimates are higher: up to 25 percent of the population at some point "depressed."[93] One federal survey put the lifetime risk of any disorder at 48.0 percent—nearly half the population![94]

These numbers are grotesquely disproportionate to the estimates of psychiatric illness in the population before DSM-III appeared in 1980. There once was a view that there were two very different kinds of psychiatric illnesses: the showstoppers and what were once called the psychoneuroses.

The showstoppers were very serious illnesses. Bernard Carroll called them the "A-list." Patients with the "major mental illnesses," he said, were" among the most gravely ill patients on the planet."[95]

Then there were the lesser illnesses associated with dysphoria, stress, and unhappiness. These were once called the psychoneuroses (also, "Shit Life Syndrome"[96]). Here, we are in SSRI country. Patients with psychoneurotic illnesses consider themselves seriously ill. For them, there may not be anything minor about it at all. But they are not curled into melancholic balls on the bed awaiting a hoped-for death.

Among the psychoneuroses is much "depression." And this great mass of so-called depressive illness would doom to failure any concept of psychopharmacology that pretended to treat real disease. The new drugs were drugs for unhappiness, anxiety, fatigue, and a kind of vague dysphoria, not for serious psychiatric disease. This is not science. It is the commercial exploitation of people's willingness to convert stress and unhappiness (for which they might be responsible) into an illness called depression (for which they certainly aren't responsible). The companies knew quite well what they were doing, as they encouraged doctors to prescribe for symptoms, which everybody has, instead of syndromes, which only a few will have.

DSM and the Decline of Psychopharmacology

DSM dumbed down teaching by essentially removing the study of psychopathology from the curriculum. The number of psychopathological entities in the DSM was limited, consisting mainly of such terms as "depression," "anxiety," and "psychosis." As stated, the whole European tradition of making fine differentiations among kinds of presentations was lost—and this is important because finely differentiated entities can lead to highly specific treatments, not just blunderbuss approaches like "antidepressants" and "antipsychotics." (These were, however, categories beloved of industry because each term created huge markets.)

Distinctions? Richard Shader of Tufts University said in 2008, "It is very discouraging to me to see clinicians who don't know the difference between being demoralized and being depressed, who don't really recognize that some kinds of anxiety can be dealt with by reassurance." He deplored programs for intervening in "prodromal" schizophrenia, "when we really don't know that those people are going to turn out to have schizophrenia."[97] It is not uncommon to hear senior clinicians deplore the loss of the differentiation between "dysphoria" (feeling lousy) and "dysthymia" (depressed mood). Does it really matter?

Yes, it does. They may respond to different agents, not everything responsive to SSRIs.

Industry played no role in creating the DSM-III diagnoses. But it did ensure that the diagnoses were turned into profitable entities. Profit is always bad news for science. Industry made billions of dollars on the back of major depression and bipolar disorder. As David Healy observed, "Companies are not simply confined to finding drugs for diseases. They have the power to all but find diseases to suit the drugs they have. The effective incidences of depression, of obsessive-compulsive disorder, of panic disorder, and of social phobia have all grown a thousand-fold since 1980."[98]

Well, then, how are we supposed to draw up diseases? There is a social model and a medical model. The social model goes back to the tradition of Alfred Meyer, professor of psychiatry at Johns Hopkins University in the 1920s, which basically sees everything as relevant in the causation of a specific patient's illness: stress, family environment, previous psychological history, and so forth. And these circumstances are doubtless all relevant in explaining why someone falls ill, but they serve us poorly in identifying disease entities that might have specific treatments.

Opposed to the social model is the medical model, otherwise used in medicine, that insists on a careful description of the characteristics of a disease, on the verification of that disease with biological tests, and the validation of the entity by response to a specific treatment. Max Fink and Michael Alan Taylor used the medical model to define melancholia and catatonia as specific diseases. Fink wrote to a correspondent in 2011, "The medical model asks the physician to listen to the complaints (symptoms), their history and development; examines the body of evidence of faults; seeks objective evidence in tests; offers a diagnosis and prescribes treatments. Successful treatment validates the diagnosis; unsuccessful treatment offers a 'test' of the diagnosis."

The DSM, continued Fink, offered the exact opposite of the medical model. "DSM-III rejected all tests and treatment-responses in diagnosis. Physical examination is omitted and we no longer record weight, blood pressure, or temperature. The cortisol abnormality in melancholic depression and the dexamethasone suppression test were rejected by the APA in 1986. The EEG is no longer essential nor is it considered part of psychiatry so that various hidden seizure disorders are not discovered. The lorazepam test for catatonia and the lactate infusion test for panic disorder are considered 'research' and not part of the examination."[99] Under such conditions of scientific poverty, how could the DSM diagnoses possibly be considered "scientific"?

"I see the core problem as an amateurish approach of psychiatry to objective verifiable evidence," said Conrad Swartz in 2010, at the time at the University of Illinois. "Psychiatrists have nothing in common with Sherlock Holmes, save arrogance. In place of evidence, psychiatry substitutes consensus, as if the APA were the U.S. Congress. The DSM is legislated, just like the IRS tax code. The result is . . . related more to special interests than to life's reality."[100]

Just as in Congress, at the APA it was a committee that came up with the DSM. Diagnoses created by committee consensus reflect committee dynamics and not the world of nature. Herman Van Praag, one of the grand old men of biological psychiatry and professor in Maastricht, said in 2000, "The DSM-III was a consensus-based document rather than an evidence-based proposition. After its publication, a moratorium should have been declared on new editions until the proposed constructs had been sufficiently validated."[101] But it wasn't.

Thus, the issue of validity concerned many observers. Were these diagnoses valid? Did they exist in nature? The judgment of Nancy Andreasen, a premier schizophrenia researcher at the University of Iowa, was piercing: "DSM diagnoses are not useful for research because of their lack of validity."[102] Why has there been so little progress in genetic research in psychiatry? asked van Praag. "The irreproducibility of almost all genetic findings in psychiatry is probably the consequence of diagnostic inaccuracy. We need new diagnostic conceptualizations, to even try to follow the biological express train."[103]

Successive editions of DSM continued to grind out new diseases. Looking back, Allen Frances, as editor of DSM-IV in 1987, confessed to having created gigantic problems. "We made mistakes that had terrible consequences," he told interviewer Gary Greenberg. Greenberg then paraphrased, "Diagnoses of autism, attention-deficit/hyperactivity disorder, and bipolar disorder skyrocketed, and Frances thinks his manual inadvertently facilitated these epidemics—and, in the bargain, fostered an increasing tendency to chalk up life's difficulties to mental illnesses and then treat them with psychiatric drugs."[104] DSM-5 has created such diseases as "disruptive mood dysregulation disorder" (which was confected to take some of the pressure off "pediatric bipolar disorder," which DSM-IV created) and "premenstrual dysphoric disorder" (which was promoted from Appendix B of DSM-IV). This is sort of like a party game in which each team of disease-designers has a go at inventing neat diagnoses.

The DSM had sailed under the flag of "specificity of response." New diagnoses were needed because different diseases responded differentially to different medications. English psychiatry critic Charles Medawar said in 1997, "Nowadays, perhaps the most unifying definition of 'depression' is that it is a condition to be treated with antidepressant drugs."[105] How do we know major depression exists? Response to SSRIs! And bipolar disorder, how do we know that exists? Response to mood stabilizers! And schizophrenia? Response to antipsychotics—here the traditional assumption was that only schizophrenia responded to antipsychotics, whereas in fact they were panaceas. We could continue through the childhood disorders: response to Ritalin! None of this had anything to do with science. "The designation of a drug as an antidepressant," said David Healy, "is a business decision."[106]

The scientific bankruptcy of this approach soon become apparent. With the exception of lithium, there was really very little specificity of response. And even lithium turned out to be beneficial for everything in the mood basin as well as for acute schizophrenia. The benzodiazepines for anxiety? Kraepelin didn't even think anxiety existed as a separate diagnosis, and of the ten separate anxiety diagnoses that DSM-5 elaborated, all responded to more or less everything. Under these circumstances, specificity of response was a myth, and psychopharmacology, as a scientific doctrine that depended on specificity, became a sleight of hand. (If you carve up depression into its various forms, there is, in fact, specificity of response—yet DSM does not recognize this.)

Michael Alan Taylor's judgment of the DSM enterprise was devastating. "The APA and the creators of DSM have lost the forest for the trees that they have planted. The purpose of a diagnostic system is to achieve more than uniformity of language. It must identify homogeneous groups of patients so that the best treatments for them can be prescribed and common pathophysiologies identified so that treatments can become more specific, etiologies determined, and prevention strategies formulated. The DSM provides none of this."[107]

8

Science

London doctor Edward Sutleffe wrote in 1824 of a case of "uterine imbecility" that, "The case was scientifically treated by venesection."[1]

There was a strong desire within psychopharmacology to find a firm scientific basis for the field. Proponents wanted it regarded as a science and wanted to ensure that it was regarded as one. At a meeting of the Psychopharmacologic Drugs Advisory Committee (PDAC) of FDA, Carl Eisdorfer, professor of psychiatry at the University of Washington, said, on the subject of prescribing for the elderly, "We don't have good data on drug efficacy in older people, all of which makes it a little tough to prescribe for them in a rational way, and most of us, while we accept an empirical medicine, would prefer a rational medicine, and by the term rational, by the way, I mean a scientific basis for what it is we do, rather than it has worked for 100 years, and why the hell not."[2]

Chemical Imbalance

No pseudo-scientific proposition has proved more profitable than the notion patients are suffering from "chemical imbalances." Industry leapt on chemical imbalance from the beginning because it sounded so plausible and so scientific, and patients could easily grasp it. "You mean, doctor, that my serotonin is low. Do you have anything that can fix that?" Oh, boy.

From the get-go, industry capitalized on the reuptake-blocker story. A 1976 ad for USV's tricyclic antidepressant Pertofrane (desipramine) promised "higher norepinephrine levels" through "reuptake blockade." "Some, if not all, depressions are associated with an absolute or relative deficiency of catecholamines, particularly norepinephrine," explained the hype. A nifty sketch showed norepinephrine granules about to pop out of the neuron's end bulb and into the synapse, where they would work mental-health wonders.[3]

The SSRI ads aimed at the public were radioactive with talk of chemical imbalances. Citalopram (Celexa): "Helps to restore the brain's chemical balance by increasing the supply of . . . serotonin." Fluoxetine (Prozac): "When you're clinically depressed . . . the level of serotonin (a chemical in your body) may drop." Paroxetine (Paxil): "Paxil . . . seeks to correct the chemical imbalance believed to cause the disorder [chronic anxiety]." Sertraline (Zoloft): "Zoloft works to correct this imbalance [in brain chemicals]."[4] The ads directed at physicians were not that different. Doctors and patients believed in chemical imbalances.

So did psychiatric social workers. One study in 2020 found that a majority of mental-health social workers "reported using a chemical imbalance explanation of depression" with their clients. It was only for antidepressants that this mantra was invoked.[5]

Doubts about the low-serotonin hypothesis of depression started to be voiced as early as November 1974, when, at a conference on depression at Tulane University sponsored by Ciba, several discussants expressed great dubiety about the "biogenic amine hypothesis" in depression. Carlo Perris, from Umea University in Sweden, said the biochemical findings supposedly specific in depression were found in normal individuals and across the board in psychiatry. Joe Mendels at Penn said that you could profoundly deplete serotonin and norepinephrine in normal people "and in most instances not produce a syndrome that looks like depression."[6] In 1978, three investigators at the Section on Clinical Neuropharmacology at NIMH reviewed the evidence, casting doubt on the "serotonin hypothesis" and urging "great caution."[7]

Now the blows landed fast and firm. Alec Coppen, at West Park Hospital in Epsom, who in 1963 had proposed the serotonin–depression link and arguably was the wagon-driver of psychopharmacology in the United Kingdom, said in 1979 that "The lack of any correlation between the supposed mode of action of these drugs (reuptake inhibition) with clinical improvement is striking."[8] Bernard (Barney) Carroll stated flatly in 1984 that chemical imbalance theories were "discredited."[9]

Yet industry clung for years past its sell-by date to the chemical imbalance theory, simply because it seemed so convincing. It made such a good story. At Lilly, executives coached one another in 1991 on the points to emphasize in TV interviews: "Low serotonin levels leave patients vulnerable to tragic behavior." (Also, "absolutely no evidence indicates Prozac as a cause of [suicidal] behavior.")[10]

In the 1960s, academic psychiatry played its part in the propagation of this error, in the belief that the chemistry of synaptic transmission was the central mechanism in the action of antidepressants. Joseph Schildkraut at Harvard was first out of the box in 1965, with his famous article on the "norepinephrine hypothesis" of depression."[11] This would rank among the most influential articles ever written in psychiatry. Meanwhile, in 1969, Leningrad psychopharmacologists Ira ("Slava") Lapin and Gregory Oxenkrug countered with a "serotonin hypothesis" of depression.[12] For a while, serotonin and norepinephrine dueled across the

Atlantic. The dopamine hypothesis of schizophrenia was still a contender, and the "low serotonin" argument staggered along for decades, upheld by cupidity on the part of industry and a hyper-suggestible kind of credulousness among many academics (see lower in this chapter).

Scoundrels all? Bernard Carroll said rather defensively, "Those were the days of disinterested [impartial] clinical science. Back then, the whole point of experimental therapeutics, backed up by preclinical psychopharmacology [animal research], was to give us a point of leverage into the proximate mechanisms of these successful new drugs. The follow-on goal was to advance our understanding of the mechanisms of clinical depression. The 'business of psychiatry' was never a consideration in the construction of the catecholamine [norepinephrine] or the serotonin theory of depression in the 1950s–1960s."[13]

To be sure, the chemical imbalance theory suffered from a kind of intrinsic implausibility that only large amounts of advertising could overcome. Jeffrey Lacasse and Jonathan Leo noted the large number of indications that SSRIs like Zoloft and Paxil were accumulating. "Serotonin regulation," they said, "would need to be the cause (and remedy) of each of these disorders. This is improbable, and no one has yet proposed a cogent theory explaining how a singular putative neurochemical abnormality could result in so many wildly differing behavioral manifestations."[14]

In scientific circles, low-serotonin and chemical-imbalance theories ceased to be taken seriously from the 1970s on. Yet such was the imprint of corporate advertising that the myth continued a zombie existence among the less well informed. Sandra Steingard, a psychiatrist in Burlington, Vermont, said in 2015, "I fairly recently had the experience of sitting in my office with a patient, family member, and his psychologist. For many reasons, I was less than eager to prescribe an SSRI. The psychologist brought in beautiful, colorful printouts from McGill University's website that demonstrated the abnormal serotonin levels in the brains of people who were depressed to educate me on the serotonin hypothesis of depression. He wanted to make sure I knew about this important scientific knowledge. From McGill! How could a lowly community psychiatrist question that source of knowledge?"[15]

Robert Whitaker, a noted critic, indicted psychiatry as well as industry in furthering this urban myth: "Those psychiatrists who were 'well informed' about investigations into the chemical-imbalance theory of mental disorders knew it hadn't really panned out, with such findings dating back to the late 1970s and early 1980. But why, then, did we as a society come to believe that mental disorders were due to chemical imbalances, which were then fixed by drugs?" Answering his own question, Whitaker said, "Psychiatry, all along, knew that the evidence wasn't really there to support the chemical-imbalance notion, that it was a hypothesis that hadn't panned out, and yet psychiatry failed to inform the public of that crucial fact."[16]

Early Science

As the science of psychopharmacology lay aborning in the 1960s, there were basically two competing approaches: One was neurotransmitters (namely, studies of serotonin in the United Kingdom), the other was norepinephrine (studied in the United States). Opening up research on neurotransmitters had immense importance for neuroscience, as it demonstrated the existence of brain chemistry, and showed that the bits of neurochemistry that one could actually study—namely reuptake and receptor blockade—fit somewhere in the larger picture of pathogenesis of brain illness. As neuroscientist Alfred Pletscher later said, "The original monoamine hypothesis initiated the neurotransmitter era in neuropsychopharmacology, introducing a new paradigm in psychiatry."[17] Yet it was never demonstrated that these bits had a central role, that they constituted *the* explanation of psychiatric illness.

The second approach was endocrinological, namely the study of the axis that led from the hypothalamus to the anterior lobe of the pituitary gland, to the adrenal gland, called the HPA axis.[18] Here the object of study was changes in cortisol (secreted by the adrenal gland) in the course of illness. Many biochemical changes in this axis would converge upon lowering or raising cortisol. Now, writing in 2020, we know how this story came out. The neurotransmitters won, resulting in a long period of scientific sterility and a virtual cessation in drug discovery. The endocrine approach lost, and by the 1990s, endocrine psychiatry was dead.

All the science had availed little in psychiatry. Barry Blackwell's judgment was that, "Over the next four decades (1972–2012), the complexity of mental function and the difficulty of translational dialogue became increasingly clear. Receptors, enzymes, and transmitters, often with manifold functions, were modulated by multiple messengers. Genes, like Shakespeare's sorrows, came 'not as single spies, but in battalions,' expressing themselves in uncertain ways and frustrating fifty years of wasted effort on the DSM fantasy that phenotypes, derived by political consensus, might be linked to drug function and specificity. In short, neuroscience prospered while psychopharmacology dwindled."[19]

Then there was a feeling that all the progress in neuroscience had contributed little to clinical care. In 2014, Allen Frances wrote, "The neuroscience and genetic revolutions have been astonishing in their technical virtuosity . . . but to date have not helped a single patient."[20]

Edinburgh psychiatrist John R. Smythies told a depression symposium at Cambridge University in September 1959, "At the moment no one has any really scientific explanation for anything in psychiatry."[21] Almost 60 years later, the situation had not changed that much. Thomas Insel, in stepping down in 2015 from the leadership of NIMH, conceded that the $20 billion spent on his watch had accomplished little: "I spent 13 years at NIMH," he said just after leaving Bethesda, "really pushing on the neuroscience and genetics of mental disorders, and when I look back on that I realize that while I think I succeeded at getting lots of really cool papers published by cool scientists at fairly large costs, . . . I don't think we moved the needle in reducing suicide, reducing hospitalization, improving recovery for the tens of millions of people who have mental illness. I hold myself accountable for that."[22] It is painful to read of the waste of these vast sums that could have gone into productive research.

Industry and Science

The research community is experiencing an unprecedented "privatization of science" in which knowledge is no longer free.—David Korn (2005)[23]

Wyeth had a problem. In 1993, they were about to launch their new antidepressant Effexor (venlafaxine) and needed to cook up a snazzy class name for it, comparable to SSRIs, a class name that had sold billions of dollars of Prozac clones. So Wyeth polled the academics who consulted for them. One was Barney Carroll, then chair of psychiatry at Duke University. "Dear Doctor Carroll . . . We would like to develop a class name that effectively communicates to the average clinician that venlafaxine is distinct and different from the tricyclic antidepressants (TCA), and the selective serotonin reuptake inhibitors (SSRI)." They proposed various options: "NESRI, norepinephrine serotonin reuptake inhibitor," "SCRI, selective combined reuptake inhibitor," and so forth. Carroll voted for "SMRI, selective multi-reuptake inhibitor."[24] In fact, the company opted for none of these and announced in 1995, a year after the launch, "the world's first SNRI— serotonin noradrenaline reuptake inhibitor."[25] We are accustomed to thinking of these class names as scientific descriptions, not marketing tropes. In fact, all the antidepressants act on all the amine neurotransmitters, and enlisting academic talent like Dr. Carroll on behalf of a commercial jingle was done purely as a sales exercise (which does not alter the fact that venlafaxine was probably the most effective of the post-TCA antidepressants).

Indeed, it was because the acronyms made such convincing stories (not because they were ever important in drug discovery), that industry leapt upon neurotransmitter explanations for the actions of their drugs. The first airing of neurotransmitters at the Psychopharmacologic Drugs Advisory Committee (PDAC) occurred in 1979 when Ciba, presenting its new antidepressant maprotiline (Ludiomil) for approval, argued that the drug "has relatively specific norepinephrine reuptake-blocking properties and has little effect on the serotonin system."[26] (At that point, FDA permitted them to advertise the presumed neurotransmitter mechanism, later it did not.)

In the conflict between research and marketing, marketing always won. There is nothing recent about this. Paul Hoch, a chieftain at the New York State Psychiatric Institute, said in 1960, "The scientific divisions of these companies are influenced, and not always positively influenced, by the sales departments, and sometimes the struggle which goes on between these two things is rather strong, but you can easily pick who wins. . . . I was witness to several such things, and invariably, of course, the sales department won."[27] In 1961, A. Dale Console, medical director of Squibb in the 1950s, told the Kefauver Committee that the "medical director" of a firm was often a figurehead. "In some companies the medical director is more or less a . . . smokescreen. He merely throws a cloak of respectability over what are really business decisions. Usually if the investment in a product has been large, and if it has great potential for sales, and particularly if the underground indicates that another company is going to market it, the medical director will be overruled. He has one vote."[28] Console, a psychiatrist by training, had resigned from Squibb in 1957, and 12 years later, in 1969, he returned to the Senate to testify about the perfidy of the industry and its detail men—"extremely expensive parasites." He had resigned from the New York Academy of Medicine "because it began to sponsor obviously biased 'symposia' which were nothing more than grandiose promotion programs intended to push a particular product."[29]

In 1997, an academic researcher wrote to AstraZeneca executive Jeffrey Goldstein for help in funding his work on Seroquel in rat research. Goldstein replied, "I think it is fair to say that the decision to fund any preclinical work will depend on the competitive advantage that the work can demonstrate for Seroquel. . . . This is primarily due to the fact that R&D is no longer responsible for Seroquel research—it is now the responsibility of Sales and Marketing. So preclinical research studies aimed at mode of action . . . do not translate to marketable messages that will impact sales."[30] This was a quite clear statement of the company's position on science. There was nothing new about this. The companies had never aspired to being small-bore NIMHs. What was new, of course, were the KOLs.

David Healy clarified at a meeting in 1998 the difference between psychopharmacology and neuroscience: "Neuroscience is about the development of techniques and great men and great women who've got great ideas. Psychopharmacology inevitably involves itself with the culture of the period, the market, what is feasible. It is involved with the marketing of ideas, and the marketing of the evidence in a way that neuroscience isn't."[31] If Healy was right, this news was shattering; neuroscience was ideas and investigative techniques; psychopharmacology was, at the end of the day, marketing.

There is a debate here. Was industry uninterested in science, using lab results merely as a means of selling drugs? Or did genuine science flourish amid the precincts of industry giants like Merck?

Healy and likeminded scholars took the former viewpoint. In 2012, Healy wrote, "Pharmaceutical companies have no interest in what molecules might reveal about how humans work. Molecules are only interesting insofar as they can be used to capture market niches."[32] Yet this view may be overdrawn.

In contrast, Mark Kramer, who spent many years at Merck as head of research in psychopharmacology, had an exchange in 2016 with colleagues. Kramer first quoted George Merck, one of the company's founders, "Profits will follow when we produce medications that are of true value to patients." Then Kramer wrote of his own experiences, "All I know is that Merck and Co. awarded me an internal $50m grant to develop NK1RA [neurokinin-1 receptor antagonist] antidepressants based on my original ideas. Merck allowed me to publish my findings as a first author academic and without interference."[33] Merck and Lilly counted as the two Pharma firms that were science-driven. Many at these firms would have shared Kramer's experience.

"Evidence-Based Medicine"

Who could have imagined that simple ideas like randomized clinical trials or evidence-based medicine could've become vehicles for so much corruption, creating a virtual superhighway for the commercial contamination of our literature?—Mickey Nardo (2016)[34]

Psychiatry is a clinical discipline, not a basic science, and nobody expects it to become wrapped up in abstract theories. But psychopharmacology was, at least, supposed to be "evidence-based medicine" (EBM).[35] Evidence-based sounded good, but what did it mean? In theory, it meant that the efficacy of medications should be tested in the light of randomized controlled clinical trials (RCTs). The problem with this blue-sky aspiration was that industry-funded trials were easy to corrupt—"vulnerable to manipulation and distortion"[36]—so that one didn't have judiciously weighed evidence at all, but instead the corporate story.

The judgment of Glen Spielman, a psychologist at Metropolitan State University in St. Paul, Minnesota, and industry critic, was that the acronym was slightly wrong. "One could argue that rather than EBM, we are actually now entrenched in is *marketing-based medicine* (MBM), in which science has largely been taken captive in the name of increasing profits for pharmaceutical firms."[37]

Thus, the entire evidence-based project had been corrupted. Des Spence, a GP in Glasgow, offered in the same year, 2014, a view from the trenches. "Today

EBM is a loaded gun at clinicians' heads. 'You better do as the evidence says,' it hisses, leaving no room for discretion or judgment. EBM is now the problem, fueling . . . overtreatment." And how about screening patients, let's say teenagers at risk, Dr. Spence? "EBM screening programmes . . . are the combine harvester of wellbeing, producing bales of overdiagnosis and misery."[38]

EBM became the banner under which the KOLs moved forward, paladins of the voice of science and why it called for their patron's drug to be number one. For Nardo, this represented a downgrading of clinical judgment:

> Back in 1980, the people who brought the DSM-III revolution in psychiatry to my own neck of the woods [Atlanta] saw themselves as the prophets of evidence-based medicine. They were specifically disdainful of anything that slightly smacked of clinical judgment (as in "How do *you* know that?" or "But that's just what *you* think" ad nauseam.) They were followed by a second wave who were even worse, in the range of contemptuous—the generation that became what we now call the KOLs. They came at a time when psychiatry may have needed an encounter over its reliance over matters subjective [psychoanalysis], but in the process they turned clinical judgment into an object of ridicule.[39]

Neurotransmitters?

> The known biochemical pharmacology of psycho-pharmaceuticals neither explains their mechanism of action in stereotypical disease phenotypes, nor points the way yet to the pathophysiology of mental diseases.—Mark Kramer (2016)[40]

Knowledge about dopamine as a neurotransmitter seemed best fortified of all. It was Swedish psychopharmacologist Arvid Carlsson, who received a Nobel Prize in 2000, partly for his work on dopamine, who first put dopamine on the map. He had spent a half-year fellowship in the late 1950s at Bernard Brodie's lab in the National Heart Institute in Bethesda. It did not go well. Carlsson later said, "There are two things you should not mention, because then Brodie would be upset: You should never say 'Carlsson,' and you should never say 'dopamine' (laughter)—because he was the serotonin man, and I stole the show from him, and that's of course terrible. I came there, and I was there for five months, and he had this terrific story about serotonin—and a few years later, it became dopamine, all of it. So that was understandable."[41]

With dopamine in schizophrenia, the situation is slightly different from serotonin and norepinephrine. There is a lot of good evidence that blocking the dopamine receptors does relieve psychosis. But asserting that dopamine blockage relieves schizophrenia is a slightly different proposition, if only because schizophrenia, as a postulated disease, doesn't really seem to exist. Yet in the world of chronic mental disability, which "schizophrenia" has somehow come to stand for, the observation of Robin Murray, professor of psychiatry at the Institute of Psychiatry in London, must be weighed seriously: "The excess of presynaptic dopamine in the striatum is supported by high-quality evidence showing a large effect size, thus solidifying the claim that dopamine dysregulation is the final common pathway underlying much of psychosis."[42]

Yet, there are dissenting voices that may not have received quite the airing in trans-Atlantic science that they merit. At a meeting in 1983, Oleh Hornykiewicz, professor of biochemical pharmacology at the University of Vienna, indicated discomfort with the dopamine hypothesis of schizophrenia, although he did not disprove it outright. Rather: "Whatever the mechanism of antipsychotic effects may be, neuroleptics may influence secondary biochemical [dopamine] phenomena, and not the primary biochemical disturbance in schizophrenia."[43] This was not a rousing affirmation of the dopamine hypothesis of schizophrenia.

In 2006, Oldrich Vinar, the head of psychopharmacology at the Charles University in Prague, found that the negative symptoms of schizophrenia worsened with the administration of antipsychotics. For the positive symptoms, the dopamine hypothesis held up.[44] When Ross Baldessarini at McLean Hospital was interviewed in 1998 by David Healy, he added an American voice to these cautionary remarks. Baldessarini began by saying that US psychiatry was subject to enthusiasms. "We have long been a fad-prone group of professionals. Whatever new trendy thing comes along, we not only buy into it, but we package it, market it, push it to extremes and overdo it." He mentioned the overdoing of psychoanalysis, of deinstitutionalization to the point of using the prison system as the main facility for psychiatric care, and the overvaluing of drugs in biological psychiatry. "In turn, this view has encouraged massive but largely fruitless efforts to support a dopamine-excess hypothesis of schizophrenia."[45]

The research of Philip Seeman in Toronto and Sol Snyder in Baltimore in 1976 seemed to clinch an increase in dopamine receptors in the brain as the key to schizophrenia—and blocking them as the key to its treatment.[46] But not all were on board. Leslie Iversen, a neuroscientist at Merck who had been at NIMH, said that after Seeman's work appeared [in 1993],[47] "We went for it. The Merck chemistry team in Harlow did a magnificent job in coming up with a highly selective, high-affinity dopamine D4 antagonist in a very short space of time." But the drug didn't work. "The patients didn't show any improvement, in fact there was a tendency for them to get worse."[48] The Merck team realized that Seeman's claim that there was a sevenfold increase in this receptor in schizophrenia was "a very contentious claim. There's something about schizophrenia research that

impels people to make extraordinary claims. If you look over the history of schizophrenia research, it is littered with the skeletons of chemical hypotheses."[49]

The point of these doubting voices is that a supposedly scientific field will end
up quickly discrediting itself if it nails itself to the mast of theories of dubious validity. The dopamine hypothesis of schizophrenia, while doubtless capturing an
important piece of neurochemistry, has made it appear as though blocking dopamine receptors held the key to curing madness.

There was trouble ahead when Melvin Kohn, a sociologist at NIMH in the
mid-1950s, started attending the biochemistry seminars: "I may hold the
world record among sociologists for attending seminar presentations about
catecholamines [dopamine, norepinephrine neurotransmitters] and for being
able to spot where any particular biochemical agent stood in the seemingly inev-
itable course from being *the* hypothesized cause of schizophrenia, to becoming
a hypothesized genetic marker for schizophrenia, to perhaps being the cause of
what was then termed manic-depressive psychosis, to perhaps being a genetic
marker for that disorder."[50]

Kohn was in at the very beginning of the triumphal onslaught of the receptors
in taking over almost all of psychiatric science. The number of mentions of
"neurotransmitters" in the *New York Times* soared from zero in 1955–1960, to
108 in 1981–1990, to 171 in 1991–2000. Mentions of "dopamine" over that time
rose from zero to 112. These were clearly media concepts to conjure with.

But media concepts are not the same thing as real science. The world of neurochemistry is much more complex than the handful of biogenic amines, such
as serotonin, norepinephrine, and dopamine; the world of the brain and mind
is much more complex than the domain of the neurotransmitters, a reductionist
theory at the very best. When Robert Cancro arrived at New York University
as chair of the department of Psychiatry in 1976, "I found to my chagrin that
residents could talk confidently about hypothetical receptor activities which had
not yet been demonstrated. They spoke of upregulation, downregulation, hyper-
sensitivity, proliferation, etc. All of these conclusions could be made on the basis
of a clinical interview. When these same remarkable observers were asked simple
questions, such as: 'Does the patient have children?' they often did not know the
answer." Cancro concluded with a devastating indictment of this version of biological psychiatry: "Psychiatry had been reduced to a primitive form of derma-
tology. If it is wet, make it dry. If it is dry, make it wet. If the patient complained
of anxiety, you gave an anxiolytic. If they complained of depression, you gave an
antidepressive. It seemed pointless to have four years of training when everything had been reduced to such a simple matter."[51]

Observers have been stunned by the obvious lack of progress in drug discovery and development over the last 40 years. With each supposedly promising
molecule that comes along, the neurotransmitter profile is carefully traced, as

though that were the secret to the drug's mechanism of action. The drugs have all failed in trials. Is there a problem with our focus on neurotransmitters? Max Fink and Turan Itil say Yes.

Max Fink, Turan Itil, and Pharmaco-EEG

> Pharmaco-EEG is a quantitative science that yields direct images of ongoing biochemical and neurophysiologic brain events that are intimately connected to human behavior.—Max Fink (2018)[52]

One scientific sprout did not depend on neurotransmitters: pharmaco-EEG, the study of the impact of drugs on the electrical activity of the brain. The study was done with the electroencephalograph, hence the term pharmaco-EEG.

Hans Berger, a professor at the University of Jena in eastern Germany, introduced EEG in 1929. As early as 1931 he was using it to study the impact of cerebral lesions on the brain's electrical activity and the impact of sedatives on the dominant electrical oscillations, which are called alpha-waves.[53] The EEG records continuing waves with frequencies from 3 to 30 Hz (Hertz, or cycles per second) and with varying amplitudes. In the clinic, waves are described as alpha (8–12), theta (5–8), delta (less than 4), and beta (more than 13).

After the Second World War, it was Martin Roth, then at the Crichton Royal Hospital in Dumfries, Scotland (and later, at Newcastle as one of the grand figures in British psychiatry), who in 1951 revived the study of drugs on the EEG. In 42 patients undergoing ECT, Roth endeavored to discover the mechanism of convulsive therapy. (He acknowledged Willy Mayer-Gross as his mentor.) He reported that, after administration of the barbiturate thiopental, increased slowing was associated with better clinical outcomes. This linked EEG patterns to a measurable physiological or chemical effects.[54]

In 1954, Charles Shagass at McGill University devised the first biological test in psychiatry with his use of EEG to define the "sedation threshold" in different diagnoses. With two EEG leads recording frontal electrical activity, Shagass would slowly infuse sodium amytal into patients. At first, the EEG showing fast-wave activity would rise swiftly. Then the acceleration of the fast waves would stop and plateau out. This point was called the sedation threshold. Clinically, it was sometimes measurable as the point at which the patient started to develop slurred speech or nystagmus. The essential finding was that the threshold varied from diagnosis to diagnosis: for "conversion hysteria," it was at 2.79 mg of sodium amytal for every kilogram of patient's body weight; for "anxiety states," it was at 5.27 mg/kg. There were some differences in sedation threshold among the psychoses as well, ranging from 2.81 mg/kg in psychotic depression to 4.7 mg/

kg in "borderline schizophrenia." As a demonstration that different psychiatric diagnoses corresponded to real differences in brain physiology, the test was startling. It is an incredible commentary on psychiatry that in the 1950s, the age of psychoanalysis, the sedation threshold was lost sight of.[55]

At the end of the 1950s, Dieter Bente, a staffer at the University of Erlangen-Nuremberg, later a professor in Berlin, together with his student Turan Itil (who had received his MD from Istanbul University in 1948), began the systematic EEG study of the effect of drugs on cerebral electrical activity.[56] Bente's pioneering role in this work has been widely unrecognized. Bente also introduced the idea that classes of psychoactive drugs could be recognized on the basis of their EEG signatures.[57]

Simultaneously, in the United States, Max Fink at Hillside Hospital in Glen Oaks, New York, began research on pharmaco-EEG to study the new treatments, such as ECT and insulin therapy—and shortly thereafter chlorpromazine and imipramine—that were sweeping psychiatry. In 1958, he and the Bente-Itil team all gave papers on the subject at the CINP meeting in Rome. This crystallized relationships.

At a symposium at the Third World Congress of Psychiatry in Montreal in 1961, the relationship among drug response, EEG changes, and diagnosis ("changes in behavior") started to clarify. At this point, the idea began to emerge that not just specific drugs but entire drug classes had specific EEG signatures and that one could determine what drug class a new molecule belonged to by studying its EEG signature. At the San Juan meeting of the American College of Neuropsychopharmacology (ACNP) in 1967, Fink and Itil reported on this for the drug class hallucinogens.[58] Max Fink later said, "Changes in EEG following psychoactive drugs are drug-specific and directly reflect the drug-induced changes in brain chemistry. Changes in behavior are predictable sequelae of the chemical changes. Changes in brain chemistry are systematically reflected in patterned EEG changes." He called EEG changes "the Rosetta stone" of predicting which drugs will induce which behavioral changes. Pharmaco-EEG was thus the most powerful instrument in the toolkit of psychopharmacology. No other technique provided a blueprint for knowing which drugs would be effective. A corollary of this was that drugs that did not produce EEG changes were more or less inert."[59]

In 1962, George Ulett at Washington University in St. Louis persuaded Fink and his family to move to St. Louis and set up an EEG lab on the grounds of the St. Louis State Hospital. Turan Itil joined them from Germany, and Sam Gershon came from Australia. These investigators formed what was probably the most dynamic center in the world for research on pharmaco-EEG—but not the only one. In 1964, Fink compiled a bibliography of 580 articles on pharmaco-EEG since 1951 by more than 900 authors.[60]

In the mass of EEG squiggles, the eyeball may miss important variations. EEG was a technique that cried out for quantification. Doing the analysis with a ruler and calipers, said Fink, "was tedious, made imprecise by fatigue and boredom." In 1957, Fink learned of an electric analog frequency analyzer that Ulett had built on the basis of the designs of Grey Walter and the Burden Neurological Institute in Bristol. Ulett agreed to build such a device for Fink's EEG lab, and the computer quantification of EEG began. The practical analysis of EEG data did not take off until the advent of more powerful IBM computers. MIT scientists demonstrated the technique's utility at a meeting at UCLA in 1960. And in 1964 the EEG lab in St. Louis was up and running with an IBM 1710. The technique became known as quantitative EEG (QEEG).

Now drug testing began. A new agent, fenfluramine, reduced appetite. Was it more like a barbiturate or a stimulant? The EEG analysis suggested that fenfluramine patients would be sedated, and indeed that is what happened.[61]

Animal pharmacology seemed to show that doxepin (Pfizer's Sinequan) would be effective as an anxiolytic, but clinical results were disappointing, and Pfizer's marketing failed. Pfizer convened an investigators' meeting with Herman Denber, Turan Itil, and Fink, where they looked at EEG recordings of the doxepin patients and "agreed that the patterns were similar to those of TCA antidepressants and not to the known anxiolytics."[62] Pfizer rebranded doxepin in 1975 as a tricyclic antidepressant, with great success—that is, until the advent of the SSRIs put an end to the entire previous generation of antidepressants.

With the aid of several English pharmacologists, Organon (in Oss, the Netherlands) developed a series of drugs that the firm hoped would be serotonin antagonists with antidepressant activity. GB-94 (later mianserin) was the most active of this series, but preclinical (animal) pharmacology was disappointing. Yet Itil predicted on the basis of EEG that it would have antidepressant activity similar to that of amitriptyline.[63] "Organon's pharmacologists and neuroscientists scoffed at his prediction," said Fink. "But Jack Vossenaar, director of medical research, gambled on Itil's prediction and supported clinical trials," which confirmed that mianserin was an antidepressant.[64]

Itil recalled these events in an interview. "Organon went to Max, who was by that time in New York, with a potential psychotropic substance and Max sent them to me in Missouri. I found it showed a similar profile to amitriptyline. To celebrate the discovery, Max gave a party at his house in Long Island and invited me from St. Louis." At the party was an intellectual property lawyer who suggested that Itil obtain a US patent for the drug—which he did not. (Organon holds the US patent.)

At that point, Itil and Marty Katz at NIMH flew over to the Netherlands to consult with Vossenaar. "Do you really think mianserin has antidepressant effects?" he asked. To confirm that it did, Itil gave the drug to his old psychiatry professor in Turkey, who administered it to a number of patients and saw that it had no apparent anticholinergic side effects and seemed convincing. Itil showed the findings to Vossenaar.

"What do you want?" asked Vossenaar. "Nothing," said Itil. "I just want appreciation, that's all." (Can you imagine this happening today!)

Itil concluded, "That was the first time in history that the antidepressant property of a drug was discovered by quantitative EEG."[65]

In 1976, Organon brought mianserin out as the antidepressant Bolvidon in the United Kingdom. (Organon retracted its NDA at the FDA because some of the trial data turned out to be cooked.) Mianserin had mild anticholinergic side effects and less overdose risk than the tricyclics; its efficacy was a matter of dispute.[66] Mianserin's direct lineal descendant—mirtazapine (Organon's Remeron)—did reach the US market. These stories suggest how vastly superior pharmaco-EEG was to animal pharmacology.[67]

Pharmaco-EEG labs developed internationally at many sites. In 1982, the first formal meeting of the International Pharmaco-EEG Group took place in Hannover, and the group designated *Neuropsychobiology* as its official journal.

Yet some of the news from pharmaco-EEG was quite unsettling for those who believed in the centrality of neurotransmitters (neurohumoral doctrines). Fink wrote in 2004, "Compounds classified as anticholinergic, serotonergic, and MAO-inhibiting *elicit similar EEG profiles* and similar behavioral effects [emphasis added]. This variety in measurable pharmacology and chemistry argues that another system in the brain, not the neurohumoral effects, is the basis for the common EEG pattern and behavior changes."[68]

The neurotransmitter people found all this electrical talk just too incredible for words and turned their backs.

Thus, just as pharmaco-EEG was on the threshold of producing convincing results, it was almost discarded! (But, for a rebirth, see *JAMA Psychiatry*, in the first week of 2020.[69]) There are so many of these stories in psychiatry: the DST, one of the very few biological markers in psychiatry, discarded! ECT, the most powerful treatment in the field, (almost) discarded! Pharmaco-EEG really did disappear, except for among a small handful of convinced scientists.

It was the triumph of the neurotransmitters that caused pharmaco-EEG to be prematurely discarded. Fink said, "Government support for pharmaco-EEG studies effectively ended in the mid-1980s, a casualty of the nation's unfunded wars and the rush to close long-stay psychiatric hospitals and their research centers. Funding shifted to large-scale multicenter clinical trials, the STAR*D, STEP-BD and CATIE studies."

Moreover, Fink continued, FDA licenses psychoactive agents "without evidence of brain effects, flooding the public markets with ineffective treatments. . . . Pharmaco-EEG offers a quantitative methodology that is safe, repeatable, and reliable. It was prematurely rejected by a neuroscience community enamored [of] expensive electronic and magnetic equipment."[70] Carroll added, "I have long thought that the sidelining of pharmaco-EEG work occurred because it didn't fit easily with the prevailing neurotransmitter ideas about depression. Plus, it was empirical and observational rather than experimental [animal research]. It didn't have a clear basis in known brain mechanisms. Plus, psychiatrists training in the 1970s were clueless about the theory and practice of EEG."[71]

When EEG was unable to identify distinctive EEG profiles for the various enhancements of serotonin, dopamine, and epinephrine, it was EEG that was discarded, not the neurotransmitter doctrines. The story is incredible.

9

KOLs

Most academic advisers to industry today are advisors to marketing departments and not, as in my time, to research departments.—Karl Rickels (2011)[1]

There have always been physicians who advised industry, often gratis and in the interest of bringing an effective compound to the attention of the profession. Roland Kuhn, the Swiss asylum psychiatrist who in 1957 discovered the effectiveness of imipramine in depression, advised Geigy about how to market the drug, about what dosages were effective, and indeed about which marketing strategies to use.[2] Kuhn was a ramrod of integrity and would have dismissed the suggestion that such collaboration was somehow corrupt.

Yet there is another bridge, perhaps one too far. Industry has always had physicians willing to testify on behalf of a drug. A. Dale Console, former medical director of Squibb in the 1950s, told Congress in 1960, that "The true nature of these testimonials is well known to the industry and its own contempt for them is shown by its vernacular for sources from which they are easily obtained. These are called stables."[3]

In the 1980s and after, the stables became KOLs, or Key Opinion Leaders. The sardonic term "KOL" was used as an insider expression in industry correspondence for the academics we can persuade to flack for us. Technically, a KOL is an academic leader whom industry pays to praise specific products to unsuspecting colleagues, who are unaware that they are being rolled. The KOLs receive large payments from drug companies, which, as Sergio Sismondo at Queen's University pointed out, "are primarily intended not to affect their prescriptions, but rather to purchase their influence on other physicians' prescriptions."[4] Here's a rough-and-ready definition: ""Key Opinion Leaders—physicians in high places who became high-priced detail men."[5]

The Rise of the KOLs

The notion of a key opinion leader was introduced by Columbia sociologist Paul Lazarsfeld in 1944 as "opinion leadership" regarding the influencing of elections.[6]

It's not that pharma executives were students of Lazarsfeld, but the term hovered in the air, ready to be plucked. KOL started to appear in industry discussions as early as the 1980s. Medical writer "Talbot" said in 2011, "This stuff goes back decades. Anyone who 'told' what was going on was black balled."[7]

Mickey Nardo reflected, "In my first 20 years in medicine (1963–1983), I can't recall any physician I knew or worked with having a financial relationship with a pharmaceutical company." A grand rounds at Emory in 1983 was the turning point. "Checking back in 25 years later [in 2016], it seems like everyone had multiple such connections. . . . It was the same with industry-sponsored clinical trials in mainstream academic journals—from *never* to *every*."[8]

The first decade of the twenty-first century marked the take-off. Sismondo reported that "the number of articles in the industry journal *Pharmaceutical Executive* that mention 'opinion leader' roughly triples between 2000 and 2010."[9]

For industry, the "management and clinical development" of the KOLs was a fine art. In 2003, Johan Hoegstedt at AstraZeneca briefed colleagues on some key points:

- Rotate the attendance and add maybe 10%–20% of the group yearly so that a few KOLs/physicians are not seen as AZ employees/puppets.
- Open up and share our plans, demand confidentiality, and make the participants feel like they are part of the organization for the day(s) and also between the meetings.[10]

Part of the organization! The KOLs basked in the attention and the payments they received from industry, but behind closed doors they were often viewed as useful idiots whose cooperation could be bought and whose reputations could be monetized. Tom Ban, professor of psychopharmacology at Vanderbilt University, told David Healy that industry "treated the profession with handouts, the opinion leaders of the profession as puppets, and their collaborators from the profession as 'call girls.' "[11]

And if the "author"-KOLs got in the way, out they went! At a meeting in 2004 with Parexel, an agency that ran and reported trials, AstraZeneca executives were fretting about getting the results out as soon as possible "to support key claims for the brand. Therefore, if the authors recommend anything that will slow up this process, AZ should consider asking them to step down from this project."[12] Asking the author to step down! The message to authors: Keep your mouth shut when you're on industry's dime.

Sismondo called attention to a hierarchy of KOLs. At the bottom were "ordinary physicians . . . who are paid to speak to other physicians." Sales representatives organize local lunchtime talks and the like for them. Then there were the "researcher KOLs," who were paid to speak at Continuing Medical Education sessions. They served as authors of articles or initiated trials. In other words, there was "a continuum from KOLs employed primarily to change their own prescribing patterns to those employed primarily to change other physicians' prescribing patterns." Researcher KOLs might get $2500 a lecture (as of 2013), low-level physician-KOLs maybe $500 for local presentations. The companies trained them to be effective speakers.[13] As of 1980, there was no APA policy restricting the payment of industry honoraria to members.[14]

Physicians scarcely had to be coaxed to join speakers' bureaus. They were clamoring to get in. In one Janssen federal case tried in Pennsylvania, the prosecution said, "Sales representatives identified local doctors to be trained as speakers based on their potential for writing Risperdal prescriptions. Sales representatives told doctors that if they wanted to speak, they had to increase their Risperdal prescriptions. . . . One sales representative told her district manager that a doctor in her district wanted to be a speaker for Janssen, but only 16 percent of his antipsychotic prescriptions were for Risperdal. The representative [told] the doctor that he could qualify to speak the following year if he wrote 50 percent of his prescriptions for Risperdal. The doctor subsequently increased his Risperdal prescriptions and became a paid speaker in 2004."[15]

Some of the sums are truly eyewatering. The *New York Times* reported in 2008 that AstraZeneca paid Melissa DelBello of the University of Cincinnati more than $238,000 to flak for Seroquel. "The University of Cincinnati agreed to monitor those payments more closely."[16] (See also the section on Charles Nemeroff below.)

We might well add on a third category of "hanger-on-KOL-breakthrough-freaks," such as those who cluster at NIMH and at APA: breakthroughs are just around the corner![17] We heard much of this in the run-up to DSM-5. Of course, the great breakthroughs never materialized, but they are still just around the corner.

The KOLs were not scientific advisors. They were "employed by the marketing departments to do marketing," as Roy Poses put it. He described companies that were "entirely devoted to the adoption, care and feeding of KOLs, plus numerous companies, including some medical education and communication companies (MECCs), that provide KOL-related products and services." Guideline development—as in the Texas Medical Algorithm Project (TMAP, see Chapter 19)—organizing Continuing Medical Education (CME), signing on as "ghost" authors: all were the function of KOLs. Poses concluded, "It looks like there has been a massive campaign by healthcare corporate marketers to make useful idiots out of . . . medical academics. . . . This appears to be a massive, cynical effort to hollow out our once respected healthcare institutions and professionals in the service of marketing."[18]

To be sure, there is a long history of academics working with industry, as for example Abraham Myerson, a neurologist at the Boston State Hospital who had a long relationship in the late 1930s with Smith, Kline & French over its stimulant Benzedrine, which Myerson put into clinical trials, reaping research grants from the company. Historian Nicolas Rasmussen found this a "scientifically respectable" example of "the Friendly Expert's relation with a sponsoring firm. The relationship depended on a genuine and deep convergence . . . one that redefined both the intellectual program of the investigator and the commercial agenda of the firm."[19] Myerson, in other words, was not a KOL. He was not a member of any speakers' bureau (speakers' bureaus did not then exist), nor did he sponsor enthusiastic satellite sessions at medical society meetings on the firm's latest offering.

Money Needed

What happened? Did everybody just become evil?

No. There are several explanations for the shift from scientists to stables and KOLs, some related to the structure of the industry, others to the peripeteia of financing academic departments of psychiatry.

For one thing, the percentage of drug research money flowing from industry to the academy for trials declined from around 75 percent in the early 1990s to 34 percent by 2000. The actual decline seems to have begun in the 1980s. Instead, industry began funding private trials firms.[20]

In response, universities started active programs of outreach to drug companies, soliciting trials. Columbia University had an Office of Clinical Trials (OCT) that included as an affiliate the Psychiatric Institute. "The sense is that you come to Columbia University and we will get your drug approved," said one source. The OCT made about $10 million a year for the university and offered industry "quick access to lists of schizophrenics, manic-depressives and other potential human guinea pigs," said a (hostile) source.[21] Clearly pressure on clinicians to be helpful would arise from this university office. One psychiatrist at Brown University ran a private company that conducted clinical trials. Consisting of a principal investigator and two other psychiatrists plus office staff, the company actively solicited Pharma business. "For any given clinical trial we can recruit up to 100 patients per year," the principal investigator told Kali-Duphar, a potential client.[22] Here, the pressure to conduct quick, successful trials was clearly monetary.

This story was not really driven by venality, although among individual psychiatrists that might have been present. The basic motor was the fact that, around 1980, "academic psychiatry was broke," as Mickey Nardo put it. Medical deans had become much more reluctant to fund individual departments than previously. Third-party and public funding was shrinking. And hospital incomes had never been handsome in psychiatry. Nardo: "The solution to the funding of academic departments in psychiatry was funding from Pharma. The departments desperately needed support. Pharma needed academicians to author articles, be PIs [principal investigators] for clinical trials, act as KOLs, etc. [Thus] the academic–industrial complex emerged in its current form by the late 1980s."[23]

But once the money began to flow to departments, it started to run into individual bank accounts as well. Mark Kramer, from his perch as head of neuroscience at Merck (which did not have an SSRI) was horrified at the parade of KOLs through the CME sessions and satellite lunches at the meetings: "Those succumbing to the corporate sirens are far more numerous, scattered, obsequious [and] deceitful than the handful of wily choir directors of big pharmaceutical industry. Thus, those who warrant maximum retribution for our mess are right under our noses, i.e., within the academic ranks."[24]

Competition intensified. A new wind began to blow at FDA in the early 1970s with the arrival of energetic young people like Bob Temple and Richard Crout. Temple set out to speed up drug approvals with Fast Track,[25] a positive development that backfired. Several years after his retirement in 1991, Kenneth Feather, a senior FDA executive, explained how this played out: In olden days, "the industry had a lock on the market. In other words, you came out with a new cardiac drug. You basically had the lock on that drug for a dozen years. So you didn't have to be so aggressive in your advertising, and you could be a little more laid back in your advertising schemes. That changed with two developments. One was the increased speed of NDA [New Drug Application] review, and the competition within the field of new drugs [that] began to appear. I mean, you came out with your new cardiac drug and he came out with his six months later." So quickly, because reviews were now more rapid.

As well, continued Feather, there was more generic competition "coming into what were well-established old products that were kind of cash cows. You [the brand maker] had little outgo other than production costs, but you were getting lots of money in because of the sales. Now they were threatened by the generic competition."

Feather said that, "as a consequence, the market life of your product shrank from a dozen years to maybe three years or less. I mean, the real viable market life. So you had to start to recoup your money quickly." How to do that? Step on the gas. "You wanted it to shoot up right away as soon as it hit the market." You had to advertise aggressively to doctors. "You do that by scientific meetings. You do that by seminars, by workshops, by peer influence groups." Enlist community leaders, Feather said. "You hit the ground running with your product."[26] The helpfulness of KOLs here is obvious.

When Cyberonics of Houston, Texas, brought out its new device for curing depression through brain stimulation, it had a full court press of academics ready with praise. There was a scandal surrounding Charles Nemeroff at Emory and a puff-piece publication in his journal *Neuropsychopharmacology* (see below in this chapter), but Dennis Charney of Mt. Sinai Hospital was helpful with the journal he edited, *Biological Psychiatry*. And A. John Rush, professor of psychiatry at the University of Texas Southwestern Medical Center, not to be outdone, actually sat in the Cyberonics booth at a meeting of the American Psychiatric Association in May 2006, "describing the benefits of the therapy to curious psychiatrists," as the *New York Times* related. All these individuals, and many more, were on the payroll of Cyberonics.[27]

And make no mistake: once you accepted industry's dollar, *they owned you*. They owned your public persona and would control vigorously what you said at CME sessions under their sponsorship. Carroll described the experience of Consultant X, an internationally recognized clinician who was asked to be on the speakers' bureau of the [redacted] company. Consultant X said, "In a large audience . . . I departed from the script I was given for the published data to note that the effect size . . . was significantly lower than the [redacted] treatments. Since most [of the audience] had no idea what 'effect size' is, I gave a brief explanation. That evening I received a phone call in my hotel room from the [redacted] company's director about the problem. He chastised me for being off message and warned me not to make intrusive statements. I told him that I did not work for the [redacted] company, and that presumably I was asked to give these talks because I was a respected researcher in the field. . . . I repeated my performance the next day, and was never asked to talk for them again."

Consultant X said that, "Over the years I have given many talks sponsored by corporations, but I gave *my* talk, using *my* slides, and choosing *my* topic. . . . About five years ago I was informed that henceforth I must use the company's topics and slides, with no deviations allowed. The corporate material provided was mediocre in quality and infomercial in tone. That is when I stopped giving company-sponsored lectures in the U.S."[28] (In 2012, Nardo registered with disbelief, "The notion of KOLs giving talks using a drug company's slides? I never even imagined that until a couple of years ago."[29])

Yet, independence was unusual. Kimberly Elliott, who repped for several global companies from the late 1980s to 2007, liaised with the firms' "thought leaders." They would typically get $2500 per lecture, the company supplying the slides. "These people are paid a lot of money to say what they say," she said. "I'm not saying the key opinion leaders are bad, but they are salespeople just like the sales representatives are."[30]

The Academic–Industrial Complex

> Corporate interests have fused with academic medicine to create an unhealthy alliance that works against the objective reporting of clinical research [and] sets up meetings and symposia with the specific purpose of selling the participants to the sponsors.—Giovanni Fava (2016)[31]

As described above, the initial alliance of industry and the academy was cordial to science. Don Klein, recalling the studies of Geigy's antidepressant drug imipramine (Tofranil) that he and Max Fink had conducted at Hillside Hospital in the early 1960s, said, "Our Geigy contact was a scientist who never interfered. Things deteriorated sharply once drugs got profitable. But it still galls me that when I quite naively called Geigy (1962) with the exciting news that their antidepressant also blocked spontaneous panics, I was met with stiff incredulity."[32]

Then, as Klein said, things really did deteriorate. This happened in part under the guise of evidence-based medicine (EBM). Roy Poses, an internist at Brown University and editor of an influential blog, slammed the whole nexus of the KOLs and the trials they administered, massaged, and promoted. "What is often touted as 'EBM' is really pseudo-evidence based medicine, a mélange of manipulated, biased studies done to serve vested interests, while studies that provide inconvenient results are suppressed, hawked by conflicted 'key opinion leaders,' compounded by other KOLs into 'evidence-based' guidelines that are also meant to promote commercial interests, then promoted by various kinds of stealth marketing, including marketing disguised as various kinds of medical education."[33]

As a testimonial to a field in scientific bankruptcy there can be no more eloquent evidence than the willingness of the field's leaders to become part of industry's promotional machinery in exchange for cash payments. The fish rots from the head. The biggest money-grubbers of all were the medical deans and academic department heads who sat on the boards of Pharma. In 2013, the average compensation of these medical factotums for serving on industry boards was $313,000. Eli Lilly, for example, paid med-school executives $309,500 to sit on its board.[34] Under these circumstances, it was quite unrealistic to expect the academic medical leadership to ride herd on the lowly KOLs among their faculty, whose compensation was much less.

The men and women who became KOLs were not necessarily wicked. What factors drove these otherwise honest and upright people to sell out to industry? We have reviewed the drying up of *industry* funding for trials. Yet *government* funding for psychiatric research also began to shrivel in the 1970s and after. Edward Domino, an instructor in psychopharmacology at the University of Michigan in the late 1950s and early 1960s, later told an interviewer, "Basically,

I have to survive, and at the University of Michigan the name of the game was then, and still is, either you bring in grants or get out."[35] Given this stark choice, the temptation to court drug money was irresistible.

In the 1990s, Nardo said, this worsened. "There was something I'd never seen before, long lists of industry affiliations and conflicts of interest appended to the end of their publications. [The KOLs] authored most of the clinical trials, but they didn't do very many of them (industry did them). Our literature was choked with their scientific papers about patients that most of the authors had never even met, and in fact had never even seen the data itself."[36]

Thus, special arrangements developed between firms and psychiatry departments. Otsuka patented its big new antipsychotic aripiprazole (Abilify) in the United States in 1990 and shared the marketing with Bristol-Myers Squibb. By 2000, the drug was in Stage III trials, and the authorities were at North Shore–Long Island Jewish Health System (earlier called Zucker-Hillside). John Kane said, "There is plenty of room on the market for aripiprazole. . . . Only one out of every three patients with schizophrenia remains on their initial therapy after one year of treatment."[37] Kane and others wrote one of the first clinical reports, in September 2002, in the *Journal of Clinical Psychiatry*, describing Abilify as "a safe and well-tolerated potential treatment for schizophrenia and schizoaffective disorder."[38]

The Kane piece, however, bore some of the hallmarks of an industry-sponsored report. The study was done in 36 sites, with an average of 12 subjects per site. Only Pharma can organize so many sites. At least two of the authors were Otsuka or Bristol-Myers employees and the corresponding author had a Bristol-Myers address. Kane acknowledged receiving honoraria from Bristol-Myers. In November 2002, the FDA approved aripiprazole for marketing.

As with all the other atypical antipsychotics, there were reports about aripiprazole's efficacy as augmentation therapy in "treatment-resistant depression" (see Chapter 18). The first was in 2007. The first author was a Bristol-Myers employee and the article was the subject of rigorous criticism.[39] The aripiprazole patent then expired in 2011, but because of a pediatric extension, generics weren't permitted on the market until April 2015.

Happily, Otsuka had a clone waiting in the wings: brexpiprazole (Rexulti), developed by Otsuka and Lundbeck and approved by the FDA in July 2015. Here again, the Hillside–North Shore Long Island Jewish group had been of great service. Of the first published trial in May 2015 for "acute schizophrenia," led by John Kane, all ten authors were at Zucker-Hillside, Otsuka, or Lundbeck.[40] The next trial for "acute schizophrenia" in September 2015, once again, was led by a Zucker-Hillside staff psychiatrist, Christoph Correll, and all ten authors were either at Zucker-Hillside, Otsuka, or Lundbeck.[41] For both articles, Otsuka and Lundbeck funded "writing support" that was provided by QVX

Communications in the United Kingdom; in other words, the studies were presumably ghosted. Kane was, moreover, the principal investigator on a big NIMH study on recovery after the first schizophrenia episode (NIMH RAISE-ETP), and senior investigator with a commercial interest in another Otsuka project to show that Otsuka's aripiprazole depot treatment (Maintena) warded off relapse in first-episode patients.[42] I have to declare an interest here, having lectured in psychiatry at Zucker-Hillside and having been the recipient of Dr. Kane's hospitality. But readers may draw their own conclusions about a possible academic–industrial complex at work here.

In terms of organizing meetings—which cost money—there was a slippery slope, starting with seeking industry support for the cost of coffee and concluding with a bang by selling branding opportunities, such as the name tags or the cover of the program. Preparing for the CINP congress in Munich in 2008, the two organizers sent out a letter to national representatives of the CINP ("CINP Ambassadors"), seeking aid. "It would be of great help if you could try to convince national pharmaceutical companies . . . to bring participants to the CINP congress or to support the congress in other ways." This request seems rather unexceptional, but it does involve academic psychiatrists' picking up the phone and asking that the company in question shell out for air tickets, accommodation, and registration fees. There would be a quid pro quo. One of the "Ambassadors," who wishes to remain anonymous, commented, "In the late 1950s and all through the 60s people in close contact with industry were kind of looked down on in academic departments. It was pretty stupid but this is how it was. Then in the 1970s the situation slowly started to turn around. And now the professor of pharmacology in Stockholm and the professor of psychiatry in Munich [the two organizers] are organizing a meeting which they intend to support with handouts from industry."[43]

Peter Whitehouse, professor of neurology at Case Western Reserve University in Cleveland but with one foot in psychiatry, tried to find his balance on that slippery slope. He began by consulting on dementia and found himself at more and more head offices. Lilly flew him back from Germany on the corporate jet. "As more drugs came onto the market over the past decade," he wrote in 2008, "my concern about being a KOL grew. I became interested in the management of KOLs by industry and suspect that Big Pharma . . . has extensive databases on all of us." He did not know the half of it. "I began to realize that they were trying to manipulate my opinion as much as I was trying to give them mine. I came to see that marketing was replacing science as the dominant conversation. Instead of questions about drug efficacy and patient benefit, I heard questions such as, 'How do we get doctors, especially primary care physicians, to prescribe more of our drug?'"

So he bailed. He had been earning $50,000 a year from industry. Now, "I have recently moved as close to zero income as is possible from drug companies." He no longer consults for industry "because I do not want to help them control not only our healthcare system but our very conceptions of health and ill-health."[44]

The KOLs were the cherry on top of the cake of corruption. Marlon Brando once said he didn't want to be on his deathbed wondering, "What was *that* all about?" Bernard Carroll picked up on this theme:

> What was that all about? It was about the illusion of ramping up clinical re-search to an industrial scale . . . [the] dumbing down of diagnoses through checklists, dumbing down clinical assessments through structured interviews; it was about a belief that efficiency could be achieved through recruiting symp-tomatic volunteers rather than real patients; it was about imputing validity to online and telephone assessments; it was about treating patients as commod-ities whose opinions on efficacy were disregarded. Oh, and it was also about money for the corporations and for the opportunistic helper academics and of course for the satellite industry of CROs and the like that sprang up. That is the dismal record of academic psychiatry over the past 30 years.[45]

"Biedermania"

Psychiatric illness in children is not a myth dreamed up by the pharmaceu-tical industry. Children and adolescents do get serious illnesses. And then what happens? As one anonymous psychiatrist said: "Medications are going to be used no matter what, because the families are desperate. The children are failing out of school; they're doing horribly at home; they're using substances; they're not able to function; they don't have any friends. They're completely derailed from a developmental standpoint, a psychological standpoint, a social standpoint, an academic standpoint. They're going to get medications."[46]

Yet pediatric psychiatry as a professional field was a hothouse of mischief. Diseases were spun off and then treated with powerful drugs that should never have been given to children. And the shifting winds of pediatric fancies—one day, autism, the next day, hyperactivity—illustrate Liverpool psychiatrist Michael Göpfert's observation, "Generally my impression of DSM changes is that they are not the result of determined efforts at creating meaningful commu-nication systems but follow some other influence, just like sailing with prevailing winds. Sailing with winds solves the problem of wind direction but not the issue of charting territories and seas. The prevailing winds on a particular day have little to do with that."[47]

The whole saga of "pediatric bipolar disorder" is a case in point. The bi-polar diagnosis began with bipolar II in adults, conceived in DSM-IV in 1994. Bipolar disorder as such has, in a sense, always been with us, going back to the mid-nineteenth century as a form of severity, not as a distinctive form of illness. As a mixture of mania and melancholic depression, bipolar disorder was considered to be a severe brain illness.

Bipolar II, however, was much milder, a mixture of major depression—which could mean anything—and "hypomania." So much behavior could qualify as hypomanic that, when DSM-IV proposed bipolar II in 1994, many, many patients qualified for it. "Pediatric bipolar disorder," not in DSM-IV, was only a skip and a jump away from adult bipolar because children can so easily be seen as "depressed," the garden-variety mood fluctuations of childhood can qualify as "illness," and outbursts of anger can substitute for "hypomania." This is a slippery slope, and pediatric bipolar was already halfway down a slope that earlier would have been considered normal behavior.

Children can be trying under the best of circumstances, and so it was with the eye of faith that parents and doctors alike started seeing otherwise ill-behaved children as having pediatric bipolar disorder. These are diagnoses that have degraded the entire field of pediatric psychiatry and led to a great tide of powerful medications that has washed over children who don't have the ability to say no.

On the psychiatry side, pediatric bipolar disorder is usually treated as a rock-solid diagnosis, comparable to chickenpox: There is little awareness of industry manipulation, of the question of the "eye of faith," in making the diagnosis, or of the intrinsic unlikelihood that millions of the nation's children should have a terrible psychiatric illness only slightly less awful than schizophrenia. An analysis of the literature found that the average prevalence rate for pediatric bipolar disorder was 3.9 percent, with a "confidence interval" of 2.6 percent to 5.8 percent."[48] Yet the pharmaceutical industry has so poisoned the entire literature that all these figures are meaningless.

Joseph Biederman, who furthered the diagnosis of childhood bipolar disorder, was born in Prague in 1947 and graduated in medicine from the University Medical School in Buenos Aires in 1971. He completed his training in psychiatry at Hadassah University Hospital in Jerusalem in 1977, then migrated to the United States and trained in child psychiatry at the Children's Hospital in Boston and at the Massachusetts General Hospital (MGH). In 1981, he became director of the Pediatric Psychopharmacology Clinic of Mass General. This was an impeccable psychiatric background.

Biederman's work from 1976 to about 1995 had been straightforward studies of the pediatric versions of such disorders as obsessive-compulsive disorder and attention-deficit/hyperactivity disorder (ADHD). Much of his work was on the forefront of science, such as his interest in the dexamethasone suppression test (DST) in 1990[49]—he continued use of this valuable endocrine measurement after the rest of psychiatry had unjustly abandoned it.

Biederman was not first to broach the concept of bipolar disorder in youth. The diagnosis, as David Healy explained in his overview, goes back to the early 1990s.[50] Yet it was in 1995 that Biederman and his team began the *popularization* of the pediatric bipolar concept with their first article on "childhood-onset bipolar disorder." The point of the article was that "mania" was really very common in children under 12, often was confused with ADHD. And because childhood mania was often "comorbid" with depression, the phrase "childhood bipolar disorder" practically leapt to the lips. Yet there was a problem: The criteria for mania were fairly straightforward, and most bipolar children did not meet them. The solution? "Irritability, rather than euphoria, is the essential disruption-of-mood characteristic of childhood mania."[51] The Biederman team proposed substituting regular outbursts of anger—"explosive moods" (or just mood changeability)—instead of the classical mania symptoms like euphoria, hyperactivity, and bouncing thoughts. The pediatric symptoms would occur continuously, rather than episodically, as in real mania.[52]

Work advanced so quickly that in that same year, 1995, Biederman was able to elaborate "subtypes" of the illness.[53] A steady stream of articles on pediatric bipolar now began to issue from Biederman's prestigious Pediatric Psychopharmacology Unit of the Child Psychiatry Service of MGH. In 1999, Biederman's service penned the first report linking the therapy of juvenile bipolar disorder to Johnson & Johnson (Janssen's) drug Risperdal.[54]

At this point pediatric bipolar held promise of being such a lucrative diagnosis that a number of companies that made antipsychotics were licking their chops. In 2000, for example, Eli Lilly sponsored a conference in Scottsdale, Arizona, on bipolar disorder, at which Biederman and colleagues presented on "pediatric mania, a developmental subtype of bipolar disorder."[55] Yet it would be much more promising to nail a firm like Johnson & Johnson to the bipolar mast.

Biederman's clinic had been the recipient of grants from a wide list of firms: one in the mid-1980s from the Merrell Dow Pharmaceutical Company let them study ADHD; a long grant beginning in 1991 from Pfizer allowed them to study sertraline in the treatment of pediatric OCD; and there were grants from Lilly, Glaxo Wellcome, Solvay, Novartis, and many more. Fateful, however, was the grant he received in 2001 from the Stanley Foundation to establish a "Massachusetts General Hospital Center for the Treatment of Pediatric Bipolar Disorder." In 2002, this segued into the "Johnson & Johnson Center for Pediatric Psychopathology Research."

The Johnson & Johnson Center was of particular import because it involved such a glaring conflict of interest. As David Rothman, who prepared the TMAP report for the Texas court, noted, "The overt purpose of the agreement with Biederman was to give J&J access to a team which would carry out research on bipolar diseases in children and adolescents. The latent purpose . . . was to have the Center's research promote the use of Risperdal for children and adolescents. J&J calculated that the fact that the research on the drug was conducted by a leading child psychiatry researcher at a very prestigious academic medical center would give the findings more authority." But the impetus came from Biederman, not J&J; Biederman is said to have "approached Janssen [a J&J subsidiary] multiple times to propose the creation of a Janssen-MGH center for children and adolescent bipolar disorders." J&J supported the Center to the sum of $500,000 a year.[56]

The Center's 2002 annual report stated baldly that assisting the "company marketing efforts" was a primary goal. The Center "will move forward the commercial goals of J&J." And the Center said that it would "test the effectiveness and safety of Risperdal, Concerta . . . and new products as they emerge from the pipeline."[57] It is inconceivable that any of the Deans at Harvard saw this document, with its stunning conflicts of interest. Alex Gorsky, the Johnson & Johnson CEO, said in a deposition in 2012, that "Dr Biederman would have been considered a key opinion leader in this field."[58] Thus, the epidemic of pediatric bipolar disorder that Biederman's Center spawned occurred primarily in aid of Johnson & Johnson's commercial interests.

Biederman had a prickly reputation at Janssen. In 1999, apropos a check that should have reached Biederman but didn't, Janssen executive John Bruins told colleagues that Biederman had not yet been paid the $3000 he had been promised for a Grand Rounds program. "Let me start from the beginning so that it is crystal clear with everyone involved: Dr. Biederman is not someone to jerk around. He is a very powerful national figure in child psych and has a very short fuse." Previously, Biederman had submitted a proposal to Janssen that amounted to $280,000. Janssen dragged its feet and finally sent him "a standard ding letter." "By the time I found out about it a week later," said Bruins, "and went to see him, his secretary advised me of his fury. . . . I have never seen anyone so angry." Since then, Janssen's business with Biederman had been non-existent. "He now has enough projects with Lilly to keep his entire group busy for years."[59] Then things were patched up.

Internal Janssen documents produced at litigation show Biederman's imbrication with the company to have been much deeper than he ever admitted publicly. In June 2002, J&J executive Gahan Pandina wrote Biederman, copied to colleagues, "I am sending the most recent draft of the abstract for AACAP, 2002."[60] J&J had written "Biederman's" draft. Pandina attended a bipolar seminar that Biederman organized in March 2002 at MGH: "He was very balanced in his approaches to treatment, and not perceived to be aligned with any company in particular. Evidently, he made quite a point regarding the metabolic issues related to [Lilly's] olanzapine [weight gain], to the extent of stating that the drug should not be used in the treatment of children and adolescents."[61] In the industry, this was known as "counter-detailing," but it was being done by the head of pediatric psychopharmacology at one of the nation's leading hospitals.

This "bipolar kids" story has one final chapter. How about those children with bipolar disorder who are also "disruptive," especially those in the Medicaid system? We'll calm them down with antipsychotics. In 2006, Biederman wrote an article that almost bankrupted the Medicaid system. Reanalyzing data from a previous trial that Janssen had sponsored,[62] Biederman concluded that in those children who had bipolar disorder, together with "disruptive behavioral disorders" (DBDs) and subaverage intelligence, "risperidone was effective in treating the factors of explosive irritability; agitated, expansive, grandiose; and depression." Disruptive behavior in autistic and developmentally handicapped children had been converted into a new disease, treatable with the antipsychotic Risperdal. It required only a small leap to conclude that even children with normal intelligence who manifested any of this wide range of behavior could profit from treatment with risperidone.[63]

The conceptual leap was highly remunerative. Of 389,000 children and adolescents treated with Risperdal in 2008, 240,000 were 12 or younger. Many were treated off-label for "attention deficit disorders" (read: troublemakers). A panel convened by FDA said, in a journalist's paraphrase, "Risperdal is not approved for attention deficit problems, and its risks—which include substantial weight gain, metabolic disorders and muscular tics that can be permanent—are too profound to justify its use in treating such disorders." Of the children treated off-label with Risperdal, 11 had died. Prescription rates for atypical antipsychotics were said to have increased fivefold in the decade from 1997 to 2007. The journalist's piece fingered Biederman and his pet diagnosis pediatric bipolar disorder.[64]

Pediatric bipolar was already a stretch, as far as new diagnoses went. But to add onto that children who were somehow difficult to manage, who cut up in class, who wouldn't clean up their rooms, who talked back to their parents, was to make most of the pediatric population into candidates for treatment with atypical antipsychotics. Janssen thus led the charge in diagnosing irritable children as "bipolar."

Were these drugs successful in taming the target population? Well, yes. You can sedate any kind of out-of-control behavior with the atypical antipsychotics—but at the cost of serious side effects, such as big weight gains, diabetes, and gynecomastia ("titties") in young boys.

Childhood bipolarity was suddenly everywhere. According to the National Center for Health Statistics, the "annual number of youth office-based visits with a diagnosis of bipolar disorder increased from 25 per 100,000 population in 1994–95 to 1,003 per 100,000 in 2002–2003.[65] That is an increase of 4,000 percent. The *Wall Street Journal* reported that in 2008, 2 years after the Biederman article appeared, Medicaid, the federal poverty program, spent $3.6 billion on antipsychotic medications, up from $1.65 billion in 1999. "An analysis . . . found that in 2008, 19,045 children age 5 and under were prescribed antipsychotics through Medicaid."[66] This may well have been the high point of Biedermania and is a shocking testimonial to the power of a single influential KOL.

2008 was a watershed year for another reason as well. Harvard found out that Biederman had lied to them about the amount of money he had been accepting from Janssen. Sen. Charles Grassley's (R-Iowa) Senate Finance Committee learned that, as the *New York Times* reported, Biederman and his colleagues Timothy E. Wilens "had reported to university officials earning several hundred thousand dollars apiece in consulting fees from drug makers from 2000 to 2007 when in fact they had earned at least $1.6 million each."[67]

Grassley's letter to Harvard and MGH pulled no punches. He found it curious that Biederman seemed to be promising results to Janssen even before doing the studies. Was there "a predisposition to specific findings and conclusions prior to the studies' being commenced?" Curious as well was Biederman's promise to Janssen to "find new uses for J&J products." Still worse was the opinion of an independent academic researcher whom the committee had consulted that "the slides discussed in this letter were nothing more than marketing tools, as opposed to discussions of independent scientific research." Finally, Grassley asked the presidents of Harvard and MGH, "Is it typical in your experiences to include the marketing division of a sponsor company during discussions of possible collaboration with your institution?"[68]

Harvard reviewed the situation and required that the investigators "refrain from all paid industry-sponsored outside activities for one year."[69] Draconian!

But Janssen's payments had been well spent. The Harvard pediatric psychopharmacologists had created an illness to medicate. Thanks to Biederman, Risperdal was well situated to become the drug of choice. An expert report in 2012 to the Court by David Kessler, former FDA Commissioner, documented how aggressively Janssen was promoting Risperdal for what was at the time an off-label indication. (FDA accepted pediatric schizophrenia and bipolar disorders in 2006.) The call notes of one sales rep for January 2005 said, "Continue to promote the Risperdal M-tabs for the child to use in the treatment of aggressive behavior." The note of another sales rep for the same time states, "remind him [the psychiatrist] that patient agitation and irritability at being back at school get under control fast in 3 days with ris[perdal] which is reliable and easy to dose." Another sales rep said on August 13, 2004, "Doc still using risp[erdal] 1st line for children."[70]

The experience of this particular rep was general. A government survey found that, in the years 2005 to 2009, disruptive behavior disorders were the commonest diagnoses in the pediatric visits where antipsychotics were prescribed, accounting for 63.0 percent of all child antipsychotic visits and 33.7 percent of all adolescent antipsychotic visits. In those years, antipsychotics were prescribed in fully *31.1 percent of all youth visits to psychiatrists.*[71] Antipsychotics had passed from being considered "reversible chemical lobotomies" in the 1950s to a kind of aspirin for the young brain in the new century.

Bipolar disorder became the object of savage criticism. Sam Gershon, a very senior figure in psychopharmacology, penned sarcastically, "This tiny article is packed with ideas of absolute brilliance so that one can readily see why they are the leaders of our profession. In the 'olden days,' bipolar disorder was not diagnosed in children but it became apparent at the ages of 40 and 50. Now, it is not only diagnosed in children, there are many varieties up to a bipolar spectrum and soft bipolar." Ah, but then it turned out that the bipolar children really had the new DSM-5 diagnosis, "disruptive mood dysregulation disorder." "Now having cleared this up, we can save all those that were wrongly labeled BP and avoid poisoning them with antipsychotics and lithium. [A prominent study] makes me feel like these are the minutes taken in a mental hospital."[72]

Allen Frances, who had edited DSM-IV, called childhood bipolar disorder "the most dangerous current bubble, with a remarkable fortyfold inflation in just one decade." Biederman et alia had ignored the DSM-IV definition of mania "in favor of a new and largely untested idea that bipolar disorder presents very differently in children. . . . The prophets were 'thought leading' researchers who encouraged child psychiatrists to ignore the standard bipolar criteria and instead to make the diagnosis in a free-form, over-inclusive way. Then enter the pharmaceutical industry—not very good at discovering new drugs, but extremely adept at finding new markets for existing ones."[73]

Arnold Relman, former editor of the *New England Journal of Medicine* and professor emeritus at Harvard, spoke up in more moderate yet decisive tones about Biederman and team, telling the *Boston Globe* in 2008, "These psychiatrists are nationally known for advocating the 'off-label' use of powerful antipsychotic drugs in the management of children believed to have childhood bipolar disorder, a new but controversial diagnosis that they themselves have done much to publicize." Relman noted that the FDA had approved antipsychotics "only for the treatment of adults."[74]

Relman's was the voice of Copley Square in Boston. Here is the voice of the Georgia backwoods: "Sometimes you see a kid who is so out of control that there's really no other choice except to use antipsychotics for behavior control," said Mickey Nardo of his charity-clinic experience in Georgia's Appalachia. "I've seen one such child in the three plus years I've been seeing kids in this rural place—only one." Nardo said of Biederman, "He used his prestige . . . and the prestige of Harvard and Massachusetts General Hospital to put forward a diagnostic category, the bipolar child, that gave people a license to use these medications at will in difficult children. And the child psychiatric community bought it hook, line, and sinker."[75] The last statement is the most deplorable part. Biederman and his group indulged their venality. But that US psychiatry could have so mindlessly taken up this bogus diagnosis, and applied it to young children, does not speak well of the collective judgment of the field. As one psychiatrist commented to the blog *FeedBlitz* in 2008, "Biederman is the undisputed King of Bipolar in kids, and I'm still awaiting any impressive outcome data on the 'bipolar' kids being treated with antipsychotics. Especially the young kids. 4 year olds on Seroquel. [Biederman had dismissed the critics as "not on the same level"]. I'm glad I'm not on Joe's level. Are we better off now that the diagnosis of bipolar has run rampant in kids?"[76]

As the *New York Times* noted, tongue-in-cheek, about industry efforts in the Biederman saga, "As corporate research executives recruit the brightest scientists, their brethren in marketing departments have discovered that some of these same scientists can be terrific pitchmen."[77] Risperdal and Janssen did not initiate the treatment of aggressive, challenging children with antipsychotics. That started already in the 1950s with chlorpromazine. The Biederman story is important because it shows how easily distinguished academic psychiatrists can be bought—and this cupidity doomed the scientific pretensions of child psychopharmacology.

The Boss of All the Bosses

At a meeting of the American Psychiatric Association in December 2006, Max Fink and I had arranged to interview Charlie Nemeroff, then chair of psychiatry at Emory University, for our book. We met him on one side of the convention floor, and we proceeded to walk with him across the floor to the interview room. He was bombarded with "Hi Charlie's" and "Hey Charlie's" from all sides. People were even reaching out to touch his jacket. I have never seen anything like this display of sheer charisma in an academic setting. Nemeroff was perfectly gracious in the brief interview, appeared not to dissemble, and half an hour later rose from his chair to rejoin the milling throng. Whatever one might say about Nemeroff, he has something about him—something that helps explain his success even had he not received enormous amounts of pharmaceutical money. This is called "presence."

But he is known in the industry as "the boss of all bosses," borrowing a Mafia phrase, because he sits—or sat at that time—at the center of a great vortex of money, ghostwriting, and pharmaceutical marketing that spelled doom for psychiatry's claim to be a "science of the mind." It was Nemeroff, probably more than any other individual, *il capo di tutti i capi,* who helped turn academic psychiatry into the sales arm of the pharmaceutical industry.

Nemeroff was born in the Bronx in 1949, was educated at George Washington High School and City College of New York (BSc 1970), and then earned a PhD in biochemistry from the University of North Carolina (UNC) in 1976. He graduated with an MD from UNC in 1981 and trained in psychiatry at UNC and at neighboring Duke University, finishing his residency in 1985. These were sterling credentials. In the coming years he rose in both the department of pharmacology and the department of psychiatry at Duke, chairing psychiatry at Duke in 1991. In these years, he was enormously productive. His cv lists over 350 publications between 1975 and 1991, spanning the entire range of clinical psychiatry, pharmacology, and neuroendocrinology. (He wrote 639 publications in the period 1975–2011, which averages out to "an article and a half every month for over 30 years."[78] This is a volume of activity that is almost impossible without a team of ghostwriters and guest-authorships standing by.)

The Bayh-Dole Act of 1980 made it possible for universities to patent discoveries made with government funds. This opened the door to wide-ranging academic consulting with industry—and all with the Dean's approval because any profits that flowed from consulting would accrue to the university.

This puts in perspective Nemeroff's extensive involvement with the pharmaceutical industry; his cv lists membership on 30 company "advisory boards" from 1990 to "present" (around 2007), beginning with Lilly in 1990 and SmithKline in 1991. Significant amounts of money were connected with these board memberships: toward 2011, $50,000 a year from Novadel, $20,000 from Cenerx, and from AstraZeneca, $50,000 "for two in-person meetings."[79]

Recalling his days on the faculty at Emory, Nardo said, "In 1997 we still believed what we were told. We thought that the Brave New World of atypical antipsychotics would liberate our patients from fear of tardive dyskinesia. . . . I thought the then chairman, Dr. Charlie Nemeroff, was a self-promoter and extremely naïve in his blind adherence to some simplistic biological models of illness. I had no idea about how much he was in bed with the industry, or about his 'poster-child' status, or that he was raking in personal money, or that many of his colleagues were, too. I guess I thought he actually believed what sounded to me like drivel. I didn't know the drivel was a cash cow."[80]

Cash cow, indeed. Late in the 1990s, SmithKline paid a ghostwriting company, Scientific Therapeutics Information of Springfield, New Jersey, to ghost an entire textbook in the name of pseudo-authors Charles Nemeroff and Alan Schatzberg, chair of psychiatry at Stanford University. Aimed at family physicians, the book, *Recognition and Treatment of Psychiatric Disorders: A Psychopharmacology Handbook for Primary Care* (published in 1999 by the American Psychiatric Press Incorporated),[81] paid the "authors" a 15 percent royalty of the $120,000 sales, or about $18,000. In the preface, the "authors" acknowledge an "unrestricted educational grant" from SmithKline Beecham Pharmaceuticals to

Scientific Therapeutics Information, where Diane M. Coniglio provided "editorial assistance." The book was, as Daniel Carlat put it, "like an advertisement for Paxil," a SmithKline drug.[82] David Kessler commented on this order of magnitude of ghosting, "I've never heard of that before. It takes your breath away."[83]

Other critical eyes were starting to scan as well. In 2003, Bernard Carroll and Robert Rubin, the latter then at Drexel University College of Medicine in Pittsburgh, published a letter in *Nature Neuroscience* on several of Nemeroff's conflicts of interest, among them praising mifepristone as an agent in psychotic depression—never confirmed in reliable RCTs—while serving on the advisory board of Corcept, the company holding the mifepristone use patent, and while possessing an option to purchase 72,000 shares of Corcept stock.

Furthermore, Nemeroff played a major role in the development of SmithKline's SSRI Paxil (paroxetine), and in 2003 he organized a special issue of *Psychopharmacology Bulletin*, celebrating "the first 10 years' experience with paroxetine." In academic medicine one wouldn't normally celebrate the anniversary of the launching of a drug, and Nemeroff's introduction, which gave pride of place to paroxetine, claimed that "the last half of the 20th century witnessed remarkable advances in the field of psychiatry."[84] Carroll called this issue "a put-up job, paid for by GSK." The authors included one ghostwriter and several of Nemeroff's residents at Emory. Only one author "had the decency to disclose"—as Carroll put it—that he had received an honorarium for participating in the program![85]

The year 2006 was anything but magical for Nemeroff. In 2006, *Neuropsychopharmacology*, the journal that Nemeroff edited, published an enthusiastic article about the efficacy of Cyberonics' vagus nerve stimulator (VNS) in "treatment-resistant depression." The article failed to disclose that Nemeroff himself and six of his co-authors had commercial ties to Cyberonics. The paper was also evidently ghostwritten, as the authors acknowledged Sally Laden "for editorial support in developing early drafts of this manuscript."[86] Associate Dean Claudia Adkison at Emory was furious about the sell-out appearance of this paper. She wrote Nemeroff, "I can't believe that anyone in the public or in academia would believe anything except that this paper was a piece of paid marketing."[87]

Pushback was not delayed in coming. The editorial board of *Neuropsychopharmacology* discovered the conflict of interest and in July 2006 published an embarrassed acknowledgment. This was significant news and resulted in big articles in the *Wall Street Journal* and *New York Times*.[88]

Also in 2006, Nemeroff and colleagues published an "experimercial" (Carroll) on the success of risperidone (Risperdal) in "treatment-resistant depression" in *Neuropsychopharmacology*.[89] Janssen had funded it. In the following year, 2007, Bernard Carroll, who was acquiring a reputation as a fierce critic of intellectual deceit in psychopharmacology, published a takedown of the risperidone article. The results had not in fact reached the 0.05 level of significance. Weight gains on risperidone had been hushed up. "The claim that risperidone significantly prevented relapse in a subgroup should be retracted."[90]

Yet these were peccadillos compared to what was to come. In 2008, Grassley's Senate Finance Committee investigated academics holding NIH grants who had been receiving large amounts of drug money. "In psychiatry, Mr. Grassley has found an orchard of low-hanging fruit," the *New York Times* said, including such KOLs as Melissa DelBello of the University of Cincinnati and Alan Schatzberg at Stanford. As for Nemeroff, the committee found that "from 2000 through 2006, Dr. Nemeroff received just over $960,000 from Glaxo, but reported to Emory that he received no more than $35,000," Grassley said. He referred the file to the inspector general of the Department of Health and Human Services for investigation.[91] Interestingly, while Nemeroff was collecting all this money from GlaxoSmithKline as a speaker and flack, he was also, as Daniel Carlat pointed out, "the principal investigator of a 5 year, $3.9 million grant from NIMH *to study five Glaxo drugs*."[92] The story was a colossal embarrassment for Emory, which deposed Nemeroff as chair of psychiatry.

In October 2008, in a Page 1 story, the *New York Times* called Nemeroff's extra income, which was an egregious violation of NIH rules, a scandal "that is shaking the world of academic medicine and seems likely to force broad changes in the relationships between doctors and drug makers."[93] In the world of academic medicine, this is as awful as it gets.

In 2009, Nemeroff resigned as editor of *Neuropsychopharmacology*, his reputation as a KOL weakened—but not destroyed! He had resigned his appointment at Emory in 2008 because of the nondisclosure issues and in 2009 became chairman of psychiatry at the University of Miami Miller Medical School. In 2018, he joined the Dell Medical School in Austin, Texas, as director of its Institute for Early Life Adversity.

Nemeroff and Paxil

In 2000, SmithKline Beecham (SKB) became GlaxoSmithKline (GSK). In 1994, the drug house commissioned a large trial (#352) of its agent Paxil for bipolar depression in 117 outpatients who had been stabilized on lithium at some 19 different centers. (The study was very underpowered and could not have shown much of anything.) Paxil was compared to the standard antidepressant imipramine and placebo. The results were mediocre: Neither imipramine nor Paxil beat high-dose lithium, so the conclusion was, simply upping your patients' lithium levels will serve them better than either Paxil or imipramine. In the main analysis, the two drugs did not beat placebo, and Paxil had as many side effects as imipramine (the whole logic for Paxil and the other SSRIs was that they had a "favorable side effects profile" compared to the tricyclics).

SmithKline sent this rather unsavory brew of results over to abovementioned Scientific Therapeutics Information (STI), where Sally Laden was associate editorial director. (From 1998 to 2008, STI would ghost over a hundred papers for SmithKline, all composed with the names of pseudo-authors on every title page.) In March 1997, the STI people produced the first draft of a paper that had, as Jack Gorman at the *American Journal of Psychiatry* later observed, "a very biased tinge to it."[94]

So, in this particular paper about Paxil and bipolar depression, the question was, who should the authors be? (There were no names on either of the first two drafts.) The original concept was that the authors would be Laszlo Gyulai at the University of Pennsylvania and Gary Sachs at MGH.[95] But then, in May 1997, Muriel Young, the medical director of CNS at SmithKline, decided that she wanted the names of Charles Nemeroff at Emory and Dwight Evans, then at the University of Florida at Gainesville, on the title page.[96]

Evans was a curious choice, given that he seems to have recruited only one or two patients for the study.[97] Nemeroff was already a familiar figure at SmithKline, having worked since 2000 as a "guest speaker who trained PsychNet doctors [a SmithKline program] in the advocacy of GSK's Paxil product," as the Emory student newspaper commented.[98]

With Young's 1997 decision, Nemeroff became the main player, handling all communications with SmithKline about a paper that was soon to be published with him as the pseudo-author. It is unclear if Nemeroff had any patients in the study, and Jay Amsterdam, who led the Depression Research Unit at Penn (and was unacknowledged for his contribution of patients to the study), later argued that Nemeroff was chosen on grounds of being a prominent KOL.[99] Nemeroff later claimed that "All [STI] did was help collate all the different authors' comments and help with references. We wrote the paper."[100] The statement is clearly false.

The major problems with the paper soon became apparent and the *American Journal of Psychiatry* was hesitant about an early version. Sally Laden drafted "Nemeroff's" reply to these criticisms. Alas, as Gorman told Nemeroff in June 2000, the journal's statistical reviewer "adamantly recommend[ed] rejection." Gorman was displeased with this decision and praised the paper as "important as one of the only, if not the only one, of its kind."[101] As an *American Journal of Psychiatry* insider, Gorman functioned throughout as a cheerleader for Nemeroff and SmithKline, enjoying his post of considerable editorial power while at the same time working as a paid consultant for SmithKline in promoting Paxil.[102] (Gorman was to become known as a friend of the industry, and an article in the *New York Times* in 2002 suggested that Forest Labs had influenced him to write a favorable piece on their new antidepressant Lexapro in the journal *CNS Spectrums*, which he edited.[103]) In the same year, *Mother Jones* described Gorman's efforts on behalf of Paxil, as well as his appearance on the television show *Good Morning America* on behalf of the SSRIs in treating what the show described as the "hidden epidemic" of compulsive shopping—90 percent of the sufferers female![104]

What to do? Nemeroff told Sally Laden that he could publish the paper "relatively quickly" in his own journal *Depression and Anxiety*. Or maybe the *British Journal of Psychiatry*?

STI had many irons in the fire with Nemeroff: doing the slides for a presentation he was to give in March 1999 in Florida[105]; ghosting a letter for him on sexual dysfunction; preparing a whole "Neurobiology Teaching Module for the Hidden Diagnosis CDROM project"; and organizing a symposium for the APA meeting in 2000 that SmithKline was to sponsor. Sally Laden said to Nemeroff: "Topics for your symposium are not yet decided, but candidates for yours might be Women's Issues or Biological Basis for Comorbidity in Depression." Sally Laden would decide about "Nemeroff's" symposium.[106] For the Paxil paper, there had been no correspondence at all with any of the paper's other "authors." As Jay Amsterdam said in a later legal brief, "Academics in the trial never reviewed or even saw the submitted manuscript."[107]

Things dragged on and on. Sally Laden was now on Draft XI of the paper, of which everyone now was completely sick. The brass at SmithKline were said to be "disgusted" with Nemeroff and wanted to forget about the *American Journal of Psychiatry* (until Nemeroff persuaded them to try once again). John Romankiewicz, the CEO of the ghosting company, was ready to "take a loss on this just to get it over with."[108] But finally all the exaggerated claims in the paper were dropped, distortions were lessened, and the paper came out in the *American Journal of Psychiatry* in June 2001.[109] Jay Amsterdam's later view was that, "The published manuscript was biased in its conclusions, made unsubstantiated efficacy claims, and downplayed the adverse event profile of Paxil."[110]

Nemeroff had a big conflict of interest with SmithKline, although in 2001, the year of the paper's publication, he did work for 17 other companies as well. In 2001, he made 44 paid trips for SmithKline "to give 'talks' as part of their Speakers' Bureau," as Nardo pointed out in his blog *1 Boring Old Man*, calling the paper "yet another example of malignant pseudo-science."[111] STI billed SmithKline $13,286 for its labors,[112] and all was well that ended well.

Or not.

Back in Philadelphia, at the Depression Research Unit of the University of Pennsylvania, Jay Amsterdam was highly displeased that his name had been omitted from the credits. His own clinic had contributed 19 patients to the study, which was apparently the largest number of patients from any site. But Amsterdam had had no role in the analysis, and his colleague Laszlo Gyulai at Karl Rickels' anxiety clinic was made to seem the principal investigator from the University of Pennsylvania. (Amsterdam later argued that SmithKline had excluded him from the data analysis and authorship because "GSK and the other 'authors' knew Dr. Amsterdam's professional ethics would not allow him to lend his name to a ghostwritten work . . . and would not allow the other 'authors' to turn a failed study into an undisclosed promotional marketing manuscript for the sponsor."[113])

Amsterdam complained to Dwight Evans, now the department chair at Penn, about the role of STI, not knowing that STI had ghosted an editorial in 2003 in *Biological Psychiatry* for Evans himself and Dennis Charney, then at the NIH Intramural Program.[114] This saga had several subsequent chapters that will not be reviewed here but are ably charted in the *Chronicle of Higher Education*.[115]

The shocking story of SmithKline, Paxil trial 352, the medical ghostwriters, and the so-called "writers" themselves illustrates the bankruptcy of the notion that much of the "scientific literature" in psychopharmacology has anything to do with scientific truth. As Robert Rubin, chief of psychiatry at the VA Hospital in Los Angeles, said in looking back over this whole sordid story, "The saddest part of all is that, in order to enrich themselves, these corrupt academics have tainted at least two decades of scientific literature, leaving the rest of the scientific community in limbo regarding which drug studies to take seriously and which to reject. . . . It will take a long time to rectify the reporting biases purchased by pharmaceutical companies and to produce a scientifically valid psychopharmacological literature."[116]

Connoisseurs of the academic–industrial complex will absolutely savor the "initiative" that Nemeroff assembled with his friends Tom Insel and Dennis Charney at NIMH and his paymaster GSK: "The Emory-GSK-NIMH Collaborative Mood Disorders Initiative." The deal was that this consortium of pals was to "scrutinize" several new antidepressant drugs that GSK was developing. The $5.3 million grant began in 2003 and finished in 2015—with no new antidepressant drugs in view. Despite this lack of productivity, Insel continued the grant for another 5 years. When Charles Grassley got wind of the "initiative," he asked the president of Emory if he knew that Nemeroff was receiving all this additional money to promote Paxil.[117] This scandalous example of best friends shoveling money into one another's pockets led Carroll to conclude, "that the chatter by federal scientific administrators (Hyman, Insel) about translational research strategies and innovative models of drug discovery is mostly vacuous rhetoric."[118]

Unsurprisingly, all this frenetic KOL activity came to the attention of the FDA as potentially deceiving the public. Was Dr. X speaking on behalf of a drug because he believed it superior or because the maker was paying him? Kenneth Feather, who led the FDA's Division of Drug Advertising in the late 1980s, said in an interview, "You go to a scientific meeting, you go to a medical meeting, and there are four or five doctors up there discussing the drug, and you don't know that those guys are on the payroll of the company." Feather said the FDA was about to insist that possible commercial connections be divulged in meeting programs. People needed to realize, "Well, this guy might not be unbiased. You know, he's being paid for by the company whose drug he is talking about. So what he's saying, I've got to take with a grain of salt."[119] The policy was, however, never implemented at psychiatry meetings. The KOLs continued to sail under the false flag of science.

10

Trials Begin

> Most of our knowledge about disease, drug treatment, and drug tox-
> icity has, in fact, come not from controlled trials, but from natural-
> istic observations by smart physicians using their past knowledge
> and experience as control.—Louis Lasagna (1975)[1]

Do we really need controlled trials to tell if a drug works? Paul Leber, chief of psychopharmacology at FDA, made a career out of saying Yes in public. But in private, his view was Not Really. He told David Healy in 2008, "If a drug really works, you don't hear any complaints [about FDA] at all. I remember when we first looked at clomipramine [the tricyclic drug Anafranil] on the Y-BOCS [Yale-Brown Obsessive-Compulsive Scale]. I mean the placebo group didn't budge and the patients on clomipramine all got better. Not completely better but there was a 10-point improvement on the Y-BOCS. Well, you didn't need statistics. One was on a 45-degree line [upward curve on the graph] and the other wasn't. So you knew the drug worked."[2]

The history of clinical trials is important because it is they, more than any other concept except neurotransmitters, that have given psychopharmacology the appearance of science. This is part and parcel of the general triumph of numbers within medicine. Medical historian Harry Marks at Johns Hopkins University wrote, "As late as 1950, few would have imagined the central place statistics now holds in medicine."[3] And the numbers—in drug trials, in neurotransmitters, and for receptors—are evidence of science.

The reason clinicians have been so ready to prescribe medications of doubtful efficacy to patients with such questionable diagnoses as "major depression" is that the voice of science—which is to say, the voice of numbers—seems to speak from the doctor's chair. A general practitioner from Wales said at a 1972 meeting on psychopharm for GPs, "We have reached a point now where we have to guess at the similarities between drugs, and the genus of drugs to which they belong by the sound of the name. This is really all that is left of pharmacology for many of us after we have left medical school for about 15 years. We are groping about, hoping that the title of the brand name will give us a clue as to action and possible chemical relatives. We may reach a point where, if a drug has an easily remembered, cleverly chosen brand name, then we remember it, and prescribe it. This is a really terrifying situation."[4]

How to Know If a Drug Works?

How to know if a drug works? There are two approaches: look for the "wow" factor or run a randomized controlled clinical trial (RCT) and look at the numbers.

In the early US trials, it was the NIMH, not industry, that funded the trial. Jonathan Cole founded the NIMH's Psychopharmacology Service Center (PSC) in 1956, and the PSC paid for dozens of trials run by academic investigators at their home institutions.

Cole, a delightfully off-hand figure, said it's not that hard to spot winners. "If you're working with a drug in 100 patients and a few of the patients hadn't said, 'Wow, do I feel better', then . . . the drug probably isn't going to turn out better than the placebo."[5] So, listen for the wow factor. This would be an observational, or anecdotal, approach.

The other approach is the regulatory approach of the Food and Drug Administration, which, after the FDA Act in 1938, had to approve all new drugs before they reached the market. The story is that the FDA was obliged by Congress in the Kefauver-Harris amendments of 1962 to apply the standard of "well-controlled trials." This meant evaluating questionnaires and numbers. But this may not really be what Congress had in mind and represents a bit of bureaucratic overkill. In an interview William Rankin, then general counsel of FDA, said that in the first committee report on the bill, "We would have authorized the use of claims to some extent based upon clinical experience. . . . That was some give on our part to the effectiveness claim. But that resulted in everybody focusing on, how do you really approve a new drug claim? And that was the adequate and well-controlled studies, and we adopted that and put that language in, that effectiveness would have to be proved, and we defined what was inadequate in well-controlled studies by regulations thereafter."[6] So the whole RCT mantra that followed was not the will of Congress, but the will of a few administrators in the FDA's "BuMed," as it was called. (The Bureau of Medicine was created only in 1957.)

Kefauver-Harris was not FDA's first real regulatory contact with the "ethical" (regular) pharmaceutical industry.[7] Yet previously, aside from approving drugs for safety, it had been concerned mainly with toxicology and fights against quackery. (Any measure of safety is always balanced against risk; but risk for what benefit? This is implicitly a measure of efficacy.)

FDA had developed its own culture for dealing with pharmaceuticals. Paul Leber, for many years head of the Neuropharmacologic Drugs Division of the FDA, said in an interview, "I've listened to Don Klein [at Columbia] say many times, give me a drug and I'll tell you whether it works. Well I'm not sure he can tell me in a way I can hear. He may tell me he believes it works. He may, in fact, be right, but we're unable to listen to him unless he presents it in a form where we can know in a public way if a drug works"—and that's in a controlled trial.[8]

From the controlled trial would emerge a number: the average difference between the drug and placebo. People who believed in good medicine cringed. W. Leigh Thompson, a retired Lilly executive, lambasted the FDA for paying too much attention to the mean: It deflected attention from the heterogeneity of patients. "We don't treat patients in herds. Unfortunately, the US FDA thinks of patients in just that way."[9] The single number for "statistical significance" was even worse. It measured nothing meaningful (see Chapter 10). As early as 1989, Lou Lasagna criticized the FDA's "preoccupation with 0.05 probability levels [of statistical significance] as the magical cutoff point that automatically spells either failure or success, despite the repeated criticism of such an approach in the statistical literature."[10]

Toward the Randomized Controlled Trial

[The importance of the RCT] cannot be exaggerated. It opened up a new world of evaluation and control which will, I think, be the key to a rational health service.—Archie Cochrane (1971)[11]

Psychiatry has always found the pull of numbers irresistible. In 1943, Jerome Lettvin and Walter Pitts, interns at the Boston City Hospital (and headed for psychiatry), published a paper titled "A Mathematical Theory of Affective Psychoses."[12] "It was meant as a joke," said Lettvin,[13] but nonetheless it was cited thirteen times.

From the beginning, psychiatry had a tendency toward quantification. What are the causes of mental illness? An investigation in Paris in 1843 revealed, in a survey of 10,111 patients, that among the "physical causes" there were, per 100 patients: idiocy (32.1 percent), "excessive irritation" (9.4 percent), and masturbation (4.2 percent).[14]

Perhaps with such results in mind, some of the leaders of the field in France were wary of counting. Jean-Pierre Falret, chief psychiatrist of the Salpêtrière Hospital in Paris, wrote in 1864, "Statistics are, in fact, a procedure all the more dangerous because they offer every appearance of truth. Thus statistics serve to introduce into science errors that are all the more harmful because they take on the appearance of mathematics."

What was the problem? Counting apples and oranges together was one, said Falret. This will leap to our eyes in the present book when we look at trials of treatments for "depression" that were invalid because several different depressions—neurasthenic, melancholic, atypical—were jumbled together. Averages of this brew would be as meaningless as averaging together mumps and tuberculosis.

A second problem, said Falret, is that the object under study is an intellectual construct, and "often does not exist in nature in the form of concrete entities, of real units."[15]

We encounter this often in psychiatry when we are told about Mr. Smith's complex dysphoria, which changes across the day and the week, which changes with his companion, and which he has trouble articulating except for saying that he does not "feel good in his body." We are invited to see this as "major depression." Falret would roll in his grave.

Yet a compelling case can be made for controlled clinical trials. Friedrich Jolly, professor of psychiatry in Berlin, laid out the logic of the controlled trial at a meeting in 1888 in Karlsruhe, commenting on the results of a colleague's trial of opium in mania: "But a final judgment about the meaning of these figures would only be possible if we were in a position to compare series of similar patients who received no treatment." So this would be a two-arm trial where one arm got nothing at all. "For obvious reasons, this is not easy,"[16] Jolly sighed.

Pace Archie Cochrane, director of the Medical Research Council (MRC) Epidemiology Unit in Cardiff, it is *not* evident that counting things in clinical trials is the best way of arriving at scientific truth. Many of he clinical trials of pharmaceuticals, from which so much of our knowledge of psychiatry seems to derive, include respondents (most are not actual patients) recruited online or in newspaper ads.[17] Sixty percent of the subjects on drug X responded, only thirty percent of subjects on placebo responded, hence drug X must be licensed (the actual differences are never this great and often require refined statistical techniques to tease out any difference at all).

Placebo-controlled trials go back to the 1930s, but there is nothing new in medicine about the concept of the placebo, or giving an inert substance in order to achieve a suggestive effect. As early as 1815, Etienne Esquirol, who had just finished a decade of leading the Salpêtrière Hospital, explained his placebo success with his female epileptic patients. "The patients were prepared in advance, exciting their imaginations by the repeated promise of a certain recovery. The head nurse and students played along with this." He said he had tried every imaginable remedy. It was always the same story. "The new medications always relieved the seizures for two weeks for some, for a month, two months in others, even for three months. After this interval the convulsions reappeared successively among all the women, with the same characteristics they had previously presented. . . . I must say that I was never able to obtain a cure. . . . If the seizures were suspended, it was less by the action of the medications than by the effect of the confidence that brought a patient to consult a new physician [himself]. This remission, or even this suspension, has been generally observed by physicians who treat chronic illnesses, particularly those disorders called nervous."[18]

Esquirol was describing the effect of suggestion combined with active (although ineffective) agents. Yet frank placebos, too, go back a long way in medicine. In 1893, John Nichols, a physician in Cambridge, Massachusetts, deplored his colleagues' practice of prescribing, or dispensing, "blank tablets," and he had recently learned that the manufacturer of "Harvard Experimental Diagnosis Tablets" had "just sold five thousand to a physician in my own town."[19]

The very first randomized, controlled, blinded clinical trial was organized in 1931 by J. Burns Amberson and colleagues in a TB sanitorium in Northville, Michigan. Amberson himself had been a TB patient in the sanitorium and then returned to it as a clinician, keen on evaluating the effectiveness of gold therapy (in a preparation called Sanocrysin). The patients were randomized to the gold or placebo groups with a flip of the coin and were blinded (i.e., kept ignorant of their treatment status), as were most of the medical staff. The treatment turned out to be toxic—but the effort was the first RCT.[20] Amberson went on to a post in the Chest Service at Bellevue Hospital in New York and became a well-known tuberculosis specialist.

Then there was silence for almost two decades.

Both Sides of the Pond

In the early days, clinical trials were scrupulously conducted, usually by a single investigator, and were largely uninfluenced by industry. This is part of the scientific narrative in the *rise* of psychopharmacology, and the corruption of trials into instruments of deceit and dishonesty is part of the story of the *fall*.

United Kingdom

The modern history of controlled clinical trials in England began in 1931 when the MRC set up a Therapeutic Trials Committee, in response to a request by the Association of British Chemical Manufacturers for "an authoritative body to arrange clinical tests of new remedies which in laboratory experiment had given promise both of therapeutic value and low toxicity," as MRC member

Francis Green said in 1954, explaining the history of such trials. The tests were to be conducted before the agent was marketed, not necessarily to ensure public safety but "so that the manufacturer might be saved embarrassment if the results of the tests were unfavorable." Drugs tested in the 1930s were used largely in internal medicine. Although untreated controls were frowned on (as lab tests were thought sufficient to ensure the efficacy of a molecule), a trial of antipneumococcal serum in lobar pneumonia in 1934 did include controls.[21]

The earliest trial in *psychopharm* was conducted by Linford Rees, who initially had a small-town practice in Wales, then after 1954 was at the Maudsley and St. Bartholomew's Hospital in London. He unquestionably pioneered controlled trials, some of them randomized. Industry occasionally paid for research assistants in the conduct of all this work, yet as far as is known, Rees never functioned in any sense as a Key Opinion Leader, never shilling for the drugs he was testing.[22] In 1951, Rees and a colleague reported a controlled trial in a Welsh hospital of desoxycortone acetate and ascorbic acid in schizophrenia. The 28 patients were distributed in 14 matched pairs, and one member of each pair received the treatment, the other placebo. The patients and physicians were blinded about who received what. Results were completely negative.[23]

Note that these independent academic investigators ran clinical trials without the financing of industry. The companies would supply the drug free but then have no further relationship with the trialists. So the trial was honest, and the investigators received no payments, no speakers' bureau fees, no . . . nothing. Thus, in the early 1930s, Peter McCowan, director of the Cardiff Insane Hospital, thought nothing of running quick, informal trials for Sandoz. Reported Ralph Gerard, a young neurophysiologist prospecting grant candidates in Europe and the United Kingdom on behalf of the Rockefeller Foundation, "McCowan is in close touch with [Markus] Guggenheim, of Hoffmann-LaRoche, and tests antiepileptic drugs for them."[24] Almost certainly, he received no money for doing this.

As for getting a doctor to run a short trial, this was often the task of the drug rep, known in the day as "the detail man." Mindel Shepo, in the Graduate School of Public Health at the University of Pittsburgh, said in 1960, "The responsibility for arranging with physicians to make the first trials on human beings is at times given to detail men."[25] The comment illustrates the low-key informality of relations between industry and clinicians.

As Daniel Shaw, Wyeth's vice-president for medical affairs, explained at a conference in 1971, the short little clinician-driven trials were known "as sales seeding or pre-marketing seeding back in the old days. . . . I learned more about the drug in terms of the side effects, adverse reactions, and misuse during that period of time than I did during all of the time that I was doing so-called controlled studies."[26] Distributing the drug to a large number of local doctors might garner more in the way of useful information than a six-week controlled trial, with questionnaires and the rest of the quantitative apparatus. People felt blindsided by the issue of sexual impotence that suddenly surfaced with the SSRIs; sexual function had simply not been queried in the questionnaires, but local docs would have picked it up in their patients.

The *randomized* clinical trial was popularized in drug research in 1948 by Austin Bradford ("Tony") Hill, professor at the London School of Hygiene, in an MRC study of streptomycin in tuberculous meningitis.[27] The innovative principle was the concept of "randomization," to rule out extraneous factors that might affect the results (the factors would affect the treatment and control groups equally). This has been widely held as the origin of the modern RCT in general, not just in England.[28] (The principle of randomization does antedate Hill, and it is said to have been introduced as early as 1923 by Ronald Aylmer Fisher in agricultural research.[29])

Industry was quite involved in the English controlled trials. In 1949, Alan Broadhurst had just started working for Geigy at Rhodes near Manchester, where the Geigy drug company in Basel had a local office, the Geigy Dysestuffs Warehouse. It was Broadhurst's job, as a nonphysician, to organize trials of some of Geigy's products.

Q: "When you say clinical trial, what did that involve at this stage?"

Broadhurst: "Oh, this was way back in 1951. There was almost no question of doing double-blind studies—strictly controlled trials at this time. These were 'suck it and see' trials." (Overcome by his sense of bottomless ignorance, Broadhurst went to medical school, then commuted between Manchester and Basel, working with Geigy on the development of the first antidepressant, imipramine.)[30]

Then trials moved beyond suck it and see. Some of the trials resembled the Wild West. Early in 1956, clinicians at one London hospital wanted to evaluate Lundbeck's phenothiazine antipsychotic Pacatal (mepazine, later renamed perazine). Unfortunately, at their hospital there were no wards with fresh patients not on anything, "so the plan was made of taking two identical wards where chlorpromazine was already in use. In one ward Pacatal was to be substituted for chlorpromazine." The behavior of patients in the two wards could then by compared. "The plan of the experiment was kept secret from the nursing staff." The clinicians just went ahead and changed 50 patients from one drug to the other. The Pacatal patients responded beautifully. "In the ward where Pacatal was used, there was a much warmer spirit. The visitors were greeted cheerfully by the patients and made to feel welcome," as opposed to patients' smearing and tearing their clothes into bits on the chlorpromazine ward.[31] Despite the patients' spirited clinical behavior (and an experimental approach that today would result in the clinicians' loss of their medical licenses), Pacatal did not turn out to be quite the wonder drug the authors claimed. It had unacceptable side effects and was registered only in Germany (where a generic version remains on the market). The disarray on the chlorpromazine ward was doubtless due to the patients' having catatonia rather than schizophrenia: catatonic patients would get worse, if anything, on chlorpromazine.

The most famous of the early controlled trials in psychopharmacology in the United Kingdom was reported in 1954 by Charmian Elkes at the Winson Green Hospital in Birmingham, together with her husband Joel Elkes, professor of experimental psychiatry at the University of Birmingham. On the basis of the chlorpromazine trial, in which the patients served as their own controls (blindly switched from drug to placebo and back), the researchers definitively established the efficacy of the agent.[32] (Charmian Elkes, whose role as an early female psychiatrist has been almost entirely unstudied, conducted in 1957 a trial of reserpine and associated alkaloids in chronic psychotic patients, demonstrating their effectiveness.[33]). May and Baker, the company that had the British license for chlorpromazine, furnished the drug and placebo tablets; the trial itself was funded by several regional charities. Michael Shepherd at the Maudsley conducted several other early trials, which almost certainly were paid for from the hospital budget. Industry played virtually no role in these undertakings save furnishing the compound and the placebo tablets. Yet Aubrey Lewis, professor at the Institute of Psychiatry, had little use for drugs, preferring social treatments, and drug trials never really gained a footing at the Maudsley.

In 1954 or early 1955, Linford Rees and Carl Lambert at the Maudsley used a cross-over procedure in a study of chlorpromazine in anxiety, switching the blinded patients back and forth between drug and placebo. They reported this in the *Journal of Mental Science* and again at Jean Delay's big international chlorpromazine conference in Paris in October 1955. Fifty-four percent of the sample improved, and two-thirds of those relapsed.[34]

It was David Lewis Davies and Michael Shepherd at the Maudsley who in 1955 reported one of the earliest placebo-controlled, double-blind randomized trials. It was of reserpine. This MRC trial was a "huge feat," as Shepherd later said. Industry had no role in it. The patients were in parallel groups rather than serving as their own controls in a cross-over trial. (The problem with cross-over studies is the large carry-over effects of the drug once the patients are switched to placebo; furthermore, in depression trials, many patients recover before they cross over.) This reserpine trial was the gold standard. In 67 outpatients from various clinics, "troubled in the main by anxiety and depression for which they had been referred to hospital [the Maudsley]," 64.3 percent of the reserpine patients improved, as did 34.6 percent of the placebo patients.[35] Reserpine later stood accused of causing as much depression as it cured, but this was the first modern trial.

Shepherd's 1955 trial was part of a larger MRC effort to gin up trials. Shepherd recounted that 40 or 50 physicians "from all over the country" were invited to MRC headquarters, and "George Pickering [then an academic investigator at St. Mary's Hospital in London, later Regius Professor at Oxford] came in and made a speech. What he actually said to them was, 'I want you to understand that you are privileged to participate in an MRC study. It's going to be a lot of work for you and you're not going to be paid and we expect a high standard but do remember that this is an honor.' And they took it. I remember sitting and thinking surely somebody is going to have the guts to get up and say, 'Who do you think you're talking to?' which is what would happen now. Because all these people now would be paid by the industry to do trials for money."[36]

In fact, Pickering presided over one of the most impeccable trials in the history of psychopharmacology. Entirely uninfluenced by industry, the trial was reported in 1965 by the Clinical Psychiatry Committee of the MRC. Two-hundred and fifty patients 40 to 69 years old who were hospitalized for depression were enrolled and randomly assigned to four groups: imipramine (a TCA), phenelzine (a MAOI), ECT, and placebo. ECT and imipramine beat phenelzine (which had no effect at all beyond placebo).[37] The trial cemented the reputation of imipramine and ECT as the treatments of choice in serious depression and remains even today a model of how to investigate drugs scientifically.

United States

In 1922, two investigators at the Ward's Island asylum in New York found that patients who were operated on for infected teeth and tonsils ("focal infections") recovered from psychosis no more rapidly than patients who were not operated on. This might have been the very first controlled trial of any kind in US psychiatry.[38]

The first controlled trial of a drug in US psychiatry took place in 1938, at Longview Hospital in Cincinnati. Benzedrine was interchanged with placebo in 48 female patients who were in the "depressed phase" of various psychotic illnesses. The trial used the patients as their own controls, alternating Benzedrine and placebo in a single-blinded manner over a period of months. The behavior of the women improved spectacularly in the treatment phases: 25 percent showed "lasting improvement," 50 percent showed improvement only while receiving the drug, and 25 percent did not respond. Reported in an obscure state medical journal, the trial remained widely unknown and exerted little influence.[39]

The modern North American narrative of RCTs in psychiatry begins in 1954 with two workers, Leo Hollister and Lou Lasagna. Hollister had trained as an internist but was later the acknowledged Dean of US Psychopharmacology. In

1953, he had just joined the staff of the Veterans Administration (VA) hospital in Palo Alto, California. (He was also on the faculty at Stanford.)

Just after the Second World War, the VA set up a network for RCTs of tuberculosis drugs. The VA then decided that MAOIs, such as iproniazid, were important, and Hollister became the delegate of the Palo Alto hospital to the central office at the Perry Point facility. Here, he met John Overall from Perry Point and was exposed to psychiatric trials for the first time. Hollister ended up leading the VA collaborative trials in psychiatry, the first in the United States.[40]

The VA hospitals had psychiatric patients in the majority, and Hollister thought he would compare chlorpromazine and reserpine against placebo in this very ill population. So he set up four studies: one of reserpine in anxiety, one of combined chlorpromazine and reserpine in anxiety, one of reserpine in "chronic schizophrenic reactions," and a final one of chlorpromazine in such "reactions."[41] Each trial had a placebo group, and all were double-blind studies, although the patients were not randomized. Hollister presented the findings in December 1954 at the meeting of the American Association for the Advancement of Science at Berkeley. "So there was a chance, for the first time, to publicize my work," he later told an interviewer. Dick Roberts from Ciba accompanied him to the Berkeley meeting (reserpine was a Ciba drug). "So Dick introduced me to Nate [Kline]. Nate's attitude toward both of us was like we were peasants beseeching the emperor; I was put off by it and remember saying to Dick, 'Who in the hell does that son-of-a-bitch think he is?' "[42] To be sure, Hollister was involved with industry but was only dragged along by a company person to an academic meeting. Hollister definitely did not tour on behalf of Ciba nor—as far as is known—get payments from them. This whole generation of investigators would have found such an idea grotesque.

In the United States, the first proper randomized and placebo-controlled trial was conducted in 1954 by Louis Lasagna, then in the department of anesthesia of Massachusetts General Hospital (MGH) and considered, along with Leo Hollister, a founding figure of US psychopharmacology. He ran a study of hypnotics given to patients the night before their surgery. The study was randomized and placebo-controlled, and chloral hydrate was found to be the best agent for inducing sleep, although the patients awakened during the night as often as on placebo. The other drugs did not improve on placebo.[43] In 1954, Lasagna then joined the department of pharmacology of Johns Hopkins, and in 1956 he reported another controlled, randomized trial of hypnotics: secobarbital and pentobarbital were found to be the most efficacious.[44] These two trials initiated the full-fledged RCT in the United States. In 1954, three investigators at Johns Hopkins reported a very small trial of mephenesin (Tolserol), across a variety of psychiatric diagnoses, in which the 24 patients were randomized to various treatment sequences.[45] The placebo outperformed mephenesin. Interestingly, Lasagna, in the pharmacology department at Hopkins, would have had these investigators in psychiatry as colleagues, but he seems never to have mentioned this trial, possibly because he considered it an embarrassment, or because of internal politics.

Hollister, Lasagna et al. did not, it appears, undertake trials for any drug company. They were motivated by scientific curiosity. Yet the drug companies, keen to know if their products were safe and effective, often commissioned trials of their own. In June 1955, Smith, Kline & French convoked in Philadelphia a conference of researchers who had been investigating chlorpromazine. It is unclear to what extent the researchers were indebted to the company for their work—yet the conference increased considerably the number of placebo-controlled trials. Alas, most not randomized.[46]

Comparable to the Pickering trial of depression treatment in the United Kingdom was a big US trial begun in 1961 in nine different VA hospitals for patients with "acute schizophrenia." Conducted under the auspices of NIMH's PSC, which was led by Jon Cole, the trial investigated three antipsychotic drugs set against placebo in the 344 randomly assigned patients who completed the trial. The drugs were chlorpromazine (Thorazine), thioridazine (Mellaril), and fluphenazine (Prolixin); although chlorpromazine had already proven its value in a number of investigations, many psychiatrists, still heavily oriented toward psychoanalysis, were not convinced that the "pills" actually worked. The results were encouraging: At the end of six weeks, 75 percent of the drug patients showed marked to moderate improvement, versus 23 percent of the placebo patients. There were few side effects. The three drugs seemed equally effective.[47] The trial was a landmark in the acceptance of psychopharmacology in the US psychiatric community.

The PSC then organized a number of collaborative trials. In 1964, for example, Milton Greenblatt, superintendent of the Boston State Hospital, conducted under PSC auspices a three-hospital study of ECT, two MAOIs, and imipramine in inpatients with depression. The study found ECT highly effective, the MAOI phenelzine (Nardil) and the TCA imipramine (Tofranil) moderately so, and isocarboxazid (Marplan) inferior to placebo.[48]

There is one outlier that, although it remained almost entirely unknown, may merit the title of "first randomized controlled trial." The story is this: In 1951, a French-Canadian investigator had conducted a rather unsatisfactory trial of nucleotides in schizophrenia. (Nucleotides are the building blocks of DNA.) Unconvinced by the results, the Mental Health Division of the Canadian Department of Health and Welfare in Ottawa asked a group of eager investigators at the Saskatchewan Hospital in Weyburn, Saskatchewan, to run the study over again—but with strict attention to the rules. Ottawa assigned each patient in the study a number. Treatment and control groups, the authors said, were "selected at random." Thus, there arrived in the mail in Weyburn a shipment from Ottawa containing 40 individual packages; half the packages had nucleotides, the other half placebo, and nobody in Weyburn had any idea which was which. The trial clearly occurred before 1954, although the results were not published until then. None of the patients improved on the nucleotides or the placebo and that was that. But this seems to have been the very first trial conducted with patients randomized to treatment and control groups, although the recounting of the trial was so loose-limbed that it is impossible to be sure.[49]

All of the above-described relations with industry seem to have been unproblematic. Don Klein said of the experience that he and Max Fink had testing drugs in the late 1950s and early 1960s at Hillside Hospital, "When we did our imipramine and mepazine studies—as I recall, our contact with industry was to request the drug, which they freely sent with no requests but the implicit scientific attitude that we should communicate to the public whatever we found. These included the findings that mepazine did not work, the antidepressant effect of chlorpromazine, [and] the serendipitous discovery of panic disorder and its imipramine treatment."[50]

Klein and Fink described the effectiveness of imipramine in arid clinical language. But Rachel Klein was part of that trial, too, as a Hillside psychologist (who would shortly marry Don). She had to evaluate the patients before and after they started treatment. "These were patients whom I will never forget; severely depressed individuals with retarded or agitated depressions. People I wanted to run from because they were in such pain, causing me pain. Yet, six weeks after the initial evaluation, when they had been on medication, they walked into my office and they were well; I get chills even now thinking about them. They talked with me the way you [David Healy] and I are talking now. One could not dismiss that sort of event. It seemed miraculous."[51] Miraculous. This is "wow" evidence. You don't need an RCT for it.

Europe

The European story: Simultaneously with Lasagna at Hopkins, Mogens Schou, professor of psychiatry at Aarhus University in Denmark, reported in 1954 the first randomized placebo-controlled clinical trial on the Continent, which was of lithium in psychotic mania. The patients served as their own controls and were shifted "in a random manner from lithium to placebo and vice versa." (Schou said he randomized whether to put the patients in the next switch on lithium or placebo by flipping a coin.[52]) It was this paper that initiated the modern treatment use of lithium in psychiatry.[53]

One is at pains not to say, "*This* was the very first RCT," because four investigators, within 12 months or so of one another, headed RCTs: Linford Rees, Michael Shepherd, Louis Lasagna, and Mogens Schou. These details are of some importance, not for their own sake about trial minutiae but because *they show that individual clinicians are perfectly capable of conducting valid trials without the assistance of the pharmaceutical industry.* Later, when industry took over the running of trials, the door to mischief was opened and academic independence was lost.

One more trial illustrates the point about the integrity of the early investigations: In 1959, Richard ("Dick") Ball and Leslie Gordon Kiloh reported an RCT of imipramine in "depressed states." They had been students of Aubrey Lewis at the Maudsley and now, in 1959, they were finishing their training in the north of England, Ball at Newcastle, Kiloh at Durham. (They were friendly with Alan Broadhurst at Geigy, who donated the drug.) They recruited their depressed outpatients from two hospitals in Newcastle, and the hospital pharmacist randomized the patients to the treatment and placebo groups. But what is interesting is that they differentiated between two kinds of "depression," endogenous and reactive, and argued that in both kinds imipramine was to be preferred to ECT. The conclusion of the trial was impactful: "The real importance of these new antidepressive drugs appears to be twofold. Firstly, they provide an effective, easily administered, and readily acceptable form of treatment in most cases of depressive illness. . . . Secondly, the modes of response to these drugs indicate lines of research which may well lead to the elucidation of the etiological factors which play an immediate part in determining the onset of depressive illness."[54] The trial was not, in other words, conducted for purposes of registration and was not scientifically barren. All this was to change. (Ball and Kiloh shortly migrated to Australia, where they became major figures, Ball a specialist in transgendered sexuality.)

In recent years, the whole concept of the RCT as the gold standard of drug evaluation has been challenged, but not because it is technically deficient. ("It minimizes the biases that we don't know about," as Paul Leber put it.[55]) The challenge has occurred because the trials can be easily gamed. Tricking the trial, plus elevating to God's Truth the concept of "statistical significance," with its misleading p-values, have called into question much of the supposed psychopharm wisdom garnered from the trials.

Looking back over the history of clinical trials, Lasagna doubted that RCTs were the only way to study efficacy. "Most of the early discoveries were serendipitous. They weren't science marching down a pathway in a straight line but lucky observations by people in studies where the controls were really historical controls [patients observed to get better] and not randomized controlled trials." So, Lasagna continued, he found himself conflicted between arguing to colleagues about the importance of RCTs and "having to face the fact that the breakthroughs were not achieved that way. So it is interesting that so much of that was serendipitous and maybe will continue to be that way."[56]

11

Trials

Fantasy Patients for Fantasy Diseases

The wonderful influence of imagination in the cure of diseases is well known. A motion of the hand, or a glance of the eye, will throw a weak and credulous patient into a fit; and a pill made of bread, if taken with sufficient faith, will operate a cure better than all the drugs in the pharmacopoeia.—Charles Mackay (1869)[1]

In the years after 1980, drug trials departed increasingly from the concept of treating real patients. In psychopharmacology, the trials began treating fantasy patients for fantasy diseases. Clinical trials thus accompanied psychopharmacology on the upswing and on the downswing. Clinical trials are the basic means of gathering evidence in the field, and they can be conducted reliably and scientifically. They can also serve as the premier means of evasion and distortion and can be used fraudulently and covertly to corrupt the evidence base of the field.

Before around 1990, it was common for academics to run trials on their own, to analyze the data, and to publish the results, letting the blows fall where they may. In the late 1980s, Lederle Labs asked a group of researchers at Cornell University Medical College to run a trial of their new antidepressant amoxapine (Asendin) against amitriptyline, the standard tricyclic antidepressant. The investigators, including Allen Francis and James Kocsis, found amoxapine not at all superior: "Amoxapine does not offer any clear advantage over amitriptyline."[2] At no point did the collected data disappear into Lederle's headquarters in Pearl River, New York, for a massaged analysis behind closed doors.

Then, in the early 1990s, the new SSRIs began pouring onto the market, producing billions of dollars in profit that would not brook the possibility of failure. Amoxapine was instantly forgotten.

Not All that Depressed

The fundamental problem in running clinical trials of depression therapies was that the "patients" were so heterogeneous. Many were, in essence, "fantasy patients" who really had nothing.

But endogenous depression was real. To identify a specific treatment effect, in 1975 Leo Hollister recommended that depression trials be confined to patients with serious ("endogenous") depression. "These types of depressions represent the minority of patients encountered both in hospital and clinic practice." So trials should be done in them because an effect would be seen. "It is easy to appreciate how difficult it would be to detect the specific effect of antidepressives in a heterogeneous group of patients of whom only a relatively few could show a specific response to the drug being tested."[3] This was the problem that almost crippled the SSRI trials (see Chapter 16): The "depressed" patients were a mixture of everything.

In fact, some patients were not all that depressed. "These aren't the clinically depressed patients that come to our offices," said Mickey Nardo. "They're another breed—a heterogeneous collage of people recruited from who-knows-where to be in a study. . . . These are hardly the DSM-IV major depression patients [that industry] advertised—rather[, they are] ad responders, students, pros, characterologic patients, the curious, etc."[4] Gordon Parker, professor of psychiatry in Sydney, called them "pristine subjects with nonbiological depressive disorders, with unstable symptomatology and disorders of marginal severity, disposed to 'respond' irrespective of the treatment arm." He said it was "illogical" to extend such studies to "biological" depressions.[5]

Mark Kramer at Merck greatly deplored the loss of the ability to conduct trials on really depressed patients—whom drug treatment was most capable of helping. "The further out studies are conducted from deinstitutionalization [outpatients], the more we lose the ability to identify and enroll the most drug-responsive patients." Look, he said, at the difference between pre-1970 patients and patients in current antidepressant studies. "The latter studies generally are not required to enroll patients on the basis of their vegetative signs and symptoms [sleep, appetite, sex], or endogenous (vital) quality." Also excluded in outpatient studies are "patients who are a danger to themselves or others, who are grossly agitated or retarded, and who are incapable of getting to appointments regularly." These rules, he said, "preclude investigators against enrolling patients most appropriate for antidepressant treatment."[6]

Kramer said do the math. "It only requires 10% to 15% professional patients to derail a well-powered trial into one which misses its already meager endpoint. Whereas 30–50 per arm had been sufficient to detect a strong antidepressant signal prior to 1965 [in serious depression,] . . . today's dilution of diagnosis (essentially enrolling pretty sad 'medicalized normals') requires 150 or more patients per arm, in order to obtain a difference of as little as 1.5 HRSD [Hamilton Rating Scale—Depression] between the groups treated with the antidepressant and placebo. This has not deterred the FDA from approving on this basis."[7]

Bernard (Barney) Carroll, writing in 2008, praised the early trials for their attentiveness to "clinical subtyping, stratification by severity, and the reasons for failure. That we do not generally do these things nowadays is an indication of how degraded the process has become, with the emphasis shifted from academic physicians disinterestedly asking clinical questions to corporations self-interestedly aiming just to clear the lowest bar allowed by FDA."[8]

In the early days, before RCTs became gospel, investigators were satisfied with close observation to see if the drugs worked. Roland Kuhn, a staff psychiatrist at the asylum in Münsterlingen, Switzerland, who in 1957 discovered the antidepressant effects of imipramine, prided himself on not running controlled trials; he shunned numbers and advocated the close observation of individual patients. Kuhn told David Healy, "I have never used 'controlled double-blind studies' with 'placebo,' 'standardized rating scales' or the statistical treatment of records of large numbers of patients. Instead I examined each patient individually even every day, often on several occasions, and questioned him or her again and again."[9]

Indeed, among old-timers there was a lot of skepticism about rating scales. In 1956, Fritz Freyhan at Delaware State Hospital, who was among the founders of psychopharmacology, said that he much preferred close clinical observation over "aides or attendants." "The time, we hope, has not come when the clinician abdicates and the rating-scale marker takes over as judge."[10] Malcolm Lader said in a symposium, published in 1983, "I strongly believe that the use of rating scales on their own in a clinical trial is a retrograde step." He had done a meta-analysis of a number of benzodiazepine trials. But at the end, "I had no idea whether the benzodiazepines were of any use clinically. By using the rating scale, trialists had [abandoned] the old 1950s way of counting heads and saying 'patient recovered' or 'patient did not recover.' " The clinician wants to know, "whether that patient is better . . . or is the patient going to be changed from the medication?"[11]

This reliance on close observation, then, was a European tradition. Jules Angst, head of research in psychopharmacology at the University of Zurich, said of the early lithium trials that he and colleagues had conducted, "We didn't operate with control groups. All these major drug developments in psychiatry came about without controlled trials by using accurate observation, by open trials with good observers and by [inter]-individual comparisons."[12]

Leo Hollister, from his perch in the Veterans Administration (VA) hospital in Palo Alto, where he conducted some of the first US drug trials, was among the few Americans to escape the numbers fetish. He said of the early large VA trials, "I call this a massive scientific overkill, because even my early controlled trials were not very necessary. All I had to do was give these drugs to a patient and watch him. You knew damn well something was happening. But at that time, the Zeitgeist in psychiatry was such that nobody wanted to believe it. You know, psychoanalysis was dominant."[13]

The consulting firm PricewaterhouseCoopers, in an assessment of Pharma in 1998, deplored the extent to which patient perspectives were ignored in trials. "Much of the [trial] data has nothing to do with how patients feel: few people, for example, could detect a four point decrease in their Hamilton Depression Rating Scale, yet this counts as a clinically significant outcome."[14] Healy called the RCTs "a sophisticated means to override the patient's voice. An abundance of scales means that one will surely be found that affirms the drug's efficacy."[15]

Did You See the Patient?

To credibly report a trial, you actually had to see the patients. Yet the big names on the published results were often not the ones who actually did the trials. As Paul Hoch, a leader at the New York State Psychiatric Institute, observed at a meeting in 1960, "I can quote you cases where the principal investigator never touched a patient, never saw the thing, and the name was simply on to lend the thing a great deal of respectability."

Theodore Rothman added, "It is known as a telephone investigation."[16]

We are not talking about ghostwriting (see Chapter 14), but about delegating the actual running of the trial to underlings. Paul Leber, who ultimately became the head of the FDA's Neuropharmacology Division, was fully aware of this. He told David Healy, "[The nominal investigators] are the people who are going to . . . many international meetings and are on the tour and don't have time to see anybody. I mean I doubt whether they follow up patients—they need to be seen every day, don't they, or every week depending on how sick they are. I don't think [the investigators] can do it if they are out of town."[17]

This practice made Paul Janssen furious. Janssen was shocked when a researcher in Miami reported that chlorpromazine and haloperidol were no more effective, and had no more side effects, than placebo. He got on a plane and few to Miami to verify this with his own eyes, "[The chief investigator] when he entered the State Hospital did not even know how to open the doors . . . . He had hardly ever seen the patients and . . . of course it became very clear this was 'garbage in and garbage out.' It was so crude and unreliable that even a difference between 4 g of chlorpromazine and placebo was not detected. From that day on, I have always been very skeptical when it comes to double-blind trials because the same risk exists everywhere. I don't know of any learned professor . . . who takes the trouble of doing what the protocols require in terms of observing."[18]

"Statistical Significance"

. . . a tale involving scientific shenanigans in the corporate pursuit of profit . . . with statistical significance being elevated over clinical significance.—Bernard Carroll (2013)[19]

Problems began with the question, How large should the trial be? There are statistical rules for deciding how many patients are needed for a certain "power," i.e., to detect a "twenty percent difference," or a difference between men and women, or whatever. But even beneath such considerations, Archie Cochrane, the modern god of the RCT, said in 1971, "With small numbers it is very easy to give the impression that a treatment is no more effective than a placebo, whereas in reality it is very difficult indeed to exclude the possibility of a small effect. Alternatively, with large numbers it is often possible to achieve a result that is statistically significant [but] that may be clinically unimportant."[20]

The highly mechanistic nature of an RCT—with its questionnaires and quantitative analyses—gave some observers the creeps. One was Yale's Alvan Feinstein, sometimes seen as the godparent of epidemiology in the United States, in other words, a very considerable figure. As early as 1971, Feinstein slammed the whole notion of "statistical significance," as opposed to clinical significance. "There is the appalling idea that efficacy has been demonstrated if a statistically significant difference can be shown between two agents. That is not efficacy. It means only that there is a numerically distinct difference between the agents. The difference itself might be of trivial magnitude, but if the sample is large enough, that difference can be magnified into statistical significance." The question, he said, is "How much of a difference makes a difference? This distinction, of course, cannot be decided statistically. The decision requires a judgment about what we regard as a good result or a better one."[21] In other words, at the end of the day, clinical judgment is the only thing that counts. Numbers cannot help.

On another occasion, Feinstein dwelt upon "familial factors" and such that could be less easily measured. He then added, "Until we realize that all of these important humanistic data are being deliberately ignored [or] inadvertently neglected, we will continue to engage in a dehumanized form of pseudoscience."[22] At a conference at the Smithsonian Institution in November 1972, Feinstein said, "In our current era, we have boxed ourselves into a rigid methodological approach for evaluating any kind of therapy. . . . The underlying assumption is that as long as the study was randomized, double-blind, and used large enough statistical numbers as well as a placebo group, it doesn't make any difference whether the observed phenomena can be identified . . . or whether they have been assessed properly. As long as we have carried out the doctrine of this particular ritual for eliminating bias, we need have no more thought."[23]

Thus, the first perversion of science in the chain of perversities was the concept of statistical significance. A finding is judged "significant" if the probability of its being reproduced by chance is less than 1 in 20 (this is written as $p < .05$). As William Wardell and Louis Lasagna, the two great authorities on clinical trials, remarked in their textbook in 1975, "There is a difference between statistical and biological significance. Even a 1 percent difference between a placebo and an active drug can be demonstrated statistically if one is willing to study enough patients."[24]

Statisticians have been aware of these issues for a long time. As Amos Tversky and Daniel Kahneman of Hebrew University of Jerusalem noted in 1971 in a classic article, "The emphasis on significance levels tends to obscure a fundamental distinction between the size of an effect and its statistical significance."[25] Thus, statistical significance is not a measure of strength of association, which is to say, not a measure of *effectiveness*. What it measures is: Was the sample large enough that the results weren't achieved largely by chance? Yet in the industry, and for the FDA, statistical significance became fetishized as the one number showing that your drug worked. (Indeed, the FDA Modernization Act of 1997 stipulated that one trial would really be enough, as long as there was "confirmatory" information, and Bob Temple said in 2005 that a really super-duper p-value of as low as 0.001 would be "good enough for a single trial."[26]) This was very convenient for industry because it meant that quite ineffective drugs could nonetheless have "statistical significance of less than point oh-five"—simply because the sample size was large. In a large sample, the chances that the findings were due to chance are much smaller than in a small sample.

Thus, brandishing these misleading p-values, industry strode through the halls of the FDA with one weak drug after another, all of course with trial results that were "statistically significant." Michael Taylor at the University of Michigan said of one trial that, despite the glowing ads claiming the drug's effectiveness, "The differences in depression rating scores between the placebo groups and the drug groups, although statistically significant, were clinically meaningless. A statistical difference [p-value] between a new agent and placebo is not a sufficient standard of adequate efficacy. There are several antidepressants on the market with 'proof' that they work but many clinicians recognize that these agents offer little benefit to patients."[27]

Gordon Parker, professor of psychological medicine in Sydney, found this entire dance close to meaningless. "No one gains from a strategy deriving trivial to nonexisting differences between active drugs and placebo, and which ... fails to differentiate one treatment from another. Such information is specious, while common sense is compromised."[28]

There are statistics that do measure strength of association, which is also called effect size, such as Cohen's d and the odds ratio. For the sake of simplicity, many clinicians prefer the Number Needed to Treat, written as NNT, or the Number Needed to Harm (to measure side effects, written as NNH).[29] The NNT is an intuitive and simple way of estimating how likely it is that a treatment or medicine will help an individual person. It is the number of patients who must be treated with an intervention for a specific period to prevent 1 bad outcome or result in 1 good outcome. But in the more historic trials, the NNT and NNH were rarely used because their judgment could be so devastating. By 2002, of 359 trials surveyed, only eight reported NNT.[30]

For the SSRIs, the average NNT was about 10, meaning that you'd have to treat 10 patients with your drug before you'd get one patient whose response wasn't due to placebo. Industry and FDA colluded in insisting that statistical significance was the best measure. In David Healy's analysis, "As RCTs function at the moment, if there is a minimal difference that is statistically significant, it becomes pragmatically equivalent to a substantial difference on a solid outcome measure. This gives Seroquel treatment of bipolar depression as much face validity as treatment with ECT."[31]

The FDA liked statistical significance because it seemed to correspond to the congressional mandate. Industry liked the notion of "significant" p-values because virtually any large trial would be "significant," in that the results, however weak, were unlikely to have been obtained by chance. As Don Klein put it in 2008, "The pursuit of short-term statistical superiority to placebo became industry's Holy Grail of marketability."[32] Paul Leber of the FDA's psychopharmacology division told the advisory committee in 1981, "The law of large numbers allow[s] you to reach statistical significance with relatively small changes [in efficacy]." So, Leber was critical of the whole affair but used it anyway.[33] Indeed, not until about 2015 did FDA statisticians start considering strength of association, or treatment effect, in addition to "significance."

Whom to Keep Out

The patients in trials started to become fantasy patients, quite unlike those seen in real practice. A list of exclusion criteria managed to exclude almost anyone who was really depressed (e.g., suicidal); alcoholics, who respond poorly to "antidepressants"; people who were too old or too young; and people who had serious medical illnesses. Hoechst-Roussel excluded from phase III of its nomifensine (Merital) trials patients who required ECT, thus conceding in advance that their drug wasn't for serious depression.[34] Obviously, then, the trial population bore little resemblance to the patients psychiatrists would actually see in the office.

Does that really make a difference? Yes, it does. Between 2001 and 2006, the National Institute of Mental Health organized, at the cost of $35 million, a huge trial, called STAR*D (Sequenced Treatment Alternatives to Relieve Depression) of "real world" patients,[35] and 4,041 outpatients from 41 clinical sites were enrolled. These were patients already seeking care who happened to be screened and were found to be depressed. There were few exclusion criteria, the trial had no placebo control, and the organizers' goal was to see how well antidepressants performed in the real world, and what to prescribe next if the patients did not respond to the first antidepressant prescribed (in Round 1).

The organizers, among whom were some veterans of the TMAP fiasco in Texas (see Chapter 19), were apparently so shocked by the results—the substantial failure of antidepressant medication—that they didn't publish results for the primary outcome measure: reduction in Hamilton Rating Scale for Depression. The patients had been put on citalopram (Celexa) in Round 1. (A whistleblower claimed in 2012 that Forest Labs had bribed the study's main investigator, A. John Rush, to choose Celexa as the Round 1 drug.[36])

In 2018, a group of investigators, led by Irving Kirsch at the University of Connecticut, went back to the original trial data and found that the reduction in Hamilton Depression Scale scores had only been 6.6 points, verging on trivial. This would be compared to other open trials, with no placebo, where the reduction was 14.8 points. Remission rates in Round 1 were only 25.6 percent (versus 48.4 percent in "comparator trials"). These numbers represented an almost complete failure for the SSRIs. (The numbers in the subsequent three rounds were even worse.) But what is of interest here is that there were lots of exclusions in the comparator trials, but almost none in STAR*D—and the results in the comparator trials seemed twice as good.[37] So, yes, exclusions make perfect sense if your objective is to create a fantasy world of drug responsiveness. The exclusions make a difference between "efficacy" in this fantasy trial world and "efficaciousness" in the real world: Showing that the drugs have a treatment effect of some kind is not the same as showing they will work in practice.

Resentment at all these placebo trials continued to worm away at senior people, who over the years had come to trust close observation of individual patients rather than arithmetic averages of large numbers of patients. It had been Leo Hollister who got multicentered trials going in the 1950s, when he and John Overall stepped away from the VA trials and began enlisting four or five centers on their own. But much later, Hollister was appalled at how this story had turned out. "We need to find new ways to prove [that] these drugs . . . are simpler, cheaper and quicker, because to do these massive controlled studies, with a couple of hundred patients, costs tens of millions of dollars and takes about a couple of years. Furthermore, only people with big bucks can get into the field."[38] This was a long way from Roland Kuhn, carefully observing individual patients in the Münsterlingen asylum to see if the trial drug had made them better.

What Could Possibly Go Wrong?

Nevertheless, clinical trials are the basic means of gathering evidence in the field, and they can be conducted reliably and scientifically, what could possibly go wrong?

Coming unblinded, for one thing. When pharmacologist Harry Gold and colleagues at Cornell University Medical College proposed the "blind test," together with the modern concept of the placebo, in a trial published in 1937, it was seen as a big step forward.[39] And indeed it was. The problem was that the placebo patients often quickly figured out that they weren't on the drug, which would inflate the efficacy of the drug arm. In research on panic disorder published in 1991, led by a joint team from Marburg and Stanford universities, the authors concluded, "Panic disorder patients as well as their physicians were able to rate very accurately whether an active drug or a placebo was given."[40] In 1993, after reviewing a raft of such studies, Seymour Fisher and Roger Greenberg at the State University of New York Health Science Center in Syracuse concluded that the double-blind was "vulnerable to penetration and therefore vulnerable to bias. This means that most past studies of the efficacy of psychotropic drugs are to unknown degrees scientifically untrustworthy."[41]

Then there was the problem of pseudo-patients. As Benjamin Brody of Weill Medical College of Cornell University pointed out in 2011, "Since the initial antidepressant trials in the 1960s, participants have gone from being patients who were recruited primarily from inpatient psychiatric populations to outpatient volunteers who are often recruited by advertisements."[42]

Patients recruited through newspaper ads were not patients at all but had just wandered in off the street. (It was said that they all "met the criteria" of major depression, but this could mean anything.) The first trial with "symptomatic volunteers" recruited from newspaper ads was conducted by Burton Goldstein at a Miami hospital in the late 1960s and was published in 1970.[43] Companies that contracted with industry to run trials (CROs, or clinical research organizations) quickly cottoned on that using symptomatic volunteers was a quick way of getting the contract done, and trials with symptomatic volunteers became standard. By 2002, CROs were involved in about 60 percent of all clinical trials, up from 30 percent in the late 1990s.[44]

Fast was good for industry and the CROs. But there was a tension between speed and a homogeneous trial population. The patent clock was ticking, so speed was important in terms of getting the product on the market. But the faster you moved, the greater was the temptation to recruit patients who may not ex-actly have had the disease you wanted. As Sam Gershon, then chair of psychiatry at Wayne State University and one of the leading psychopharmacologists, said in 1981, "We are all sort of aware of this dilemma. If you have the purest popu-lation, you are likely to get the best and most specific results, but once you take that data and put it into the dirty population, because of drug–drug interactions [if patients were on other drugs for other illnesses], the whole thing may either disappear or they may drop dead."[45]

Mark Kramer, who as head of psychopharmacology at Merck had had much experience with clinical trials, asked rhetorically, "Lacking enrollment of the real McCoy [real patients], why would we ever expect mainly symptomatic volunteers to exhibit low placebo responses and specific drug effects? By this, I am not saying that all industrial psychopharmacology investigators are corrupt. However, 15–20 percent must be in some manner. It only requires 10–15 per-cent professional patients to derail a well-powered trial into [missing] its already meager endpoint. Whereas 30–50 patients per arm had been sufficient to detect a strong antidepressant signal prior to 1965, today's dilution of diagnosis (essen-tially enrolling pretty sad 'medicalized normals') requires 150 or more patients per arm, in order to obtain as little as 1.5 HRSD points [difference between drug and placebo], and huge placebo effects. This has not deterred the FDA from ap-proving on this basis."[46]

Symptomatic volunteers aroused the ire of many observers. Bernard Carroll, then at the University of Michigan, told the Psychopharmacologic Drugs Advisory Committee (PDAC) in 1980, "I guess I have a fairly strong feeling about the inappropriateness of using symptomatic volunteers for drug efficacy studies. Some studies nowadays are done by placing advertisements in newspapers and getting people to come in." He said his personal preference was to "use real patients who have declared themselves through the medical referral network in the usual way." The meeting was about anxiety, but Carroll added, "The same thing applies to studies of antidepressants, too. . . . They are not really depressed patients and I think if you contaminate treatment trials with those subjects, you are getting information of a different kind than you really want."[47]

The *Toronto Star* ran this ad in 2007: "Do you suffer from major depression? I feel sad all the time. I'll never feel any better." Several other characteristics of frank melancholic illness were listed. People who sort of felt this way were then invited to phone a given number to hook up with "local researchers who have joined a national clinical trial." There were professional patients who joined as many trials as possible, asserting for each trial that they had the symptoms in question. (Participants were paid.[48]) This, as stated, became a general industry practice. (In Europe, recruiting via newspaper ads is not allowed.[49])

Recruiting trial participants through newspaper ads thus turned out to be a terrible way of constituting a clinical trial: The "patients" weren't really sick (although they may have "fulfilled DSM-III criteria for major depression"—which is a relatively low bar). Why would clinical investigators resort to such an obviously fraught move? The answer is that it was devilishly difficult to recruit real patients for RCTs of antidepressants. Bob Temple of FDA articulated this at a PDAC meeting in 2009: "We have not yet figured out how to do outcome studies with highly symptomatic conditions, because you won't find anybody willing to be untreated [with placebo] in the face of recurrent depression." He continued, "It's fine when what you're treating is lipids, which nobody feels, or the blood pressure, which nobody feels. You get outcome studies there. We don't really know how to do it [in depression, with antidepressants] against placebo."[50]

Or the patients might wise up! Why risk being put on the placebo arm when you could stay out of the trial and get the drug on demand? Herb Meltzer, who oversaw several clozapine trials, said, in a moment of frankness, "At our VA hospital all the patients who knew that they could get clozapine for sure without being randomized, rejected going into that [trial] protocol. The ones with family members who knew about it, all they had to do was make an appeal for clozapine. They kept their patients out of that protocol, so it was the subgroup who least understood the system, with no social support, in one VA hospital, who went into that study, and there are countless examples of that." This process of selection, Meltzer said, "very much limits the generalizability."[51]

A further disadvantage was that high placebo response rates meant that many good drugs could be lost: Their efficacy was simply overpowered by a huge placebo return, and the company ditched the program. Also, even in a standard drug trial, a number of the responders will have a placebo response to the drug. Yet the placebo has been elevated to an article of faith in the clinical trials culture.

These placebo problems affected mainly depressed outpatients. There were bioethical problems about leaving depressed inpatients on placebo (essentially, untreated), and trials on them came to have active drugs on the placebo arm rather than sugar pills. As Bob Temple told the PDAC in 1993, "Historically, we have had difficulty getting placebos to be used in depression trials at all. . . . We have insisted on them for outpatient settings, but for the more severe, more suicidal people inside, we have had a lot of trouble getting those trials."[52]

In 2011, the APA met in Honolulu. On the program was a session called "Why Do Antidepressant Trials Fail?" What the earnest big domes missed was that they were dealing with business, not science. There was no "scientific" answer to the question. Articles in the *American Journal of Psychiatry* indicted some of the enrollees for shopping around for trials as though it were a business. Nardo: "*It is a business.* The sponsoring drug company is in the business of getting their drug approved. The Clinical Research Center is in the business of enrolling subjects. The Clinical Research Organization is in the business of getting a successful trial on the books for the FDA for approval. The medical writer is in the business of getting a publishable paper written. The guest author is in the business of padding a résumé and pulling in some speaker fees. Why shouldn't the subjects be in business too? It stands to reason. To expect mentally ill people to seek treatment by looking at newspaper ads and chance getting treated with a sugar pill or an ineffective drug is a very unlikely scenario."[53]

In 1994, Bob Temple suggested an alternative kind of "enrichment" strategy, or what has come to be called a "randomized withdrawal study."[54] It's simple. Don Klein, a major advocate of this kind of enrichment, explained: "There would be small-scale trials that begin with long-term observation of patients taking open-label medications, titrated to give the best response without toxicity. Patients who appear to respond would then be randomized to a double-blinded course of placebo or the drug. Slowly withdrawing the drug and initiating placebo would allow investigators to look for changes in symptoms. Patients who get worse on the placebo are the real responders, not the beneficiaries of a placebo effect in the first round of treatment." The real responders are then put back on the medication, and the placebo responders from phase I stay well and are spared the side effects of further treatment.[55]

To date, there have been relatively few such trials in psychopharmacology because so few new agents have been proposed, but it is a means of sidestepping the standard RCT with its uninformative p-values. This kind of trial has the advantage of following patients over much longer periods than those used in a standard 6-week RCT (you can't leave patients on placebo for more than 6 weeks). It also creates a homogeneous population of genuine drug responders who can be further studied.

The play with fantasy patients had become a kind of game. But it was a game with hundreds of millions of dollars and the public health at stake.

12

Trials

Industry Takes Over

Even though already 14 years out of industry, I am still reeling from
the cabal's late-stage corruption of our most promising research
tool—the double-blind placebo-controlled randomized clinical
study.—Mark Kramer (2016)[1]

It is one of the great ironies in psychopharmacology that none of the later drugs
equaled those of the "golden years" of the 1950s. It is as though no subsequent
generation of railway locomotives equaled the Iron Horse of the pioneers.
But lithium remains the agent nonpareil for mood disorders, no subsequent
"antidepressants" were ever the equal of imipramine and the other tricyclics, and
older clinicians today look back with fondness upon chlorpromazine, the first of
the antipsychotics—and while clozapine is widely admired as a superior antipsychotic agent, it can also be a death sentence (see Chapter 18).

The lack of progress in psychopharmacology has been stunning, equaled no
place else in medicine. How did this happen?

It happened partially because industry took over the trials. By the 1970s, following the 1962 Kefauver-Harris amendments, drug trials had become so expensive that the incentive to try bold new experiments was minimal. (Of course
this might have happened elsewhere in medicine as well, but only in psychiatry
were the placebo response rates through the ceiling.)

Beginning at least around 1950, industry had stimulated investigators to organize trials (see Chapter 10). As for larger RCTs in psychiatry, Abraham Heller's
RCT of imipramine, desipramine, and placebo in 1971 at the Community Mental
Health Center in Denver was apparently the first trial organized by a pharmaceutical company. The authors acknowledged Geigy for the analysis and the reporting "of the statistical findings in this study."[2]

Yet in the background was the need for a larger number of patients than most
private physicians could put together on their own. As we have seen, large Ns had
a much greater chance of attaining statistical "significance" (the only measure
that counted) than did small Ns. Thus, industry recruited large numbers of

trialists, and aggregated the results at the head office. Often the trialists didn't know who one another were.

In the 1980s, a great pivot from investigator-led to industry-led trials began, and the "medical advisor" in a drug company became responsible not just for insuring quality as before, but also for collating the data as it came in from the various centers. As noted, the need for significant p-values at the 0.5 level demanded large trials. And a company might commission 10 or 20 centers each to contribute a few patients to the study. None of the trialists would ever see the overall data pool, and it would be company statisticians—and paid medical writers—who undertook the analysis, not the investigators themselves. At a meeting of the Psychopharmacologic Drugs Advisory Committee (PDAC) in 1996, Pippa Simpson, a biostatistician at Wayne State University, pointed out that some study arms at some centers didn't have any patients in them. Was this a problem for randomization? Oh, not at all, replied Bob Temple, this happens all the time, especially in Japanese studies, "which tend to have small numbers of patients and large numbers of centers."

Dr. Simpson replied, "This isn't small. This is zero in some of the arms."[3]

But in the company analysis, all these microscopic fragments were thrown together in one big pot and boiled into "significance." Note that industry preferred a large number of small trials, rather than a small number of large trials. This was, as Duncan Vere, professor of therapeutics at the London Hospital Medical School pointed out in 1976, because "Adverse reactions are too rare to be noticed in most of these trials, which therefore tend to amplify the advantages over the disadvantages of a new drug."[4]

Thus, the code was broken only at headquarters, not by the individual clinicians. Max Fink recalled a trial he did for Pfizer of sertraline (Zoloft), imipramine (Tofranil), and placebo. He evaluated the patients with pharmaco-EEG, and the subject had a certain interest: How do the EEG profiles of these drugs differ? But he needed the code for his 19 patients.

Fink: "My assistant must have said to me, 'Max, where the hell is the code' and I say to him, "What do you means where is it? Don't you have it?'"

"No."

"Well, I pick up the phone and I call the monitor at Pfizer and she says to me, 'No problem,' but eventually it doesn't come."

"So I say to her one day, 'I must have it.' I happened to know who her boss was. I call him up and I say, 'Mr. So and So, can I get the code?' He says, 'Of course, why not.' And he finds out he can't get the code. In fact nobody gives me the code."

"So I then write a letter to the president of the company, saying 'I'm going to send it to the FDA.'"

"I get a phone call saying, 'You don't want to do this, Max. All those data are sealed.'"

"What's sealed mean?"

"They're sealed. They don't go to the FDA."

Fink: "I don't care whether they go to the FDA. All I want to know is the codes for my own patients. Right? To this day, I've never gotten it."[5]

Papers began to appear written entirely by company employees. An early example of this varietal was Lilly's effort in 1991 to demonstrate that Prozac, its wonder drug, did not cause suicide.[6]

Between 1966 and 2000, the percentage of clinical trials in all fields funded by industry increased from 23 to 51 percent.[7] Industry's invasion of clinical medicine was thus not just confined to psychopharmaceuticals but occurred across the board.

By the time that the FDA approved Otsuka and Lundbeck's new drug, brexpiprazole (Rexulti) for "acute schizophrenia" and "the adjunctive treatment of major depressive disorder" in 2016, the takeover was virtually complete (see Chapter 9). The schizophrenia indication had two pivotal trials. Of the 10 authors in one trial, only one was not an employee of either Otsuka or Lundbeck.[8] Of the 10 authors in the other trial, same story.[9] The studies used 117 sites![10] In a long-term open-label study, *all* of the authors worked either for Otsuka or Lundbeck, and the assistance of Cambridge Medical Communication Ltd. (Cambridge UK) was acknowledged for "writing support."[11] This was as far away from the days of Leslie Kiloh and Richard Ball in Newcastle as it is possible to get.

Cutting Corners

I'm [not] fully paranoid, but the skepticism nuclei on my MRI are bilaterally enlarged and my trust circuits have some early atrophic changes.—Mickey Nardo (2014)[12]

Here's an idea: We'll pay the trialists if the results of the trial are positive! What better way to ensure that a trial delivers the goods. This was such a flagrant violation of conflict-of-interest principles that even the Pharmaceutical Research and Manufacturers Association (PhRMA) agreed that it shouldn't be done. At House hearings in 1996 on the "financial interests of clinical investigators," PhRMA argued that a proposed rule regulating conflicts of interest was a bad idea—increasing the regulatory burden on small companies, you know. "However, PhRMA and other witnesses did agree that sponsors should not enter into *explicit* payment schemes, i.e., where payment is directly linked to a favorable outcome, or if a company offers financial rewards if the results are favorable."[13]

A simple way of cutting corners was to compare low doses of your drug against high doses of a comparator drug (some trials merely compared placebo). Upjohn loaded the dice in an alprazolam study by doubling the dose of the comparator drug, Wyeth's lorazepam. (Bernard Carroll asked Wyeth's clinical pharmacologist if Wyeth would like him to run "a study to challenge this report."[14]) Upjohn lost its UK license for the benzodiazepine sleep aid Halcion after it came out that the company had "compared the two lowest doses of Halcion with the two highest doses of Restoril."[15] As discussed in Chapter 18, several trials for atypical antipsychotics established their "safety" profile by comparing their drug to high doses of Haldol, thus ensuring that their molecules would come off as "safe" (although they were in fact anything but).

It wasn't that patients checked into the Novartis or Janssen hospitals and company doctors ran the trials. Increasingly, the companies funded so-called clinical research organizations (CROs) to commission the work. By 2000, in the United States 60 percent of all Pharma funding for trials went to CROs, and 40 percent to academic trialists.[16] This was strictly for-profit medicine, and the CROs placed a premium on cranking subjects through as quickly as possible. Mark Kramer said, "The pressure to enroll rapidly at study mills— Garbage In, Garbage Out—has led to the staggering proportion of failed trials submitted to FDA."[17]

In 2013, Barney Carroll said of the CRO trials, "Cutting corners took several forms." One was to "fudge the inclusion criteria—rating up the Hamilton depression score to meet enrolment targets." Another "involved glossing over toxicity events. . . . In the CRO world, we have pretend physicians recruiting pretend patients into clinical trials that pretend to test efficacy while being biased for an outcome that suits the commercial sponsor."[18]

For the most part, industry did not actually make up the results in trials. Too many people would know about it and blow the whistle, and the company would be ruined. But the numbers were massaged. George Simpson, a veteran trialist, said, "You don't have to read the posters [at meetings] of these comparative studies of atypical antipsychotics. The sponsorship of the trial seems to dictate what the results are going to be. I don't think people cheat, but they are unlikely to design a study that could go against what they'd like to see."[19] In other words, as an investigation established in 2017, financial ties to industry were significantly associated with positive RCT outcomes.[20]

But it's worse than that.

The deception might not be just implicit. It was explicit. In February 1997, AstraZeneca executive Richard Lawrence wrote to colleagues about the weight-gain problem with Seroquel: "I am not 100% comfortable with this data being made publicly available at the present time—however I understand that we have little choice—Lisa has done a great 'smoke-and mirrors' job!"[21] The Lisa in question was Lisa Arvanitis.

When the note became public in litigation, it was the straw that broke the camel's back. As Jay Amsterdam explained to correspondents in May 2017, "Pharma-sponsored RCTs, in my opinion, have largely become corporate exercises in 'smoke and mirrors' with virtually all aspects of the RCT research outsourced to other stakeholder corporations and profit-motivated investigators. These factors were the prime reason that I 'bailed' from engaging in Pharma-sponsored RCTs by the early 2000s."[22]

Thumb on the Scale

One means of placing a thumb on the scale was to administer a sedative together with the trial antidepressant. As David Antonuccio and colleagues at the University of Nevada School of Medicine and Stanford pointed out, "There are at least six points on the HAM-D [Hamilton Depression Scale] that favor medications with sedative properties."[23] In many of the Prozac trials, a benzodiazepine was co-administered, essentially sedating the patients and diminishing the drugs' early effect of causing anxiety.[24]

Trialists were driven crazy by the high placebo response rates. Drugs they knew to be perfectly effective were lost because the trial was filled with placebo responders. What to do? One controversial solution was to remove the placebo responders in the "washout" phase: at the beginning of the trial. In this phase, all the patients are often put on the placebo to wash out of their systems whatever previous drugs they had been on. This phase also identifies the patients previously on an antidepressant drug who get better once they're taken off it. These patients would be nonresponders to the drugs in the trial! In 1977, the industry-friendly American College of Neuropsychopharmacology (ACNP) issued trial guidelines that said, "If after washout the patient's symptom severity has dropped below the selection threshold; the patient should be dropped."[25] The guideline proved highly controversial because it limited the generalizability of the trial to ordinary practice, and it was widely not implemented. Yet in 1990, at a symposium on depression sponsored by Lilly and chaired by A. John Rush, Wayne Katon from the University of Washington in Seattle said, "We need to know the characteristics of placebo responders and may want to pull those patients out of our clinical trials because they in fact get better whether given placebo or active drug. Therefore it is harder to demonstrate that active treatments work."[26] Did such desperate solutions to commercial problems really redound favorably upon a field that was trying to fashion itself as a science?

After one looks at all the tricks for gaining positive results, the fact that the Prozac-style drugs came close to failing their RCTs speaks volumes about those drugs being, essentially, inert.

13
Marketing

There never was an "Eden," but there now is a serpent in the psychiatric garden, and it has taken the form of the pharmaceutical industry.—Michael Alan Taylor (2013)[1]

There Once Was a Time

Today, we associate Pharma advertising with manipulativeness, even though the FDA is supposed to ride herd on it. The benefits are always exaggerated, the side effects downplayed. (That Zyprexa caused huge weight gains—Who knew?) Industry's manipulation of science did not begin yesterday. Haskell Weinstein, former medical director of Roerig, maker of the tranquilizer Atarax (hydroxyzine), told a Senate subcommittee in 1960 that the company's advertising was not untypical. Of the "200 references" the company cited in their promotional literature, "60 percent [were] not entirely favorable or pertinent."

Senator Kefauver, in the hearings named after him, wanted to make sure he had understood; ""Sixty percent were not pertinent, didn't work out, or were not favorable?"

Dr. Weinstein: "That is right, sir. . . . They [the reports] cover the whole gamut, all the way up to feeling that the drug is completely worthless, up to a complete dissent." The subcommittee seemed stunned.[2]

Yet marketing was once seen as an honorable profession. In the 1920s, John E. Powers was the dean of advertising. "He told the truth," says ad man Claude Hopkins, "but told it in a rugged and fascinating way."

A clothing concern in Pittsburgh was on the edge of bankruptcy and called in Powers. He said: "There is only one way out. Tell the truth. Tell the people that you are bankrupt and that your only way to salvation lies through large and immediate sales."

The clothing company protested. But Powers said, "No matter. Either tell the truth or I quit."

Their ad the next day read, "We are bankrupt. We owe $125,000 more than we can pay. This announcement will bring our creditors down on our necks. But if you come and buy tomorrow we shall have the money to meet them."

Hopkins related, "Truth was then such a rarity in advertising that this announcement created a sensation. People flocked by the thousands to buy, and the store was saved."

As already discussed, medical advertising before the Second World War was not a model of probity. But Hopkins saw it as a make-or-break challenge. "All [advertising people] realize that medical advertising placed men on their mettle. It weeded out the incompetents, and gave scope and prestige to those who survived. . . . Medicines in those days dominated the advertising field. The best magazines accepted them. Almost nobody challenged their legitimacy."[3] This 1927 account has a kind of eerie prescience, but the point is that Pharma advertising was not always tainted with deceit.

Do we really need marketing? As Bernard (Barney) Carroll said, "A really effective new drug will sell itself, driven by the experience of patients and prescribers. For such products, marketing is an afterthought. Our problem in psychiatry is that marketing is deployed to create the deceitful impression of efficacy and safety for compounds that offer little true therapeutic advance." He cited the campaign to sell the atypical antipsychotics (such as olanzapine). More bad news: "At the same time, marketing is deployed to trash really effective old drugs that are off patent. There is no better example of this than the desuetude of lithium in mood disorders."[4]

So, it turns out that, if what's being done is commerce rather than science, we do need marketing.

"Hard marketing"

> From the business perspective, starting around 1980 we saw the rise of the salesman. Marketing took over almost all enterprises and product was pushed to the back, way back.—Steve Lucas (2013)[5]

The "hard marketing" of pharmaceuticals is said to have begun when John Elmer McKeen became president of Pfizer in 1949, turning the small Brooklyn chemical company into a worldwide Pharma giant. His policy of "coordinated promotion" got the sales reps into physicians' offices.[6]

Does marketing to doctors really work? Surely, physicians are too smart to fall for this guff? A huge number of studies demonstrate that marketing is in fact highly effective, and even though doctors might believe their prescribing behavior is not affected, it is. Several analyses attributed the enormous increase in the diagnosis of adult ADHD—and the prescription of stimulants to treat it—to the relentless marketing to physicians of the diagnosis by companies like Shire, maker of Adderall. The *New York Times* wrote of the explosive growth of this market: "Foreseeing the market back in 2004, Shire sponsored a booklet that according to its cover would 'help clinicians recognize and diagnose adults with ADHD.' Its author was Dr. [William W.] Dodson, who had delivered the presentation at the Adderall XR launch two years before. Rather than citing the widely accepted estimate of 3 to 5 percent, the booklet offered a much higher figure. About 10 percent of adults have ADHD, which means you're probably already treating patients with ADHD even though you don't know it," the first paragraph ended.[7] In other words, the diagnosis of "adult ADHD" was being systematically flogged to psychiatrists, who responded by prescribing stimulants to adults who almost certainly didn't have ADHD and didn't need Adderall.

Thus, the rest of the marketing panoply unfolded. Sometime in the 1980s, Key Opinion Leaders (KOLs) began to multiply, and the commerce-riddled Continuing Medical Education (CME) seminars and other meetings flourished. In 2019, Jay Amsterdam, at the end of a very long career as a clinician and lab scientist at the University of Pennsylvania, told Don Klein, "In 1976, at the sunset of those halcyon days of modern psychiatry, I was able to witness, firsthand, the slow creep of the academic industrial complex (AIC) into the framework of scholarly activities. By the late 1990s, the dark curtain of the AIC had descended, and much that was vital in the process of academic research was henceforth a simple matter of the accumulation of *filthy lucre*."[8]

Mere nostalgia? These views were shared by many. Barney Carroll said in 2015, "Time was, we had an honorable tradition of interacting with industry while retaining our integrity as scientists. That tradition broke down when academic investigators morphed into key opinion leaders who spent most of their time with the marketing department of corporations—not with the real scientists. . . . As we now survey the aftermath, we should direct our anger to those opportunistic investigators whose ethical tackiness screwed it up for everybody."[9]

In Travis County, Texas, in 2012 during litigation of the Texas Medical Algorithm Project (TMAP, see Chapter 19), Tone Jones, a Janssen sales manager in Texas, was asked: "I believe you said it was about 1 percent of the population who had been diagnosed with schizophrenia at any given time?"

Jones replied: "Can't be a $2 billion product and 1 percent marketing."[10]

So, this was the problem. How to get to $2 billion?

One was through sumptuous entertaining of prescribers. GlaxoSmithKline was a past master of this with its "Paxil Forums," held from 2000 to 2002, according to a Department of Justice complaint, "at expensive resorts such as the El Conquistador Resort & Golden Door Spa in Puerto Rico." There were four such forums a year, and GSK paid the psychiatrists' expenses and a $750 honorarium. Each drug rep could attend two forums a year and "got to invite two psychiatrists to each meeting." The speakers received a $2,500 honorarium. Karen Wagner, an academic child psychiatrist in Texas, "recommended the use of Paxil for children and adolescents" at one Paxil Forum in 2000, three in 2001, and two in 2002. One actor/comedian whom GSK hired to emcee the evening shows told the attendees, "We have a wonderful and unforgettable night planned. Without giving it all away, I can tell you—you'll be experiencing a state of luxury." Paxil had not yet been licensed in the pediatric market, and such promotional tactics were as illegal as sin. They resulted, however, in a big uptick in Paxil sales.[11]

Expanding Indications

In 1974, an APA study of non-psychoanalysts found that only 29 percent of their patients received medications. By 1997, the figure had risen to around 90 percent.[12] Clearly, the indications for prescribing medication had expanded.

Expanding the indications for a drug is a natural process and not necessarily reprehensible. One discovers more and more reasonable uses. But FDA controls are something else. FDA insists that drugs be marketed for specific indications. At great cost, the makers of second-generation antipsychotics succeeded in getting their drugs approved for, in addition to schizophrenia, mania, bipolar disorder, major depression, child schizophrenia, and child bipolar disorder. The FDA logic was that these were all natural disease entities and the effectiveness of a drug in each of them had to be rigorously demonstrated. This was largely nonsense. These are not well-defined diseases that Nature had chiseled out of the granite face of illness; demonstrating effectiveness in each of these artifacts was largely a statistical sleight of hand. Nardo had this take: "Without other diagnosis-specific indications, [the manufacturers] can't legally advertise. This is all pretty crazy, because nobody thinks these drugs are diagnosis-specific—at least nobody I know."[13]

Many companies do try to step around this, knowing the FDA may turn a blind eye. As Don Kartzinel, leader of the Division of Neuropharmacological Drug Products, said at a meeting of the Neurologic Drugs Advisory Committee in 1977, "When you deal with a drug that has been on the market for a long time, or adding indications, it is clear that things get added in general practice before FDA says we have changed the indication. On many disorders, you are never going to get a controlled clinical trial; all you are going to have is a clinical experience, especially once the drug has been out there 15 or 20 years or even longer, so you can get into a bind of always adding indications. . . . We can probably add two zillion indications to an awful lot of drugs that are not on the label."[14]

The FDA starts paying attention when the expansion of the label appears to be driven solely by commercial rivalry and not by well-established clinical experience. It is here that the pollution of the science of psychopharmacology by the profit motive starts to become apparent.

In discussing these expansions, there is a fine line between genuine efficacy and rivalry-driven claims. In the mid-1970s, for example, there was a big and quite legitimate push from industry to use neuroleptics in the treatment of anxiety. The feeling was, in both the companies and the FDA, that the claim was legitimate. Yet in the absence of convincing RCTs, the FDA refused to grant the indication, thus denying patients with anxiety disorders access to a new treatment option (of course, doctors could prescribe the neuroleptics off label but risked lawsuits). In 1977, John M. Davis, who had been chief of clinical psychopharmacology at NIMH and was now professor of psychiatry at several institutions in Chicago, told the Psychopharmacologic Drugs Advisory Committee (PDAC) that the physician who wanted to prescribe neuroleptics for anxiety was really in a bind. On the one hand, the barbiturates were dangerous and had been associated with many deaths. "Borderline patients," he said, would not do well on "minor tranquilizers," meaning Valium and its cousins. But there had been no "single well-controlled study" of this anxiety, nor of any of these other indications. The doctor had only his or her "clinical experience" to go on.

The crucial point, he continued, was what the FDA permitted to go into the *Physicians' Desk Reference* (PDR) as the "label," generally considered the last word in prescribing. "Many physicians interpret the PDR package insert [the label] as in effect administrative law." But if the PDR didn't accept neuroleptics for anxiety, "this would require the physician to use minor tranquilizers in a condition [in] which he thought it would be bad medicine. . . . [He would think] that it would be illegal to use neuroleptics as the first drug. . . . It puts the doctor in an awful bind, because he would feel that to use the drug that he thinks is best, he would have to go against the PDR." Under these circumstances, there could be a lawsuit.[15]

So FDA wriggled on this hook, and finally adopted a solomonic decision. Yes, they said in a black box in the entry for chlorpromazine (Thorazine, the first antipsychotic), the drug might be "possibly effective" for nonpsychotic anxiety. But benzodiazepines would be the first choice because they didn't have some of the side effects of drugs like chlorpromazine. And if you do use chlorpromazine, it should not exceed 100 mg a day or be used for more than 12 weeks.[16] So there was some flexibility in the system. (One can see what an attorney for the plaintiff could do with this in a courtroom: "Doctor, your patient was on chlorpromazine at 150 mg a day for 14 weeks. Does this strike you as the practice of good medicine?") The phrase "possibly effective" comes from an earlier FDA drug-approval exercise called the Drug Efficacy Study Implementation (DESI), and "possibly effective" was a code phrase for the kiss of death for your drug.[17]

So, the point is that there are many layers in the issue of "expanding indications." What works in clinical practice—in the real world—may be miles away from what is officially approved.

Promoting Off-Label Indications

Victoria Starr, with a pharmacy degree from Washington State in her pocket, joined the Janssen sales force in 2001 after 6 years with Lilly. She thought, "They were serious about having people with pharmacy training sell doctors based on the chemistry of the drugs, the science of the nervous system, and all that."

Instead, the motto was "Sell to the symptoms. That [Risperdal] would calm the kids down." "The markets for kids and the elderly were called out as special priorities," Starr said, "because that's where they saw all the growth. With adults, you pretty much have to focus on the actual diseases—like schizophrenia—because adults don't end up at the doctor getting drugs for acting up. But kids, or the elderly with dementia, do."

And the Janssen reps promoted in these groups with a vengeance. "At one point, to amp up the troops, the CNS sales chief asked everyone in the ballroom to do the 'wolf howl.' "

"Everyone broke out into this weird howl," said Starr. "It was a cross between what you'd hear at a Super Bowl and at a religious cult—It was kind of fun, great team spirit and all."[18] Team spirit paid off. By 1996, Risperdal was in the top 25 prescription products in the United States, having grown 49 percent over the previous year.[19] A blockbuster drug, as Tone Jones observed, in a 1 percent market.

Competition in the atypical antipsychotic market was fierce. In 2001, AstraZeneca, coordinating the marketing of Seroquel (quetiapine) from its London office, noted that the drug had been approved in over 70 markets and was the "fastest growing atypical" in the US market, with over 10 percent of all such prescriptions. But there was a problem. The indications were limited to schizophrenia. What to do? In the "marketing plan" for 2001, the marketers said, "Broaden use of Seroquel beyond its current label in a wide range of patient groups through aggressive communication of its unique profile in bipolar disorder, Parkinson's disease, Alzheimer's disease, elderly, adolescents."[20] Promoting Seroquel for all these was illegal, of course (see Chapter 18).

But, hey, everybody else was doing it, too. In 2003, AstraZeneca surveyed its staff who had been hired away from other companies "to find out as much as we could about how, where, and why our competitors invest in IITs [Investigator-Initiated Trials]."

Lilly: "They offer significant financial support but want control of the data in return. They are able to spin the same data in many different ways through an effective publications team. Negative data usually remains well hidden."

Janssen: "High expectations are set on investigators who publish favorable results but they are well rewarded for their involvement."

Bristol-Myers Squibb: "Strategic focus is in unlicensed indications."[21]

From Diseases to Symptoms

> Not all diseases are created equal. The idea helps to avoid mis-
> taking symptoms for diseases and to avoid excessive diagnosis of
> comorbidities. Current psychopharmacology is aggressive and
> non-Hippocratic:symptom-based, rather than disease oriented.—S.
> Nassir Ghaemi, professor of psychiatry at Tufts University (2008)[22]

An internist said in 2011: "The very idea that I would see a new schizophrenia patient in my office and treat him for symptoms of 'suspiciousness' strikes me as belonging to the theater of the absurd."[23] He threw up his hands at the idea of managing the disease schizophrenia. Frank Ayd recalled, "At Ohio's Academy GP meeting one year, I gave a paper on the drugs, and in the discussion afterward, a man got up and said, 'Very erudite paper, but it isn't worth a damn to me, because when you say don't give this drug to an obsessive-compulsive, this drug is good in an endogenous depression, you are talking way over my head. The doctor sitting next to me might be schizophrenic or he may have an endogenous depression, I wouldn't know this.' " Ayd added that the reason for the popularity among family docs of meprobamate and Librium, "is that these drugs are relatively innocuous. [The doctors] won't get called out at night to see a dyskinesia. I don't have to worry about jaundice and cytosis, so they go ahead and give it."[24] Treating symptoms rather than disorders was thus not entirely self-interested hype on the part of Pharma. In any event, the new strategy of several companies became, shift the marketing from diseases to symptoms: "Schizophrenia I can't treat, but agitation I can."

Mickey Nardo explained how this works: "Primary care physicians are symptom and minor illness doctors. They sift through the everyday cases and refer people who need more. The drug companies knew that and specifically targeted them to look at mental illness as symptoms in need of meds. If they saw it as psychosis, they'd refer. They prescribe more frequently, more medicines, to more patients, and they don't take people off of anything. Lilly's Zyprexa campaign against specific diagnoses was the most blatant (and cynical example), but just part of a general trend. Even at the peak of the psychopharmacology age in psychiatry, they wanted primary care physicians writings the scripts."[25]

Carroll called this "indication creep." An agent is launched for schizophrenia. The family doctors won't go near it. So, "the name of the game is to promote a drug like Seroquel as a broad-spectrum psychotropic agent, then to push it hard in primary care. The 'broad-spectrum' message works hand in glove with the insecurity of primary care physicians about making clear psychiatric diagnoses that require differentiated or specific treatments. Instead, the message is that one drug fits all and they can feel good about it!"[26]

Psychoactive drugs have always been pitched for specific symptoms, such as insomnia, as well as for diseases, such as manic depression. There is an academic tradition in England of distrust of abstract diagnostic concepts in favor of the clinically concrete. In 1964, E. Beresford Davies, in the department of psychiatry of Cambridge University, urged colleagues to switch out disease thinking in favor of just noting symptoms and their response. "There is something to be said for adopting a cookery book method of investigation by which one records the signs and symptoms of an illness on the one hand, and its means of treatment on the other, as the ingredients of a particular dish and its preparation." He was suspicious of such larger concepts as "anxiety neurosis."[27]

Elsewhere, this became known as the "target symptom" approach and was associated in the United States with émigré psychiatrist Fritz Freyhan, who said in 1959 that Tofranil (imipramine) seemed to act selectively on the "target symptom" of an energy deficit in depression.[28] All this was long before the pharmaceutical industry invaded psychiatry, so it's not just a marketing trope. (There was substantial pushback against the target symptom approach, and Jules Angst said all antidepressants treat both agitation and lethargy. "I therefore think that the target symptom concept is a myth."[29])

Fully aware of the symptom approach, in 1998 Lilly, under its new CEO Sidney Taurel, decided to shift from marketing to medical specialists to primary care physicians (PCPs) with a newly created "retail sales force." Taurel said that Prozac was the model for its "retail" products, with its enormous sales that accounted for almost 30 percent of Lilly's $8.5 billion total sales in 1997.[30]

In 2003, family doctors prescribed 75 percent of all antidepressants, but only 30 percent of antipsychotics.[31] Clearly, there was room for growth. But how to get PCPs to step up their antipsychotics game?

How this played out internally at Lilly is interesting. In a memo in 2000, the Zyprexa brands manager briefed the sales force on the new approach: "This customer group is huge (> 250,000 prescribers, ~59,000 are key targets) and its potential in this arena is virtually untapped." Zyprexa is perfect for primary care, he said. "safe, simple, well-tolerated, effective, versatile." PCPs are nervous about schizophrenia and bipolar disorder. So Lilly was "enabling" the PCP to "take control of clinical situations that previously had led to referrals and/or poor outcomes. 'Mental disorders' is intentionally broad and vague, providing latitude to frame the discussion around symptoms and behaviors rather than specific indications." Zyprexa would be the next step in progression from SSRIs to a "safe, gentle psychotropic."[32] One should bear in mind that we are talking here about a powerful antipsychotic that family docs were to regard as a waystation en route to Lilly's next nerve pill, Cymbalta (duloxetine).

Tone Jones, a Texas sales manager for Janssen, testified at the TMAP trial in 2012 that among Janssen's "key strategies" for sales reps was, "Sell on symptoms not diagnosis." But the symptoms that the sales reps were to discuss with the physicians were those of depression, not schizophrenia.[33]

In sales meetings, Janssen made a big deal of the "SYMPTOM focus!" In 2002, Janssen created a new sales force, "the 500 Gold," to sell Risperdal to family docs. "Risperdal has a large volume of studies," the sales reps were told, "with proven efficacy in a wide variety of symptoms." Of course, if you are asked about diseases you should answer. "However, in the meantime—BRING IT BACK TO THE SYMPTOMS with ANY disease state."

"Bipolar disorder. BRING IT BACK TO THE SYMPTOMS (excitability, agitation, depression, delusions)."

"Pediatrics: BRING IT BACK TO THE SYMPTOMS (impulsiveness, agitation, aggression, depression, anxiety)."[34]

Of course, at this point Janssen did not actually have a pediatric indication for Risperdal. Indeed, around 2000, 46 percent of Risperdal sales were off label.[35]

Concentrating on symptoms was also a means of doing an end run around FDA's prohibition against off-label marketing, promoting indications that hadn't yet been approved. Lilly's Zyprexa had only been approved for schizophrenia and bipolar disorder, which many physicians in primary care didn't want to treat. The solution: convince family doctors that their depressed patients were only in the first half of bipolar disorder and that Zyprexa was perfectly appropriate.

One journalist who had studied the primary documents wrote in 2009, "As the company tried to break into the market for general depression, it came out with a formula for what it called 'treatment-resistant depression,' suggesting that doctors mix Prozac and Zyprexa. Such formulations involved a sort of pharmaceutical sleight of hand. 'You focus on the symptoms, that's what we were taught,'" said a Lilly sales rep. "'You don't focus on the disease.'"

Lilly's sales reps had in their briefcases three profiles of types of patients the company wanted their drug reps to pitch to doctors. "One was 'Donna,' a single mom in her 30s who came to the doctor's office in 'drab clothing,' complaining that she felt anxious, irritable and in need of little sleep." When the sales reps showed the docs Donna, the reps were supposed to say, "You may have some patients who are bipolar, and you've never really thought of the problem like that. Let me tell you about Zyprexa, how it can help with these mood swings." This was part of Lilly's Viva Zyprexa campaign to primary care. Within 3 months it is said to have "generated 49,000 new prescriptions for Lilly, bringing in hundreds of millions of dollars in revenue. Today, a quarter of Zyprexa's sales are in off-label markets."[36]

Mickey Nardo glimpsed this shift in the drafting of DSM-5 itself: "The DSM-5 leaders didn't like the DSM-IV. They didn't want to revise it. They wanted to change it into the biologically based manual they wanted it to be . . . that the pharmaceutical industry had been pushing toward for decades. Classify and treat mental illness by symptoms, not disorders. They wanted to move the system to meet the neuroscience and the psychopharmacology rather than fit those things to our patients."[37] Nardo, of course, was suspicious that both the "clinical neuroscience" agenda that Tom Insel had been pushing at NIMH[38] and the psychopharmacology advocacy of the KOLs were aimed at using "biology" to elevate drug sales. Spitzer, who had guided DSM-III and DSM-III-R, and Allen Frances, editor of DSM-IV, suspected the same thing, and both men turned fiercely against DSM-5. Don Klein said of RDoC (Research Domain Criteria), the pretentious effort to array symptoms into systems that Insel had brought to life, as "the transformation of a fishing expedition into discovery science—a triumph for marketing."[39]

Convincing

> The oldest consensus among the vendors of health, and other traders along the valley of the shadow of death, was that people want to be deceived and should be pleased accordingly.—Peter Skrabanek (1990)[40]

The challenge was to convince doctors to keep prescribing the brand-name drug after the patent had expired. One solution was, as Haskell Weinstein, former medical director of Squibb, told a Senate subcommittee in 1960, was to "brainwash" the physician "to think of the trademark name of the drug at all times. Even new disease states have been invented to encourage the use of some drugs"[41] (see the discussion of "treatment-resistant depression"). It was for this reason that the generic names of drugs were often long and unmemorable, the brand name brief and snappy. (Thus the benzodiazepine with the brand name Librium had the generic name "chlordiazepoxide.") This tactic paid off: Frank Ayd told the American College of Neuropsychopharmacology (NCAP) at its founding meeting in 1960 that he had surveyed the physicians in his hospital with a list of generic names on one side, trade names on the other. "When we took twenty-five commonly prescribed tranquilizers and asked all the visiting staff, three hundred and eighty doctors, to match them up, you would be amazed. Less than ten percent were able to do it accurately."[42]

Convincing physicians to prescribe the new wonder drug was a bit beyond the marketing departments of the companies. Communications agencies were brought on board that had specialized skills in this area.

How to find the physicians and convince them? A prime occasion for grabbing the psychiatrists' attention was the annual meeting of the American Psychiatric Association, a saturnalia of marketing that had been going on since at least 1944. Michael Alan Taylor described how these meetings had evolved by the late 1980s: "Most of the week-long meeting that used to be devoted to scientific presentations or workshops . . . had been co-opted by the industry to present infomercials about their drugs. Every lobby, corridor and meeting area offered video information about a drug. Drug reps were everywhere (hunk-types for the women docs, sexy young women in tight suits for the men docs). The reps held meetings to 'teach' physicians about the new drugs. They offered hospitality suites overflowing with free food and drink. And sponsored dinners at expensive restaurants for the APA members." There would be "future junkets to fancy spas." "The main convention hall that used to be an area in which new technology and textbooks were to be found was now an extravaganza of giant amusement park-style structures lauding the merits of this or that psychiatric drug."[43]

Around these meetings a whole galaxy of symposia swirled, chaired by "opinion leaders" in the field and, when directly sponsored by industry as "satellite symposiums," accompanied by a smorgasbord of wine, cheese, and sandwiches. Such symposia, financed by industry, were introduced in 1978 by a marketing company, AV/MD, as events before the meeting: The APA charged industry $5,000 for "the right to present symposia prior to the annual meeting," which, by 1980, had produced $60,000 for the APA (and the content was produced by AV/MD!).[44] Moreover, in 1979, AV/MD staged symposia at three locations to introduce DSM-III; the symposia were financed by Roche.[45]

In June 1980, the APA met with representatives from eight pharmaceutical companies to determine "guidelines" for receiving financial support from industry. At the APA annual meeting in May 1980, Sandoz had used "live speakers" at its exhibit area "'to give mini-lecture(s) and to have discussion with individuals who stopped by the booth."[46] Now industry wanted to generalize this. Mel Sabshin, the APA's "medical director," was asked "whether a drug company would be allowed to sponsor a seminar on depression if the company's major product was for the treatment of depression. Dr. Sabshin said that he believed this would be permitted."[47] The naiveté of the APA leaders concerning industry's efforts to shove a foot in the door is noteworthy. This was the beginning of the transformation of the exhibit-area "seminars" into full-fledged satellite symposia.

The symposia grew rapidly because they had the ability to deliver an audience. Healy quipped about the satellite meetings, "Hard as it is to understand how senior figures can agree to take part in such a charade, it's harder to see how anyone in the audience manages to stay awake." The companies prepared the speakers' slides. Healy: "Sometimes speakers stare at their slides in a manner that makes it obvious they have never laid eyes on them before."[48]

APA rules stipulated that commercial advertising was not to be inserted in "scientific" presentations. Yet this rule was honored in the breach. In October 1980, Henry Work, deputy medical director of APA in charge of professional affairs,

rapped Roche's knuckles about "the one-and-one-half minute commercials edited into the videotapes, and the product advertising which appears at the back
of the video program book." It was such a mild reprimand that Work ended by
asking Richard Dudley at Roche to "call me next week."[49]

A lovely touch was Smith Kline & French's creation of the "SKF Presidential
Fund," a slush fund to be disbursed as the president wished (there was a new one-
term president every year). Existence of the fund was to be kept secret from the
membership.[50]

One bridge further was meeting organizers' sales of marketing opportunities
at meetings to industry. You had to pay to get your name in front of the members,
in other words. At its Montreal meeting in 2002, the CINP organizers advertised
to industry the opportunity to offer "regular scientific symposia within CINP
program" at $14,500 a shot; "satellite symposia" were more expensive (because
they were more frankly mercantile) at $25,000; "educational workshops" went
for $20,000 a pop; "meet-the expert" breakfasts were a steal at $20,000 as well.
But sponsoring a dinner for the local organizing committee would cost a cool
$40,000. It is fair to say that psychiatric science was really the last thing on the
minds of the organizers of this "scientific meeting."[51]

In the minds of the marketers, there was no doubt about the utility of these
affairs. In 1989, one marketing professional told colleagues about symposia and
medical conferences, "The potential persuasiveness of peer influence is undeni-
able. A well-organized and well-moderated symposium can change physicians'
attitudes and prescribing habits, and these symposia are proliferating. Some
companies conduct hundreds of them annually and may actually pay physicians
to attend." The author polled drug industry executives about whether their usage
of symposia and medical conferences would go up. Of nine VPs in marketing, six
said it would go up; of seven VPs in sales, five said it would go up.[52]

What better place to convince doctors than at an expensive restaurant! Wining
and dining of physicians was absolutely standard. Melody Petersen reported in
the *New York Times* in 2002 that Forest Labs had tasked the advertising firm
Intramed, which was a branch of the advertising agency WPP, with promoting
their new antidepressant Lexapro. "Just days after the FDA approved Lexapro in
August [2002], Intramed and Forest invited Dr. Richard J. Brown, a Manhattan
psychiatrist, and about 20 of his peers to dinner at Daniel, one of Manhattan's
most expensive restaurants. Besides dining on tournedos of beef and cabernet
sauvignon, each doctor was paid $500 for attending."[53] Forest spent no money on
consumer advertising, but reached physicians over dinner and in other venues.

How about bribing doctors by just giving them money and free trips? Pretty
convincing? Ever since Senator Charles Grassley's committee discovered the
six-figure sums that industry was giving KOLs, there had been concern. As
the *New York Times* put it in 2008, "The worry is that this money may subtly

alter psychiatrists' choices of which drugs to prescribe."[54] No, that was not the main worry. If the drugs were equipotent—which is to say, if it didn't matter much which one you prescribed—the influencing of the choice would really be a matter of indifference. The danger was the marketing of *diagnoses*, not molecules. Giving the KOLs loads of money was done not with the aim of promoting Prozac, or Zyprexa, or whatever. It was done to promote such bogus diagnoses as "pediatric bipolar disorder" and "treatment-resistant depression." The real money lay in broadening the clinical population to include people who were not really sick and who didn't require anything in that drug class before they received their bogus diagnosis.

Sales Reps

It was with the sales reps that, in the task of convincing, the rubber hit the road. The enormous expansion of the pharmaceutical industry after the Second World War transformed the few commercial travelers of yore into the modern "detail man" of the 1950s. Between the 1930s and 1963, the number of detail men had grown from a few thousand in the 1930s to "13,000 to 18,000 men (and a few women)."[55] They were known as "detail men" because in office visits they gave physicians the latest details on their wares. As women moved into the sales field, the more neutral term "sales reps" was chosen. One survey found that 46 percent of physicians listed "detail men as their source of information."[56]

There was nothing free form about a sales call. It was divided into specific performance components, and companies were ranked on how well their sales people did on each: the *detail piece*, or reciting your screed about the product; *patient identification,* or painting for the doctor a picture of the ideal patient for your product (Lilly did well here); *closing,* or the "ask," getting the doctor to commit to prescribing your product. Then there were *message,* or "how compelling a brand's message is," as an article in the industry press put it in 2007; *knowledge*, meaning were you credible as a source of information (see cheerleaders, below); and, finally, *physician–rep relationship,* or how well the doc related to the rep.[57] The 2007 piece did not mention this, but being an attractive female or bringing pizza for the office staff would clearly be of assistance here as well.

Why was gaining the confidence of the physician so important? Partly to defend the company against complaints of adverse effects. William Goodrich, chief counsel of the FDA, told *The Pink Sheet* in 1970 that the job of the detail man was to stymie reports of adverse drug reactions to the FDA. "The physician often confides in the detail man, who tells him he's done nothing wrong, and the drug is not to blame, while turning around and reporting the case to the firm's medical department."[58]

In the sales visit, "friendship" counted for lots. Two students of detailing wrote, "Drug reps increase drug sales by influencing physicians, and they do so with finely titrated doses of friendship," or pseudo-friendship. When you are in the doc's office, look around. "A photo on a desk presents an opportunity to inquire about family members and memorize what tidbits are offered (including names, birthdays, and interests); these are usually typed into a database after the encounter." How do you approach a physician who seems "aloof and skeptical"? Said one sales rep, "I visit the office with journal articles that specifically counter the doctor's perceptions of the shortcoming of my drug. Armed with the articles and having hopefully scheduled a 20-minute appointment (so the doc can't escape), I play dumb and have the doc explain to me the significance of my article."[59] This is just delicious. One couldn't make this stuff up.

The emphasis on "evidence" presupposed, however, that there was genuine scientific evidence about safety and effectiveness in the literature; in psychopharmacology, this would be a bit of a stretch, as the "literature" had been so massively corrupted by industry and the KOLs. In 2014, Princeton psychiatrist Jeffrey Mattes said, "I think it's important that physicians ensure that 'evidence-based' reviews should not become simply another way for pharmaceutical companies to promote their newer, more profitable products."[60]

Detail men were thus salesmen, not proto-scientists. Frank Berger, the originator of Miltown (meprobamate), said, "Detail men are salesmen with little or no background in science and medicine that are trained by pharmaceutical companies to persuade doctors to prescribe their proprietary drugs. They should not be the main source through which doctors learn about advances in medicine."[61] But, alas, they once were. Rufus McQuillan, a sales rep in the 1920s and 1930s—possibly for Lilly—said in a memoir, "Nearly half the time a doctor learns of a new drug through the personal visit of the detail man. A doctor cannot practice medicine just as he learned to do it in medical school. . . . The time of the average doctor is so taken up with his practice that he can spend only about one half-hour a day reading his medical journals, looking over mail, and interviewing detail men." McQuillan knew how to make those minutes count. But, in his account of the industry in those days, there is no suggestion of manipulating the physicians or whispering off-label indications. It was a life of straight up hard work.[62]

It would never have occurred to McQuillan that he was somehow "invading" industry. He saw his job as education. Yet the expanding network of salespeople did have the effect of shifting medical education from the medical press increasingly to industry. This was among the earliest signs of the shift from education by academics to education by Pharma. At Estes Kefauver's hearings in the Senate in 1960, Walter Modell, a distinguished internist at Cornell University Medical College, sounded the alarm about the detail man. "One cannot teach about a drug without covering the entire field, and no manufacturer in this detail man's educational program ever discusses anything but his own drug. . . . There is a program of education which comes to the doctor's office by way of the detail man and by way of promotional literature which is completely biased as any advertising is. This, I think, is a dangerous procedure."[63]

Relatively early in the game, industry began selecting sales reps more for their allure than their science backgrounds. It was in the late 1950s that this change began. In 1959, Melvin Gibson, the editor of the *American Journal of Pharmaceutical Education,* deplored the decreasing percentage of "detail men" who had studied pharmacy, the percentage among big companies ranging from 5 percent to almost 100: at Eli Lilly, 95 percent of the sales reps were pharmacists, at Parke-Davis, 90 percent. In Gibson's view, the ideal sales rep "must have at least four years of chemistry and pharmaceutical chemistry coupled with sound courses in physiology and pharmacology, these being only basic prerequisites. . . . Who in a college curriculum has such a program except a pharmacy graduate?" How did physicians find out about drugs? Gibson said, "Less than 50 percent of the doctors read their medical journals in any regular, systematized manner. Doctors are now receiving almost 3,090 pieces of direct mail advertising per month—a 100 percent increase over 1940. About 62 percent of this mail is opened . . . [and] the other 38 percent is thrown away, opened or unopened, or examined by the doctor's nurse or secretary."[64]

Increasingly, the sales force became feminized. Mickey Nardo recalled, "The detail men were no longer a resource for 'details,' nor were they men. They were almost universally pretty young women—well coiffed. They had a habit of saying 'Doctor' (pause) followed by some leading question that started 'in your patients with . . .' I hated talking to them. It all felt like patter to me."[65]

Did industry look for pretty young women with science backgrounds? No. Companies hired former cheerleaders as sales reps! Any pretense of a scientific preparation, as Gibson desired, was thrown out the window. A *New York Times* reporter noted in 2005, "Anyone who has seen the parade of sales representatives through a doctor's waiting room has probably noticed that they are frequently female and invariably good looking. Less recognized is the fact that a good many are recruited from the cheerleading ranks. Known for their toned bodies, postage-stamp skirts and persuasive enthusiasm, cheerleaders have many qualities the drug industry looks for in its sales force."[66]

Novartis, a Basel-based company formed in 1996 by the merger of Sandoz and Ciba-Geigy, transitioned early in the new century from its "staid Swiss culture," as the *Wall Street Journal* (*WSJ*) put it, to a company based on high-pressure marketing. The trainee salespeople practiced their canned sales pitches on each other. The *WSJ* reported in 2002, "During a recent session at its training facility . . . a 25-year-old recruit practiced her technique for selling Lotrel [a blood-pressure drug] in a role-playing exercise with another trainee, who played the part of the doctor: 'And doctor, are you finding that your patients' diabolic blood pressure is getting to goal on present therapies?' she asked. She means 'diastolic' blood pressure, but that's what the training is for." Once she "perfected her pitch" she would join Novartis's rapidly growing sales army.[67] It escaped the *Wall Street Journal* completely that there was probably something laudable about the "staid' science-based Swiss culture.

The sales reps were briefed to conceal as well as to sell. At the TMAP trial in Travis County, Texas, in 2012 (see Chapter 19), child psychiatrist Valerie Robinson testified about Janssen's sales rep, who visited her 96 times while she was in Houston, from 1994 to 2002. He had not been exactly forthcoming. She testified that "80 percent or more" of her pediatric patients experienced a weight gain. She wasn't warned about that.

And how about extrapyramidal symptoms (EPS)? The Janssen rep told her "there was a lower incidence of EPS with Risperdal over neuroleptics such as Thorazine and Haldol. . . . I believed what he said. I mean, if he said it had a lower incidence, since he was the one who knew about this new drug and I was just being introduced to it, I believed him."

Q: "Do you think Risperdal is better than Haldol generally as it relates to EPS?"
A: "No."

Counsel asked about the "fair balance" that drug reps are "supposed to present to physicians when they meet with them about a drug."

Q: Did the Janssen sales reps "devote as much time and energy and attention and enthusiasm in discussing the adverse effects the drug could cause as they did their touting its effectiveness?"
A: "No."[68]

Bad News for Zyprexa

By 1999, it was apparent that Lilly had a problem with Zyprexa: it caused large weight gains and often triggered diabetes. These adverse effects would normally be death sentences for a drug. How to manage this? Alan Breier, who had trained in psychiatry at Yale and spent four years at NIMH, was in 1999 the team leader at Lilly for Zyprexa. He said to colleagues in November 1999, "Olanzapine-associated weight gain and possible hyperglycemia [are] a major threat to the long-term success of this critically important molecule."[69]

Breier consulted closely with Charles Beasley, also at Lilly Research Labs and also a psychiatrist (trained at the University of Cincinnati). Beasley vouchsafed a soft approach that did not aggressively deny the reality of the often staggering weight gains. Beasley said in October 2000, "[The] emphasis on marketing approach is to acknowledge weight gain and not underplay it, while for diabetes to be cautious until we are sure."[70]

In another communication, Beasley said there were really two approaches "the marketing approach and then the scientific analysis approach." He argued plaidoyed for the latter. In marketing, people "believed we should 'aggressively face the issue' and work with physicians to address methods of reducing weight gain." Beasley clearly was not thrilled about this, given the magnitude of the problem: "There does not seem much to say about scientific analyses of weight gain, we know it's a weighty problem. When you translate 1–2% gain of 40+ kilos into the absolute number based on 5 million patients, the number is 50,000 to 100,000. 100,000 people putting on 90 pounds of weight is a lot."[71]

There was no doubt that olanzapine was associated with a significant increased risk of diabetes, as one study derived from the UK General Practice Research Data Base involving almost 20,000 patients demonstrated.[72]

So the marketing people were told that the sales reps might even recommend a rival drug if the prescribing physician was uneasy about weight gain. "Probably won't be popular internally," said Robert Baker, another Lilly executive-scientist, "but we are exploring it."[73] Other people said that Lilly really has to speak up about the diabetes issue, which is "probably not the way Lilly typically does business."[74]

At this point, trench warfare began. Beasley left the file in 2002 and the hard men took over. Getting one's own experts on board and badmouthing the experts for the other side seem to have been the order of the day. Henry Nasrallah at the University of Cincinnati was the expert for AstraZeneca's antipsychotic Seroquel (quetiapine): He presented for Astra Zeneca at a psychiatry congress in November 2001. The Lilly executives didn't like his presentation at all, and the Zyprexa Brand Team told the scientists "We are requesting your help so that we can provide our national speakers [KOLs] 'answers that matter' in several upcoming formats."[75] Unnamed academics would, of course, constitute Lilly's "national speakers."

But then several days later a real crisis blew up. At a recent meeting of the European Congress of Neuropsychopharmacology (ECNP), Bruce Lambert had put up a poster on antipsychotic-induced diabetes in which Zyprexa came off poorly. Lilly executive Hiram Wildgust warned Neil Archer, the business unit manager, "I flag this up as almost certainly this poster will be published and raise the noise around diabetes and olanzapine."

Archer said, "Our attention needs to turn to how we can minimize its impact on both the global and the local level. . . . Can we stop it/delay it?" Archer asked, "Do we know the author? Can we exert any influence? This would be very dangerous as it would be seen as Lilly behaving unethically. Who sits on the editorial board of the target journal? Can we influence them in any way, with respect to the limitations of this methodology? Should we conduct a communications initiative aimed at all influential referees?"[76]

The exchange is banal, and entirely typical of office correspondence in the industry, but the perspective is that we can manipulate the academic game.

Later, Arvid Carlsson spoke in an interview about this situation: "Henry Nasrallah has problem with them, yes, he's a little anti-Lilly. Nasrallah said that they [Lilly] could be very aggressive, and they could also attack official people, and exert pressure upon those who have an influence on legal issues, with some success."[77] In 2004, as Lilly faced a raft of litigation over Zyprexa and diabetes-weight gain, Forbes mentioned Nasrallah as having "been critical of Zyprexa for its diabetes risk." He thought it "appropriate" that Lilly was now preparing to pay some of the legal bills of physicians sued for prescribing Zyprexa.[78] On another occasion, Nasrallah damned Zyprexa with faint praise as "a good drug that has a fatal flaw." He said that he might prescribe it after all the other antipsychotics "have failed."[79]

There was lots of cash riding on both sides. Nasrallah was identified in 2013 by Propublica ("Dollars for Docs") as being among the 22 physicians who since 2009 had earned more than $500,000 from drug companies.[80]

As Zyprexa's tendency to cause weight gain, hyperglycemia, and diabetes started to become a national scandal, Lilly's efforts to control the spin went into hyperdrive. The company put out the line that schizophrenia itself caused diabetes! A number of academic investigators echoed this story. But the story was met with dubiety by insiders. David Healy, who had conducted a major study of patients at a mental hospital in Wales at the end of the nineteenth century, said, "We looked through our database of 1200 plus psychoses or bipolars . . . and [found] not a single comorbid case of serious mental illness and diabetes."[81]

On balance, Lilly's early response to the Zyprexa weight-gain problem reflected the voice of science, but, after 2000, marketing took over. The diabetes issue cost Lilly a lot of money in litigation.

"Defend the Molecule"

The capacity of the industry to deploy its strategies and use its spoils to stifle the truth has been overwhelmingly successful.—Barry Blackwell (2016)[82]

In industry, scientific truth was not just a matter of uninterest, it was a potentially poisonous concept. In the view of "Talbot," an experienced insider, "A researcher who finds something that could harm sales, and wants to report it, is a potential menace. Experts are KOLs—people who can present biased data people will believe, that will increase sales. The KOLs get rewarded as well. The whole system is antithetical to good medicine, and 'first do no harm' is a thing of the past."[83]

The simplest way of handling bad news was to silence its bearer. Triazolam (Halcion) turned out to be a very profitable drug for Upjohn in the 1980s. But then Ian Oswald at Edinburgh did a controlled trial and found that, unlike a competing drug, Hacion increased anxiety. Bad news for Upjohn! What to do. Oswald later told Healy, "We sought to publish it in the *Archives of General Psychiatry*. It was turned down, with some vitriolic reviews that I ultimately discovered . . . were written either within the Upjohn company or by people who were funded by Upjohn. What we didn't know was that the editor of the *Archives of General Psychiatry* was funded by Upjohn and he had sent our paper to Upjohn to referee. Same story with the *New England Journal of Medicine*." There was later a court case, and Oswald discovered in Upjohn's internal correspondence their strategy for managing bad news, "So far we have been successful in having it stop." Finally, after 2 years of delays, the paper was published in 1989 in *Pharmacopsychiatry*, a journal with a far smaller impact factor.[84]

In 1961, the Senate's Kefauver Committee asked the Library of Congress to survey warnings for 34 "important brand name products" appearing in drug ads in six leading medical journals, from 1958 to 1959. "In 14 of the drugs the companies followed the approach of ignoring the subject [of adverse effects] completely. The remaining 20 drugs studied contained at least some reference to side effects. But in 13 of these products the references were entirely of the type listed above"—e.g., "side effects are fewer and milder," "minimal incidence of certain side effects," etc. The committee continued, "The language is less of a warning than a reason for prescribing."[85]

Over time, the companies became even stingier with side-effect information, dodging the FDA mandate to explain such effects. In 2005, Leemon McHenry at California State University, Northridge, explained Pharma's new marketing strategy: "The old vision allowed costly failures when reality did not cooperate with the company's plans for its new molecular entities. With the rising price of bringing a new drug to the market, a method that guaranteed success was needed. Instead of fitting the conclusion to the evidence, the industry's strategy now is to 'defend the molecule': Select the data that promote the drugs, file away the results that are unfavorable, and then buy just the right academic credentials to sign on to ghostwritten articles produced by the marketing department staff or by public relations agencies employed by the company."[86] Simply hushing up bad news and lying about it became a standard tactic in the pharmaceutical industry and marked the definitive departure of the industry from the highway of science. Over the years, many scandalized observers have reported on this, and the first whistle-blower was probably Roy Poses, a general internist at Brown University, who in 2003 began reporting on this scandalous behavior[87] and in 2004 took up the subject in his widely followed blog *Health Care Renewal.* By 2013, he had published 102 posts with the label "suppression of medical research."[88]

One example among many: In 1999, AstraZeneca's antipsychotic drug Seroquel (quetiapine) was still in trials and the company was trying to figure out how to spin the alarming data about weight gain that were emerging. They had "buried" some of the trials, deciding to mention them to no one. John Tumas, a company executive, messaged colleagues, "There is growing pressure from outside the industry to provide access to all data resulting from clinical trials conducted by industry. Thus far, we have buried Trials 15, 31, 56, and are now considering COSTAR."

"The larger issue is how do we face the outside world when they begin to criticize us for suppressing data. . . . Until now, I believe we have been looked upon by the outside world favorably with regard to ethical behavior. We must decide if we wish to continue to enjoy this distinction. The reporting of the COSTAR results will not be easy. We must find a way to diminish the negative findings."[89] Bury, diminish—this was the inside story.

Bury and diminish was certainly the way Lilly handled the investigations of its marketing of Zyprexa to the elderly. The company had formed a dedicated sales campaign called "Viva Zyprexa," later "Zyprexa Limitless," to market the antipsychotic to family docs. One of the patient profiles in the campaign was "Martha," a widow with adult children who appeared to have mild dementia. Not at all, chorused Lilly's PR flacks. "Lilly had actually intended Martha's profile to represent a patient with schizophrenia," said a PR person. Observers scoffed at this, since first-onset schizophrenia in the elderly was extremely rare.[90] The cynicism of the denials was over the top.

Ghosting

> I believe the SSRI era will soon stand as one of the most shameful in the history of medicine. . . . During this era, most publications of on-patent drugs in our best journals were ghost-written.—David Healy (2015)[91]

In 2003, Janssen gave its staffers an overview of all the articles on Risperdal that its communications agencies had commissioned, along with the proposed "authors." There were 43 such articles. The cast of characters was the leadership tier of US child psychiatry. Not surprisingly, Joseph Biederman at Harvard was listed. Robert Findling, still at Case Western University (he would shortly become chair of child psychiatry at Johns Hopkins Medical Institutions), appeared eight times, for eight different proposed pieces. Earlier, a staffer at the medical communications firm Excerpta Medica had written to Findling to tell him that her company had been working with Janssen to prepare a manuscript based on a trial of Risperdal in children with mental retardation. "You have been identified as the lead author to this manuscript which is targeted for the *American Journal of Psychiatry*. . . . Attached is a preliminary outline for your manuscript." Findling was told that, "Your input on the outline for your manuscript is appreciated." Findling responded that "some secondary analyses [might] be performed."[92] Clearly, by the year 2000 ghosting had become entirely routine in the upper reaches of US psychiatry.

The industry had long known the practice of hiring professional writers to craft articles, then attaching the "author's" name to the product. Herman ("Hy") Denber, research director at Manhattan State Hospital, said of the 1950s, "Frequently, sponsors offered to 'write the paper for' the researcher." (He stoutly refused to go along.[93]) In 1957, Nate Kline, at Rockland State Hospital in Orangeburg, New York, and a prominent early investigator, urged fellow psychiatrists, Don't let industry write your article! "It is certainly below professional dignity to have the pharmaceutical house write the article, to which the investigator merely affixes his signature."[94] So, this went way back.

As Haskell Weinstein told the Kefauver Committee in 1960, "It may be of interest to the committee to know that a substantial number of the so-called medical scientific papers that are published on behalf of these drugs are written within the confines of the pharmaceutical houses concerned. Frequently, the physician involved merely makes the observations and his data, which sometimes is sketchy and uncritical, is submitted to a medical writer employed by the company. The writer prepares the article, which is returned to the physician, who makes the overt effort to submit it for publication."[95] This would be proto-ghosting.

But plucking "authors" out of thin air who had no connection to the research was new. And fakery at this scale occurred because the stakes were so huge. GlaxoSmithKline (GSK) was determined to get Paxil into the adolescent depression market. Of course, the FDA had not approved this indication, but GSK pressed ahead anyway. In November 1997, the firm held a "Scientific Presentations/Meeting Strategy" review at their Philadelphia offices. Eight meetings were coming up. There would be posters and papers for each. Who should be the "proposed authors"?

For the Biological Psychiatry meeting in Toronto, GSK would ask Elizabeth Weller at Ohio State to be the "author." For the APA Services meeting (where

GSK might hold a symposium), Bill Kinnier, a biochemist at GSK; for the big APA meeting in May, Marty Keller; for the American Psychopathological Association meeting, GSK would assign Gabrielle Carlson at Stony Brook and Mike Strober, a psychologist at UCLA; for the CINP, it would be Bill Kinnier and Jim McCafferty, who was also on the CNS team at GSK; and for a poster at NCDEU, Karen Wagner at the University of Texas Medical Branch in Galveston. "Authors" were proposed for several other meetings as well.[96]

In promoting Risperdal, Janssen often asked medical communications firms to take responsibility for drafting laudatory articles, finding a "guest author" who would be willing to see his name on the title page, and then placing the articles in professional journals. This was completely fraudulent. The practice created the impression that a distinguished clinician had himself done the trial, penned the article, and then submitted it on his own (the majority of "guest authors" were male).

By 2002, Janssen discovered it had a significant problem: Risperdal stimulated production of the hormone prolactin (which might give males little breasts, for example). How should this be managed? Here, Wells Health Care Communications, in Tunbridge Wells, England, came to their aid and drafted an abstract for a forthcoming meeting of the American Academy of Child and Adolescent Psychiatry. On the title page of the draft it said: "Author: Robert Findling." The agency writers were listed on the cover sheet, and Findling was copied in on the draft.[97] When the creation appeared in 2003, the list of "authors" had grown considerably.[98]

In AstraZeneca's "Seroquel International Media Schedule" for 2001, things were looking pretty good in terms of choosing "authors" for topics: Siegfried Kasper for the forthcoming meeting of the American Psychiatric Association in May, and so forth. But not all was fixed! For the coming meetings of the International Psychiatric Association and the European College of Neuropsychopharmacology, the entry was "tbc"—"to be chosen."[99] They hadn't quite gotten around to figuring out who the authors would be. Is this not perfect!

Why couldn't the investigators write their own articles? Mickey Nardo explained that of course a real author could do this. "But they aren't very good at it. The kind of ghostwriter we're talking about here is such an expert—one who knows the logic and formats of science well, but also understands the loopholes and nuances of the tools of science. So they bring another set of skills to the table that are vital to the task at hand—telling lies."[100]

The need for this vital skill rose rapidly in the first decade of the new century, as the atypical antipsychotics and SSRIs were slugging it out with the competition. As Sergio Sismondo reported, "The number of articles in the industry journal *Pharmaceutical Executive* that mention 'opinion leader' roughly tripled between 2000 and 2010."[101]

In 2009, the going rates for the 182 "medical education and communication companies" in the United States were $18,000 to $40,000 per manuscript. Scientific Therapeutics Information, Sally Laden's firm, was one of the bigs.[102] (See Chapter 17.)

Excerpta Medica functioned as a kind of public relations company for Janssen, organizing CME sessions and tapping KOL experts. From 1992 on, they implemented a kind of "strategic plan" for Risperdal.[103] For example, late in 1997, Janssen/J&J need an article on how safe and well-tolerated Risperdal was in the elderly. So they asked Excerpta Medica to take responsibility for writing the piece and shepherding it through production. Excerpta Medica's billings to J&J are revealing:

On January 13, 1998, Excerpta Medica sent J&J an invoice for $15,000, "for Manuscript Development on RIS-USA-64—Risperidone in Elderly Patients with Psychotic Disorders/Madhusoodanan." (The latter was a physician at St. John's Episcopal Hospital in New York who had agreed to "guest author" the piece.) The invoice listed Excerpta Medica's services: "preparing 5 drafts and a final manuscript; coordinating all Janssen/Author reviews; securing all relevant information from a target journal; preparing the submission package including redrawn figures; obtaining permissions for author(s); and managing the project through submission to the target journal," in this case the *American Journal of Geriatric Psychiatry.*

David Rothman, the Columbia medical historian who drafted an expert opinion for the Texas court and who gave us this information, noted, "There is no indication that [Subramoniam] Madhusoodanan was a 'designated author,' not the actual author. Journal editors, reviewers, and readers would have incorrectly believed that the work was done by Madhusoodanan." There was no mention of J&J as funder or organizer. It was, to be sure, divulged that the second author, Martin Brecher, was a J&J employee, but not revealed that the third author, Ronald Brenner "was a member of J&J's Certified Speakers Bureau Program." There were further honoraria for Madhusoodanan.[104]

Henry Nasrallah, a much bigger fish than Madhusoodanan, had been professor of psychiatry at Ohio State and the University of Iowa. He was also a KOL for Johnson & Johnson and was a member of their speakers' bureau. Between 2000 and 2004, Nasrallah received $73,000 for lending his name to a piece on delirium and for his participation in regional sales meetings, "CNS Summits," and the like. Rothman noted that "It was Excerpta Medica and J&J who were primarily responsible for drafting the findings and analysis [of the delirium article], with the ostensible authors coming in at the end of the process." Janssen's funding was acknowledged.[105]

Excerpta Medica did a great deal of work for J&J. On the Risperdal file, of the 80 articles listed in Excerpta Medica's July schedule, 16, or 20 percent, were "author TBD," or "author to be determined." By December of 2003, of 65 pieces on Risperdal in the works, 14, or 22 percent had "Author TBD."[106]

To promote Seroquel, AstraZeneca organized a "European Think Tank Satellite Symposium" for June 2001 in Montreux, a select lakeside spa in Switzerland. The central figure was to be Jim van Os, a professor at Maastricht University, later at Utrecht, in the Netherlands. The anticipated "output" of the meeting: "Rapid awareness and distribution of 2-Com tool to 600+ delegates attending meeting." (2-Com was a wrinkle in doctor–patient communication that van Os and AstraZeneca had collaborated on.) An additional output: "Opportunity to further strengthen AstraZeneca's relationship with key European OLs [opinion leaders]."[107]

Ghostwritten articles had certain standard features. They would begin with an invocation along the lines of: "Depression is a major public health problem," "global health burden," or a stock phrase about "unmet clinical need." In 2011, Barney Carroll noted, " 'depression as the second global cause of disability,' [is a theme] theme has been internalized by all the professional writers who do the ghostwriting for all the too-busy KOLs."[108] Mickey Nardo quoted Sally Laden, who was suspected of ghosting an article on Cyberonics' VNS device: "Major depression is now recognized as a highly prevalent, chronic, recurrent, and disabling biological disorder."[109] Nardo mocked: "Depression was not only an epidemic. It was growing, affecting more people, arising earlier in their lives, and threatening to silently gobble up our youth. It was predisposing us to disease and suicide. Depression the disease was a spreading epidemic."[110] The acknowledgments section of the article contained the telltale phrase, "We thank Sally Laden for editorial support in developing early drafts of this manuscript."

Carroll responded to a blog comment by "Elmore," who claimed ghostwriting "was the standard for a long, long time."

"No, Elmore, it wasn't the standard for a long, long time. It was widespread but it wasn't the standard. I have been in academic psychiatry since 1967. I saw the corruption take hold. I saw the leadership of professional societies look the other way. I had plenty of consulting and teaching interactions with Pharma over the years. But ghostwriting was out of the question. That was only for sleazebags."[111]

Yet, *pace* Carroll, David Healy estimated in 2004 that around 50 percent of all journal articles on therapeutics were ghostwritten.[112] (This, he explained elsewhere, was one way of forming a paradigm—not through a convergence of scientific views but through "a common set of articles, produced in communication agencies with the name of various experts almost randomly attached as appropriate for the occasion."[113]) Healy, who had access to the Pfizer records, noted that by the start of 1999, Pfizer's ghosting service, Current Medical Directions, had 85 papers in the works on sertraline (Zoloft), of which 55 had appeared by 2001.[114] By 2013, Healy had upped his estimate of ghosting to include almost the entire on-patent literature. "Close to all of the published literature about on-patent drugs is ghostwritten. . . . In terms of ensuring the integrity of the primary source of a story and ensuring the authors are who they appear to be, we would all be safer if clinical trials were published in the *New York Times* than in the *New England Journal of Medicine*."[115]

Continuing Medical Education (CME)

Almost 400 doctors crowded into the Astor Ballroom of the Marriot Marquis in Times Square in June 2002, "for a free dinner of filet mignon and red snapper and a lecture on depression drugs," as the *Wall Street Journal* reported. Lilly was the sponsor, and psychiatrist Jay Fawver spoke on behalf of Lilly's new antidepressant Cymbalta (duloxetine). He led off, "Ever hear of Prozac poop-out?" Dr. Fawver knew how to get a crowd going, for sure.

Not all were enthusiastic about these events. A practitioner in Livonia, Michigan, noted in 2002, "There is a wide misconception that by giving and attending such lectures [at steak dinners]—which unfortunately also form the backbone of the CME lecture circuit and where a few slides from the DSM are followed by the same old discussion on neurotransmitters and receptors and expressions of regret at the well-known side effects—one becomes proficient in the practice of psychiatry."[116]

By 2002, 36 states required doctors to take an average of 27 hours of courses or seminars a year in order to maintain their medical licenses. This was "continuing medical education" (CME). Between 1998 and 2007, industry funding of CME increased by more than 300 percent.[117] At UCLA, more than 50 percent of CME activity was industry funded. Barney Carroll called the UCLA program "a concatenation of deceits," as attendees received the corporate message on such leading questions as "Treatment-Refractory Depression: Is There a Role for Atypical Antipsychotics?" Carroll said, "Overall, it is difficult to avoid the impression that this so-called CME activity is a meretricious infomercial for Dr. [Charles] Nemeroff's corporate clients rather than a balanced educational event."[118]

Offering seminars for which participants received CME credits became one of industry's preferred means of reaching prescribers. Starting in 1983 the American Psychiatric Association (APA) permitted industry to stage sponsored programs for which the APA and the invited speakers received fees. At first, in 1983, there were 10 such symposia. (They were not CME events as such.) "The number has grown significantly in this first decade of the new century," reported the APA medical director Melvin Sabshin. "Many are in the evening, and the company serves dinner for the attendees." Sabshin thought it wonderful that industry would be willing to sponsor such splendid events.[119]

Because the companies were not allowed to market off-label indications directly at CME meetings, they had to do it indirectly. One Johnson & Johnson executive was quoted in a deposition as saying, "I do a fair amount of CME programs, and I signed this letter that says I can only talk about [approved] indications. However, I always plant a shill because if I get asked a question from the audience, I can then speak off label. So you never like go to a CME meeting without knowing ahead of time that somebody is going to ask you what about dementia."

Dr. Andrew Greenspan, assistant director of medical affairs at Janssen, said, "That's good practical advice."[120]

Henry Nasrallah's argument that industry-sponsored CME speakers didn't have a conflict of interest because they often worked for several competing drug companies was treated by readers as risible.[121] (On Nasrallah's own efforts as a KOL, see above in this chapter.)

All this transpired behind the scenes. As far as the average physician was concerned, the information supplied by the companies was very helpful. Insiders were scornful of the physicians in the trenches. In 1958, Ian Stevenson, professor of psychiatry and neurology at the University of Virginia, speaking to the House of Representatives, answered John Blatnik's (Minnesota) question about manipulative pharmaceutical advertising:

BLATNIK: "Do you know the scientific mind of the profession?"
STEVENSON: "It doesn't appeal to the scientific mind, it appeals to the irrational."
A CONGRESSMAN: "Isn't the physician by training capable of distinguishing?"
STEVENSON: "No, he is not. The average physician in my opinion is not capable of distinguishing. . . . He relies more and more, I think, upon the advertising of drug firms."[122]

But maybe this cynicism was out of place. Statistically, the confidence of the average physician in drug advertising had not been high. In 1969, the Division of Drug Advertising was created in the FDA, which increased the medical audience's confidence in the ads' content: The percentage of ads that MDs were said to find credible rose from 40 percent to 75 percent by 1974.[123] In 1992, a poll asked 428 physicians if they were satisfied with the medical information supplied by industry at CMEs and the like. "The physicians surveyed believe that medical education programs sponsored by pharmaceutical companies can be trusted to provide fair and unbiased information."[124] Some, such as former *New England Journal of Medicine* editor Arnold Relman, might have considered this degree of trust excessive. (In 2001, Relman warned against the infiltration of CME by Pharma marketing.[125])

"Depression Awareness" Campaigns

Before it became possible in 1997 to advertise prescription drugs directly to the public without including long lists of side effects, industry did the next best thing: advertising the diseases directly to the public. This happened in the form of "depression awareness"—as though the public hadn't a clue about depression and badly needed to be brought up to speed about industry's concern for them. The first such campaign was Lilly's "Depression Awareness Campaign," launched in April 1993. By August, sales of Prozac had grown 17 percent.[126] "Awareness" meant dollars.

Few PR opportunities could beat having your drug mentioned in a popular movie or TV series. The public relations people at Sandoz rubbed their hands with glee when the character played by Diana Ross, the lead singer of "The Supremes," was cured by clozapine of a terrible course of schizophrenia in the made-for-TV movie *Out of Darkness* (1994).[127] The companies often insisted, with little credibility, that they had nothing to do with such "placement."

Devising "depression forum campaigns" on college campuses was a stroke of marketing genius. Going on the seat-of-the-pants figure that "as much as 20 percent of the nation's student population takes antidepressants at some point in their college years" (*Wall Street Journal*), the companies hired such patients as 23-year-old Cara Kahn, star of an MTV reality show, to tour and explain how Wyeth's Effexor had saved her. A Wyeth spokesperson explained poo-faced, "We don't look on it as a marketing plan."[128]

Invasion

"Invasion" is not too strong a word. From the early 1960s on, clear-sighted authorities lamented the invasion of psychiatric education and practice by the drug houses. In 1961, Charles May, a professor at Columbia, ridiculed the whole idea that the companies were "educating" physicians. He contrasted "the drab and prosaic legitimate journals" with "the beautiful and exciting magazines" that industry gave away. No wonder that physicians almost always referred to drugs by brand rather than generic name. Looking ahead, he said, "Sooner or later there will be a wholesale opposition to pharmaceutical invasion of the field of medical education."[129]

In time, the invasion corrupted much of the content of the "drab" journals as well—at least in psychiatry. Attending a meeting of the American College of Neuropsychopharmacology (ACNP), Max Fink said in 2008, "Leaders of this organization are intimately tied to industry and they do not provide data that would permit a reasonable clinician to evaluate the benefits and risks of the new drugs. I have stopped prescribing any drug produced after 1980. . . . The data are very strongly compromised and I am sorry that this society has not taken a stronger position."[130]

In 2016, Mark Kramer, head of psychopharmacology for Merck in the 1990s, noted "the rapidity with which professional integrity has liquified under tons of money, greed, and influence."[131] This was an epitaph for the Age of Psychopharmacology. The corruption of the field happened because psychiatry had permitted the invasion of the pharmaceutical industry. Mickey Nardo said, "Harvard, Brown, Stanford and Emory stopped meaning what [they] used to mean. Even editorials became suspect; for that matter, so did textbooks. In psychiatry, famous doctors became drug representatives with cv's that weren't even possible—like hundreds and hundreds of articles. The author byline was more like celebrity endorsements than authorship."[132] Who could trust such confections?

14
Journals

As a young doctor, I saw the medical literature as something like the Library at Alexandria in ancient history. And in my medical lifetime, a big piece of it caught on fire.—Mickey Nardo (2012)[1]

At the end of the day, the ghostwriters had to get their manufactured articles published. This was their responsibility, not the responsibility of the supposed "authors." Given the enormous leverage with the journals that ad sales gave industry, the ghosters' task was not difficult.

It started to dawn on the editors that there was something fishy about the uniformly positive results. Richard Smith, former editor of the *British Medical Journal*, said in 2005 that "It took me almost a quarter of a century editing for the *BMJ* to wake up to what was happening." He noted that up to three quarters of trials published in the major journals "are funded by the industry." "The evidence is strong that companies are getting the results they want." Studies funded by companies, he said, "were four times more likely to have results favourable to the company than studies funded from other sources." The tricks that companies used to achieve such results are found throughout this book, but Smith listed them: "Conduct a trial of your drug against too high a dose of a competitor's drug, making your drug seem much less toxic" (see the discussion of atypical psychotic trials, run against high doses of Haldol), "use multiple endpoints in the trial and select for publication those that give favourable results" (see the discussion of Paxil trial 329), and so forth. The game was worth the candle. Smith: "For a drug company, a favourable trial is worth thousands of pages of advertising."[2]

As David Healy pointed out, for psychiatry as a whole, the average number of authors per agency-linked article was 6.6, versus 2.9 for non-agency-linked articles; the average agency-article length was 10.7 pages, versus 3.4 pages for non-agency; the average number of articles that agency-linked authors had written was 70, versus 37 for non-agency authors. And impactful! The citation rate for agency-sponsored articles was 20.2, for non-agency-sponsored articles it was 3.7.[3] The message: if you want your drug to be a marketplace hit, hire an agency to get the story out. (The notion that scientific communication should be conducted in this manner is bizarre.)

Mickey Nardo said that the drug companies had always had "detail men with plastic brains and free pens." There had always been medical journals with "glossy pages of ads. I never saw that as a problem."

"But then things changed. The peer-reviewed journals got thicker and were filled with clinical trial papers. The articles about the phenomenology of mental illness were replaced with reviews of medications and endless clinical trials."

"At first we didn't notice they were industry financed. Then we didn't notice the conflict of interest statements."

"Then we found out the authors didn't write them. And before long, our scientific journals filled up with articles that looked like the scientific articles of yore, but read like the stuff formerly in the throwaways."[4]

Re the journals bulging with articles: In 2004, Bernard (Barney) Carroll coined a term for them, "experimercial," meaning "a cost-is-no-object exercise driven by a corporate sponsor to create positive publicity for its product in a market niche."[5] One could also say "clinical trials driven by marketing plans rather than scientific inquiry."[6]

"Supplements" in publications like the *Journal of Clinical Psychiatry* or *Current Therapeutic Research* had the reputation of being promotional documents, written after "meetings" in resorts.[7] These had once undergone the same rigorous vetting as main articles. This vetting began to end after the 1960s, then worsened with the flood of SSRIs and atypical antipsychotics in the 1990s and after. Said one industry critic in 2011, "Articles in supplements have been unacceptable as sources for close to a decade, simply because they are known to be so biased, and are virtually always the result of a ghostwriter. Supplements became what are referred to as 'bird cage liners' decades ago, when the ad salespeople at journals took them over."[8] An egregious example of this shift into commercialism was believed to be Supplement 8 of the *Journal of Clinical Psychiatry,* which was financed by Janssen and contained such industry-friendly compositions as Charles Nemeroff's "Use of Atypical Antipsychotics in Refractory Depression and Anxiety."[9]

The journals' assignment included not only publishing manipulated propaganda, but also keeping bad news out. In June 2018, bioethics researcher Leemon McHenry penned a devastating indictment of many journals. "Most people trust that medical and scientific journals are reliable sources of knowledge. In the age of fake news and junk science, nothing could be further from the truth. Most medical and scientific journals are owned by large publishing corporations and there is growing evidence that those corporations serve the private interests of their client corporations rather than the medical and scientific community. In other words, the corruption of science and the corruption of the journals are parts of the same phenomena. Science counts for very little when there is big money at stake." McHenry himself suffered first-hand from corporate control when he submitted an article on the dangers of a Monsanto product. Initially, the article was accepted, but its publication was then inexplicably delayed because of a "best practices review." McHenry ultimately withdrew the article and submitted it to a new journal, the *International Journal of Risk & Safety in Medicine*, published in Amsterdam without corporate sponsors. The journal quickly accepted the McHenry piece.[10]

What else to avoid? Better not try *Medical World News*, a throwaway sustained entirely by advertising. According to Kenneth Feather, former director of the FDA's Division of Drug Advertising, the journal would solicit business from companies who wanted to see their ad next to a clinical article. "We know for a fact—and I know because some people have told me this—that if they're going to run an article on a cardiovascular drug, they will call the manufacturer of that drug and say, 'Do you want your ad next to this article?' Now, *Medical World News* will violently deny that if you were to ask them that. . . . We know it goes on, but there's nothing we can do about it."[11]

Here's an even more profitable idea. In the 1960s, *Current Therapeutic Research* rocketed to leadership, up from one clinical drug study in 1961–1962 to 27 in 1965–1966, more than any other journal.[12] What could possibly explain such success? It was a pay-for-play journal, as periodicals would later be called that asked the author or the company to pay for the privilege of publication. In 1960, Haskell Weinstein told the Senate's Kefauver Committee (the subcommittee that radically changed FDA regulation after the thalidomide scandal), how things functioned at *Current Therapeutic Research*: "[The journal] appears to be devoted entirely to pharmaceutical promotion. It accepts no advertising as such. However, there is a fee per page for any article published and publication is very prompt. The publisher's major source of income presumably is the lucrative reprint market."[13]

If you wanted to get into print elsewhere than *Current Therapeutic Research*, your results might be published because they were positive. Investigators found that, only 51 percent of antidepressant trials submitted to FDA were positive. By contrast, 94 percent of *published* antidepressant trials were positive. There was thus an enormous publication bias in favor of positive trials. What was unclear was whether the authors of negative studies didn't submit articles for publication, or whether the editors rejected them.[14] Jay Amsterdam mused in 2019, "Although I may sound a bit cynical, I have always wondered over the past 45 years of my reading various psychiatry reports how few 'negative' findings were ever published in psychiatric research journals, and how vast was the surfeit of interesting 'positive' findings that were published—although it was always a conundrum to me just how little clinical progress all of these positive findings made to our field *writ large*."[15] The issue of publication bias was of such import that it boiled over into a big story in 2008 in the *New York Times*. The piece quoted Jeffrey Drazen, editor of the *New England Journal of Medicine*: "We need to show respect for the people who enter a trial. They take some risk to be in the trial, and then the drug company hides the data? That kind of thing gets us pretty passionate about this issue."[16]

But what if your results were negative? If you had a negative trial, you could file it in the wastebasket. Frank Ayd recalls, "If the company said no don't publish that or we'll stop advertising, that article was rejected. . . . Some of our prestigious journals . . . don't want to publish anything that's not going to please their advertisers."[17]

Lisa Cosgrove and collaborators, in a critique of approvals of the antidepressant drug vortioxetine (FDA approval in 2013). First named Brintellix then renamed Trintellix, slammed the "Reporting of results [that] over-emphasized marginal statistical significance and ignored the small effect sizes, indicating a failure to reach clinical significance."[18] This important indictment finally appeared in an obscure journal because Cosgrove had tried in vain to get a major journal to accept it: She introduced the concept of "ghost management," not just "ghost author," because the RCT has a kind of show-runner, an industrial sponsor who buys off participants at every stage of the approval process.[19] So, buying off the bad news is a powerful thumb on the scales, for sure.

But how glorious were the *positive* results in print! Submitting trial data to the FDA meant playing things more or less straight. But the same data in published form sang a different song. Two investigators learned what happened when Lilly submitted the fluoxetine data for publication. "Results of the five fluoxetine trials submitted to the FDA indicate that fluoxetine has limited efficacy in the treatment of depression. However, a different story emerged in the published articles based on these data." Of the nine articles submitted on the basis of these trials, seven found fluoxetine superior to placebo.[20] The data had been adroitly massaged.

Moreover, until recently, even high-quality journals were reluctant to reject articles that manifestly had been ghost-written at corporate command. Jay Amsterdam and Leemon McHenry wrote scathingly, "In our view the authorship policy of the *American Journal of Psychiatry* is largely window dressing, common for journals of the sort that publish industry-sponsored trials."[21] After Marcia Angell's editorial "Is Academic Medicine for Sale?" in the *New England Journal of Medicine* in May 2000,[22] it became considerably harder to get industry-sponsored "infomercials" into print. As Jack Gorman told Charles Nemeroff in June 2000, the ghost author of a paroxetine paper, editors were now really on the alert for jury-rigged results and fake authorship. "Journals are now under fierce scrutiny about drug company sponsored studies, thanks in large part to Marcia Angell's recent stuff in the NEJM."[23] So, tone it down, Gorman said. Fierce scrutiny or not, by October 2000, Sally Laden had roared ahead with preparing

Nemeroff's Paxil article for him. She told "Charlie" that she had now revised the draft "along the lines suggested by Jack Gorman. . . . I think this version is sufficiently noncommercial and fulfils the directives outlined by the journal." If Nemeroff approved, she would "have the complete submission package put together for you."[24]

In 2004, the *American Journal of Psychiatry* published a positive account of Lundbeck's drug citalopram (marked in the United States by Forest Labs as Celexa).[25] As Jon Jureidini, Jay Amsterdam, and Leemon McHenry later demonstrated, the study had been ghosted from the get-go.[26] The real writer was Natasha Mitchner at Weber Shandwick Communications, under instruction from Forest's marketing manager. Karen Wagner at the University of Texas Medical Branch at Galveston, who had run a site for the study, was recruited as one of the "authors" of the ghosted paper, although she had no role in its analysis or in the preparation of the first draft. Robert Findling, then at Case Western Reserve, was signed up as another author. The data in the article were completely manipulated in order to turn an essentially negative study positive and to win FDA approval of the indication. In 2009, the FDA, in a decision based in part on the citalopram trial, approved citalopram's sister drug escitalopram (Lexapro) for adolescent depression.

Behind the scenes, it was a story of deceit and manipulation as Forest Labs lied and distorted the data. It was, in other words, a fairly typical event. But what is of interest in the story is the ease with which Forest Labs placed the paper in the *American Journal of Psychiatry*, contrasted with the difficulties that the whistleblowers encountered in getting their critical study published. In 2017, the three whistleblowers published an account of three fraudulent trials in a Polish psychiatric journal.[27] Why such a curious venue? Amsterdam explained in an email, "An article of this sort has never been accepted for publication in a peer-reviewed psychiatric journal. Thus, the appearance of this article represents the first published, forensic deconstruction of research misconduct in a peer-reviewed medical journal." He commended the staff of *Psychiatria Polska* for "showing the moral compass and ethical backbone to publish such an article."[28]

Forest was no exception. A study in 2008 led by Kristin Rising at the Medical School of the University of California San Francisco found extensive prettyfacing of trial data submitted to the FDA: "Reporting sometimes differed between trials as they were described in FDA reviews and their corresponding publications. These changes included the addition or deletion of outcome changes, changes in statistical significance of reported outcomes, and changes in overall trial conclusion." Furthermore, 47 percent of the negative outcomes reported to the FDA were not published at all.[29] (One trialist who had participated in 27 trials largely before Kefauver-Harris told Congress in 1968 that in only nine of them were data submitted to FDA.[30])

Editors and referees are called upon to exercise critical judgment, but they often don't. In 2008, one group had reported results of a trial of the atypical antipsychotic aripiprazole in "refractory depression." Barney Carroll saw a number of holes. The drug had beaten placebo by only 2.8 points on the Montgomery-Asberg scale, a finding that was "statistically significant," maybe, but scarcely clinically significant. Aripiprazole is a powerful drug: How much unblinding had there been as the subjects realized what they were on? The patients had gained a lot of weight. Why was this not reported in the paper's Abstract? And there was a great deal of "akathisia" (in 26 percent of the subjects); akathisia is a kind of nervous restlessness that may conduce to suicide. The authors said nothing about suicide or suicidality. "In summary, although the drug beat placebo, evidence for the efficacy of aripiprazole in refractory depression is modest at best."[31] This is a perfect example of jury-rigging the reporting to make the drug appear in the most favorable possible light. No numbers were made up. But they were relentlessly massaged, and the "editorial support" of a medical communications company was acknowledged. Several of the authors were Bristol-Myers Squibb employees. Such an article is like a stinking fish, but the literature is full of them. They get published because editors need the favor of industry in their advertising pages.

In 2016, Amsterdam, McHenry, and Jureidini traced the difficulties they encountered in getting their exposé of the Forest Labs' scandal published. "Contrary to the commonly held belief that medical journals are trusted repositories for reliable medical information, it is extremely difficult to publish criticism of misleading, false and fraudulent reports of pharmaceutical-industry-sponsored research." They pointed to the conflicts of interest in advertising in "even the most well-respected medical journals." Over the course of a year, they had experienced five rejections. The *Journal of Affective Disorders* declined even to review their paper, and it was rejected by *JAMA Psychiatry* without peer review. The *Journal of Clinical Psychopharmacology* responded primly, "We do not share your concerns about what you term 'ghostwriting'—more properly described as manuscript preparation assistance." (!)[32]

The three whistleblowers issued this indictment of academic publishing in psychiatry: "When the probability of having a ghostwritten, fraudulent, industry-sponsored clinical trial accepted for publication in a high-impact medical journal is substantially higher than the probability of having a critical deconstruction of the same trial accepted, there can be no confidence in the medical literature. In this regard, medical journals, contrary to common opinion, are not reliable sources of medical knowledge. They are guilty of publishing pseudoscience and have become, in the words of former *BMJ* editor Richard Smith, '*an extension of the marketing arm of pharmaceutical companies.*'"[33]

How should we proceed, given this litany of obstacles to finding effective drugs for real diseases? More rigorous statistical analyses? No, said Mark Kramer, the opposite. (Keep in mind that Kramer was among the most knowledgeable of insiders, responsible for getting results from budgets of hundreds of millions of dollars.) What works really well, he said, were small trials "in 5–10 well-chosen patients." Yet industry had discontinued the small trials by 1995, just as Kramer was leading psychopharm research at Merck. (The small trials were known, he said, as Phase 1b studies.) What was established instead was "an era of biostatistical hegemony. Today, instead of fixing the fundamental problem, dilution of samples [heterogeneous populations of "depression"], we engage in endless missives from the side show barkers: biostatistical estimation of 'truth.' " He mentioned confidence intervals, p-values, and meta-analyses. "Compared with the big picture, this is just sophisticated mind candy."

So, just a few patients, observed closely: had this been done this before? Kramer continued, "Remember that the clinical effects of imipramine and MAOIs were initially large, easy to spot in small numbers of earmarked patients. . . . Yet today statistical analyses are required to discern clinically meager group-wise antidepressant effects. To do so, 5-fold more patients are required now than in the 50s/early 60s." And these large, expensive trials with their highly "diluted" clinical populations have found few new drugs, "causing Big Pharma to exit the field, at least for now."[34]

Bottom line: Through highly manipulable RCTs, journal articles made the new antidepressant and antipsychotic agents seem effective. This "evidence" trapped primary care doctors into practicing bad medicine. Healy argued that, "Because these agents have been shown by RCTs to 'work,' we have promoted a situation . . . in which primary-care prescribers and others, besieged by the mass of community nervous problems and all but impotent to do much for them, have been trapped by the weight of supposed scientific evidence into indiscriminately handing out psychotropic drugs on a huge scale."[35]

The journals, then, are the font of "the literature," a term that is invested with the solemnity of science. Yet, in the opinion of many clinicians, this "logarithmically expanding literature," with its avalanche of statistical tables and p-values, is of little assistance in the practice of psychiatry. New York psychiatrist Ivan Goldberg said, "The question of how to treat patients with bipolar depression is probably one for which a review of the literature is not likely to provide an answer." Georgia psychiatrist Floyd Garrett added, "The value of the literature for the practicing clinician is very slight—in my opinion, almost nil. The true importance of the literature lies not in the consulting room but the board room and the court room." Why, therefore, is there so much of it? Garrett said, "The literature exists for payors, plaintiff attorneys, government, journalists, and, of course, those whose business it is to produce the literature, academics & etc."

What are the consequences for patient care? Devastating? Not at all. Garrett said, "We have a generally accepted practical pharmacopeia, rules of the road, tips, pearls, and accumulated experience. Every medication in use helps some and doesn't help others and sometimes causes problems. Little or none of this knowledge derives from recent medical literature. When we want help, we go to colleagues with experience."[36]

15

FDA

The task [of the FDA] is to make sure that all drugs are safe and effective for use. But what does that really mean? No drug is safe and no drug is fully effective.—Paul Leber (2011)[1]

There was a time when industry and the Food and Drug Administration (FDA) were at loggerheads, and any view before the 1990s that FDA was somehow in industry's pocket was completely off base. As Lou Lasagna said in 1973, "[We have to] drop the adversary confrontation posture of the past, where all too often the FDA monitors looked on industry folk as evil geniuses trying to subvert them and to delude them. And for their part, the industry people looked on the FDA people as obstructionists."[2] Lasagna and William Wardell, who was the other big regulatory specialist in psychopharmacology, said in the *Journal of the American Medical* Association in 1975, "It is an extraordinary perversion of justice to accuse present FDA leadership of pro-industry bias." The authors had little use for the " 'consumerists,' who often have only a narrow interest and are obsessed by a pathologic hatred of the drug industry."[3] Later it may have been true that FDA was, more or less, a "captive agency," accommodating the interests it was supposed to regulate.[4]

But it could hardly be seen as in industry's pocket. It was too slow in approving drugs to be a handmaiden. To outsiders, the FDA seemed pokey, inefficient, and burdened with an excess of caution. Excessive review times came to be seen as a major barrier in international drug competition, and in the 1990s a number of steps were undertaken to shorten them. It is a measure of the resistance to change of this vast bureaucracy that review times, from the beginning of clinical testing to approval, remained stuck at 8 years.[5] The United States was, for example, the fiftieth country in which lithium became available (in 1970).[6] The paper load needed to satisfy the regulatory authorities about the safety and efficacy of Pfizer's ketamine was 120 pages in Mexico, 159 pages in Switzerland and Germany each, and 72,200 pages in the United States.[7]

Then there was the fixation upon a single number, the "0.05 level of significance." Paul Leber said at one point of schizophrenia trials—at a time when transcripts of meetings of the Psychopharmacologic Drugs Advisory Committee

(PDAC) were treated as confidential documents—"[We have to assume] that there is in fact a number that will stand for the effect of the drug. It is a total fiction. We all know that some drugs have whopping effects in one individual and no effect in another. So we start off with a model that is unrealistic, but we are using it because it is a way to make a decision in a public way that seems to account for something that might happen by chance. . . . It is even possible these drugs made people worse in some cases. But you are not going to approve a drug that makes people worse unless, on average, it makes more people better. So you end up using this convenience of a central measure of tendency and accept the variation."[8] (Of course this problem of variation would be acute in "schizophrenia," which is not a disease of its own but a heterogeneous mixture of different diseases, such as catatonia.)

Thus, the obstacle that stood between a drug and the market was approval by the FDA. Drug trials had turned into a kind of travesty of science: the purpose of the trial being not obtaining new information but gaining regulatory approval. Over the half-century history of the randomized controlled trial (RCT), the main narrative line was the degradation of clinical trials from instruments of scientific curiosity to mechanisms for the registration of drugs.

The FDA had assessed the efficacy of prescription agents—meaning whether the drug worked or not—long before the FDA Act of 1938.[9] But only with the 1962 Kefauver-Harris Amendments, which were a response to the thalidomide tragedy, did Congress mandate the FDA to do so formally.[10] This sounded like a good idea, but there were problems.

One was the inability of what had been a law-enforcement agency to come to terms with detailed drug applications. In 1964, 2 years after the Kefauver-Harris Amendments had mandated establishing efficacy, Joseph Sadusk, the FDA's medical director, told the Commissioner, that "At last report we had a backlog of about 800 pending supplemental NDAs on drugs for human use."[11] So we are just going to wave them through. (This would be comparable to declaring people could now wear jeans and flip-flops to work.) Especially under FDA Commissioner James Goddard (1962-66), the agency began a ninety-degree course correction in the direction of judging efficacy.[12] The new mission meant an enormous change in size: the FDA grew from around 600 employees in 1934 to 9,000 in 1974.[13] Because of the need to evaluate for efficacy all the New Drug Applications (NDAs), the share of FDA staff in field organizations fell from 78 percent around 1955 to 38 percent after Kefauver-Harris.[14]

As central control tightened, a handful of administrators in the Center for Evaluation of Drug Research (CDER) became major players. One was Thomas Laughren, director of the psychiatry drugs division. Well before his retirement in 2012, people were calling Laughren out as overly friendly to industry. In 2008, Fox News ran a special on the dangers to children of the antipsychotic medications then being widely prescribed, and in an interview, Stephen Sheller pointed the finger directly at Laughren, "who many say has been turning a blind eye to the dangerous side effects [of Risperdal] out of deference to his friends in the pharmaceutical industry." Sheller said, "He's been accused of major conflicts of interest, ghost authoring studies supporting new diagnoses to use these drugs—and he is not protecting the public health, he is protecting the drug industry's profit."[15] Confidence in Laughren's independence was not strengthened when he left the FDA in 2012 and became a consultant for firms that he had previously regulated.

The primary outcome measure, as we have seen, is usually regarded as sacred—and efforts are made to prevent massaging the data after the unblinding, as happened in the SmithKline trial of Paxil for pediatric depression (see Chapter 17). Yet changing the endpoint before the unblinding is acceptable to the FDA, and though it doesn't happen often, it's not seen as an offense.[16]

The FDA did not have its own ideas about what constituted a "disease" and generally speaking was willing to accept the sponsor's definition for something like schizophrenia. This opened the door to chaos. Ron Kartzinel, director of the Division of Neuropharmacology, told the PDAC in 1978 that the FDA almost never argued with a company over diagnostic criteria: "[As for] the criteria that FDA uses for being included as a schizophrenic in a drug trial, I don't think that is really written down anywhere in granite. The proposals that come from industry are highly variable and it partly depends on the reviewer and partly depends on the drug and what the drug company wants to do with it as to what the criteria are." Every company had different criteria. So there might be a difference between "designs for a very pure group of patients [in an] efficacy trial" and "diagnostic criteria for medical and treatment purposes, but I think those two sets of criteria are totally different."[17]

Surrounding every recent edition of the *Diagnostic and Statistical Manual of Mental Disorders* (DSM) has been a discussion about "dimensional" diagnoses versus "categorical diagnoses," and these discussions have been uniformly lost by those who preferred seeing distress on a scale of 0 to 100 rather than as an array of distinct diseases. And they have lost largely because FDA opposed the "dimensional" model of defining illness (few diseases, but lots of degrees of illness) on the grounds that it opened the door to returning to the days of psychoanalysis, when everyone belonged to the "walking wounded." Paul Leber said in an interview, "A dimensional diagnostic system allows virtually everyone to be classified as suffering from a psychiatric disorder."[18] The FDA preferred categorical diagnoses, and insisted that industry use them.

This decision was not without consequences. In 1996, David Healy described the role of the FDA in the "contemporary construction of psychiatric knowledge." Accepting the "highly categorical view of mental illness of DSM encourage[s] the impression that there are a number of discrete targets in psychiatry that the pharmaceutical industry could profitably design magic bullets to hit."[19]

FDA Swallows "Major Depression"

In theory, the FDA does not devise diagnoses. In practice, it sort of does. At a meeting in December 1981 of the PDAC, Hillary Lee, leader of the FDA group reviewing Hoecht's nomifensine (Merital), said of depression, "One of the ways we have been going here at the FDA lately, is that these are separate, not totally distinct indications, but separate indications [hospitalized vs. outpatients] and if a drug has shown effect both in inpatients and outpatients, then we so label it, and I was thinking as a point of discussion that this drug would be for outpatients." Thus, her group at FDA, at least, upheld the former distinction between melancholia, or endogenous depression (inpatients) and "reactive" depression (outpatients).[20]

John Overall, one of the founding figures in psychopharm and a member of the committee, was more emphatic in this discussion: "I would strongly plea not to restrict labeling to DSM-III criteria . . . because the major disease syndromes in DSM-III are essentially oblivious to the important phenomenologic distinctions upon which the selection of treatment is actually based in clinical practice, such as the distinction between retarded depressions and anxious depressions and hostile depressions."[21]

Yet by 2000 the die was cast: the various forms of depressive illness no longer existed as entities for the FDA. The only depression the agency was willing to recognize was "major depressive disorder."[22] Leber made it clear in private that he thought much of DSM was a pile of nonsense. He told David Healy in 2008,

> Well, hell, I know depression covers thousands of things, some of them probably endogenomorphic and driven by a gene, some of them not at all. I don't know. I don't even how many schizophrenias there are, how many dementias there are and so on. . . . How would you communicate that somebody gave you a praecox feeling—would this particular subset of phenomena respond well to this drug or not? It would be idiosyncratic and impossible to communicate and therefore we don't use it. Clearly these drugs aren't used by psychiatrists alone. They are used by GPs. We felt it would be useful if we could give them a fairly standard description. That's all it's intended to be.[23]

This passage, astonishing for its realism about official diagnosis, did not make it into print. But scientific diagnostics? Nobody home at FDA.

The Temple-Leber Show

As we know, many antidepressants came before the FDA for approval. Despite often terrible clinical performances in trials, some of them had to be approved. This was the problem Temple and Leber faced: They couldn't reject everything. Temple said, with a certain world-weariness in 2018—he had been with FDA for over 40 years—"A typical result would be, you start out at a HAM-D [score] of 24, 25. The placebo group will change by 10 or 12 and the drug group will change by 14. That's the difference." Two points on the Hamilton Depression Scale would not be a big improvement over placebo. Temple added, "But there are huge changes in both groups."[24] This was the problem in antidepressant trials. Often recruited through newspaper ads and not really depressed in the classical sense (although yes in the DSM sense), the subjects in trials were highly placebo responsive. So, although the drugs brought about big improvements, so did the placebos.

On the subject of schizophrenia, the regulators tied themselves in knots. Were neuroleptic drugs "antipsychotic" or "antischizophrenic"? Leber said in 1985, "We [have] agreed to fall back upon the idea that psychosis was the target of most neuroleptic treatment, knowing full well in the back of our minds that most examples of chronic psychotic behavior . . . are attributed to schizophrenia, whatever that really is."[25]

For any kind of scientific rigor in standardizing what a diagnosis actually meant, this was a nightmare. The FDA tried to cut through this knot later in the 1980s by insisting that industry use DSM-III criteria in trials. But since the DSM criteria were highly heterogeneous, this foreclosed any scientific possibility of indicating specific drugs for specific illnesses.

Congress had not specified that trials combine RCTs with placebos, insisting only that the assessments of drugs be "well-controlled." The FDA, however, interpreted that to mean placebo-controlled trials, and stipulated that the trial must have two arms: the active drug and the placebo. Some companies included a third arm, an "active comparator." Yet the FDA was cool to this, and outright refused psychopharmacology trials with two active drugs and no placebo.

It was Paul Leber, head of the FDA's Neuropharmacology Division after 1983, who imposed the placebo doctrine on FDA: only placebo-controlled trials could show a difference.[26] Leber said, "The problem with active controlled trials that do not show a difference is you cannot tell from the trial that you are having a drug effect." (The tied results could be a placebo effect.) There was also the problem of "assay sensitivity," maybe the clinical population was not capable of responding to your drug. (Leber used the example of dental patients not responding to morphine. Such morphine trials in dentistry would therefore lack assay sensitivity. A placebo control would show whether the clinical population was responsive to the assay.[27]) Taken with the best of intentions, the decisions nonetheless had the effect of lowering the approvals bar considerably. All you needed was two trials (out of however many you conducted) where your drug beat placebo and was safe (all trial data were supposedly used in assessing safety)—Later, it was one trial. The advantage for industry of placebo rather than an active comparator was that fewer participants were required to demonstrate efficacy. The disadvantage for psychopharmacology was that a host of quasi ineffective medications—the SSRIs—gained FDA approval.

In theory, all trials were sent to FDA for the evaluation of safety, and Bob Temple stated that this was the case.[28] In practice, it was not the case. At a meeting of the PDAC in 2004, Sam Maldonado, the industry representative on the committee and head of pediatric drug development at Johnson & Johnson, said, "I am sorry to bring you back to the BPCA [Best Pharmaceuticals for Children Act, 2002] and rule. I want to clarify the point, the failed trials that the FDA is seeing right now have been an issue of cost of doing business for the pharmaceutical industry for generations. When those so-called negative trials happen, the pharmaceutical industry doesn't even bother to come into the FDA with those trials because they know they are not going to get anything out of that."[29] So much for the rigorous submission of all data.

FDA disclaimed any effort to seek the best treatment—in other words, to compare two drugs—and if you, as a sponsor, went ahead and compared your drug to another, FDA would insist on a test "under conditions of actual use" and not just in a controlled trial. Wyeth, for example, had the trial data to show that their drug Ativan (lorazepam) beat Valium in treating status epilepticus (a potentially fatal condition). Nope, said Leber, that's not good enough. You can't advertise it.[30]

In general, FDA's insistence on trials with placebo, not with the industry standard, created conditions for declining effectiveness. Leber said, "[Our goal] is to demonstrate the efficacy of the drug. It is not to assess the comparative efficacy of two drugs. . . . We usually look at, does the drug work in some global way, and not how it works in comparison to others."[31] This stance was, alas, a recipe for a decline in efficacy of the pharmacopoeia; the proposed agents were never proved more efficacious than existing agents—and sometimes, as in the case of the SSRIs, they were clearly *less* efficacious.

Academics found maddening the rigidity of FDA's insistence on two placebo-controlled trials as essential for proving efficacy. Leo Hollister thought the requirement overblown, and told Frank Ayd in an interview, "I call this a massive scientific overkill, because even my early controlled trials were not very necessary. All I had to do was, give these drugs to a patient and watch him. You knew damn well something was happening."[32] Don Klein had similar views, but Paul Leber scoffed: "I've listened to Don Klein many times say, give me a drug, I'll tell you whether it works. Well, I'm not so sure he can tell me in a way that I can hear."

He may tell me that he believes a drug works. He may in fact be right, but we are unable to listen to him unless he presents it in a form where we really can know in a public way that the drug works."[33] In terms of regulatory logic this probably made some sense, but it was that logic that deformed the development of American psychopharmacology.

"Efficacy": A Good Idea?

At the end of the day, is assessing drugs for "efficacy" actually such a good idea? It has a kind of feel-good aura: Of course we want our drugs to be effective! Congress meant well when it inserted the idea in the 1962 Kefauver-Harris legislation. But it had the effect of diverting Pharma's scientific support "from discovery to validation," as Don Klein put it.[34] The great number of PhDs and MDs employed in industry became increasingly caught up in the drug approval process rather than the drug discovery process. Loud were the complaints about the long paper trail the FDA demanded, and "truckloads" of documents went off from places like Merck's headquarters in Rahway, New Jersey, to the Parklawn Building of the FDA. Reassuring though all the documentation might have been to the bureaucratic mind, it was scientifically pointless.

More seriously, the need to demonstrate efficacy led to such widespread cheating that the literature of the entire field became untrustworthy. Do the "antidepressants" actually work? We don't really know that. In the old system, individual physicians established their own opinions about efficacy on the basis of experience. Mickey Nardo began his medical career as an internist. He said in 2013,

> Thinking back to my days in internal medicine, most of what I learned about medications was OJT (on the job training), more on the apprentice model than from books and articles. . . . As the years passed, it was my own experience with a particular medication that mattered the most. I think I grew up with the model that we all did our own "clinical trials." Again, as strange as it sounds today, that was almost a code of honor. Learning to use medications was like learning to discriminate heart murmurs with a stethoscope or palpate the gall bladder in a jaundiced patient. And that model followed me into psychiatry.[35]

It was probably a mistake to give the FDA such control over the practice of medicine via its ability to declare what is risky and what is not. The FDA was designed to be a regulatory agency, not a scientific one. Then there was the unsuitability of a federal bureaucracy, highly sensitive to political opinion, making scientific judgments. Morris Fishbein, a real old-timer in the drug scene who was editor or assistant-editor of the *Journal of the American Medical Association* from 1913 to 1949, thought that judging efficacy was a terrible idea. He told an interviewer in 1968, "I fought bitterly as an individual against attempting to make the Food and Drug Administration pass on efficacy. I don't think they can. I don't think they are capable as a government—as a political organization—to pass on a scientific problem."[36] As Malcolm R. Stephens, then retired as Associate Commissioner, pointed out in an interview in 1984, "When I retired [in 1965] I remember saying that I hope that the people in Food and Drug will never forget that this is a regulatory agency. That's all it is, and all it will ever be. And don't let them tell you that it's going to become a scientific investigational unit. Some of that's necessary and all, but this is a regulatory agency."[37] (Stephens was doubtless mindful that a year after he himself retired, James Goddard became Commissioner, and furthered dramatically the political involvement of the FDA—Congressional and HEW pressures being incompatible, of course, with good science.)

Rolling the FDA

The trials can be gamed. The companies choose their own "dictionaries" of side effects to report to the FDA and there is room for maneuver here. When GlaxoSmithKline (GSK) was doing trials for Paxil in pediatric depression, they coded thoughts of suicide under "emotional lability." This rang an alarm at FDA. Tom Laughren told the PDAC in 2004, "The Paxil review did raise a question, in that events suggestive of suicidality were coded under the general preferred term 'emotional lability.' This struck the reviewer as rather odd, and so in responding to GSK, we asked them to separate out the verbatim terms suggestive of suicidality." The results were alarming. In one of the pediatric trials, the suicide risk on Paxil was six times higher than the risk on placebo.[38] In 1995, when Johnson & Johnson submitted the side-effects data for their antiepileptic and mood drug topiramate (Topamax), Bob Temple scolded them for having concealed serious symptoms under anodyne labels: "In some cases, the severity of the event was severely understated; a patient described as 'agitated' in fact killed his mother."[39]

There are other ways of cooking the data. (Some of which are reviewed in Chapters 12 and 13.) Patients with really nothing can be made to sound seriously depressed, then experience marvelous relief on the sponsor's drug. Michael Alan Taylor said, "I happened to pass the waiting area for [a] study when the first subject showed up. I chatted with her and could detect few signs of depression. She was animated and in good humor. Patients with depressive illness are *never* animated and in good humor. Later that day, I asked our study site coordinator what the subject's score was on the rating scale and I was told '24.' On that scale, a score of 24 meant substantial depression that should be easily identified. The industry bias is to make the subject appear as ill as possible so that the new drug being tested looks more effective than it actually is."[40]

Thus, exactly what to report to the FDA constituted a kind of fine art in cutting corners. Clearly, a patient's death during a trial would look bad, so sometimes companies simply didn't report them. In a trial of the benzodiazepine lorazepam that Wyeth Labs conducted at the Cushing Hospital in Framingham, Massachusetts, there was a patient who died, "and whose records were apparently eliminated from the study," an FDA inspector reported in 1976. Evidently, by that time it was ancient history and no further action was taken.[41]

In 1994, Upjohn suppressed a death during a trial of its blockbuster panic drug Xanax. There had been a special in-house meeting where a consultant told the firm, "We cannot have a death."

The dialogue around the table went something like this:

THE UPJOHN COMMITTEE: "The patient wasn't technically on the study when he died."
RESPONSE: "But he was on Xanax when he died."
COMMITTEE: "The study wasn't a panic study."
RESPONSE: "Yes it was a panic study."
COMMITTEE: "But it wasn't a key panic study."
RESPONSE: "It was starred as one of the key studies."

The committee finally decided not to report the death to FDA, but the agency found out about it anyway.[42]

There was little actual making up of numbers, which could be a felony and end a company's reputation. But it did happen. FDA referred to made-up information as "graphite data," as Dale Console explained, "data derived from a pencil rather than from lab studies."[43] In 1961, the FDA blew the whistle on the William S. Merrell Company of Cincinnati for having grossly falsified the data in an NDA (New Drug Application) for its new anticholesterol drug MER-29. The company was convicted in court.[44] In 1981, Theodore Maraviglia, a retired FDA regional director, recalled in an interview, "That was the earliest outstanding incident of clinical investigators falsifying data."[45] To be sure, Sen. Ted Kennedy's hearings in 1978 did uncover evidence of outright fraud in the industry as a whole.[46] Yet that covers a lot of ground. I can only say that in my own research I have seen little fraud beyond the occasional unreported suicide.

Beneath the level of outright fraud, there was a lot of massaging of results, turning nonsignificant results into significant data with various kinds of jury-rigging. Pfizer had huge difficulty getting Zoloft (sertraline) through the FDA because the trial results had been so poor. Interested, Nardo ordered the original

NDA on a disk from the FDA under the Freedom of Information Act and went back and recalculated some of the results. Pfizer had claimed in an article in 1995 that low doses of Zoloft were just as effective as high doses[47] (and would, of course have fewer side effects). Nardo's recalculation established that this wasn't true. "I'll have to say that I didn't expect this much sleight of hand that long ago, but *it is what it is,* as they say. And *what it is,* is really bad."[48]

How many side effects should the NDA report to the FDA? For industry, the answer was as few as possible. In submitting the NDA for Prozac, Lilly said the incidence of sexual dysfunction was "under 1 percent." They later "grudgingly acknowledged 30 percent," said Harvard's Carl Salzman. "Most physicians find it to be 90 percent," he noted. What were the causes of the underreporting? Bob Temple, head of Office of Drug Evaluation I, said, "When you ask questions with a questionnaire . . . you get a very distorted idea of what the adverse reactions are." Lilly used a checklist, and patients were quizzed rather than allowed to volunteer information. The FDA's own spontaneous reporting system for side effects produced much higher rates of adverse effects. "What is going on in the [medical] community can surely affect the reports [doctors' reports to FDA] by a factor of 10. After the report ascribing suicidality to Prozac, we saw a roughly tenfold increase in reports of suicidal ideation," Temple said.[49]

The Label

The various bureaucratic complexities show how greatly the regulatory system in psychopharmacology was formed by politics, by internal bureaucratic logic, and by commercial pressures. The resultant, or outcome, of these efforts was the "label," or "package insert," that the sponsor designed and the FDA had to approve. The label includes the instructions for use of the drug, and layer after layer of bureaucracy added on long sections. The label for Valium, for example, lists "contraindications," "warnings," "precautions" (different from warnings), and "adverse reactions": all before the physician's weary eyes reached "dosage and administration."[50] In 1977, Leo Hollister commented about this mish-mash, "The package insert has become a monstrosity, generally representing the least common denominator of disagreement between the lawyers of the FDA and those of the drug company. It has little to do with medical science."[51] Exactly. The FDA had turned the science of drug development into a series of rituals.

The trials were psychopharmacology's main claim to being a science. And when they turned out to be pseudoscience, the game was lost.

PART III
SCIENCE DISASTER

16

Prozac and Its Cousins

[The Prozac] branding message dumbed down clinical depression to a mostly trivial condition and removed the brakes from pragmatic prescribing for nonspecific unhappiness. That's what marketing departments do.—Barney Carroll (2016)[1]

Some things never change. People have always believed that they have something. Daniel Cathell, a family doctor in Baltimore, wrote in 1882: "Almost everyone is filled with the belief that he is debilitated. Say to the average patient, 'You are weak and need building up,' and you will instantly see that you have struck his key-note. . . . Many of the sick, fully impressed with this idea, will want you to treat them with tonics and stimulants."[2]

Today, it requires no great stretch of the imagination to substitute "depressed" for "debilitated," and to substitute Prozac for "tonics." The World Health Organization (WHO) has sped things along with their questionable statistics on "the global burden of depression."[3] Bernard Carroll commented, "Every Pharma-commissioned, ghostwritten article on antidepressants highlights those dubious WHO estimates—it's like a ritual genuflection in the service of disease mongering."[4] (It was true that Sally Laden's articles often began by evoking the fearsome "global burden.")

There has always been a need to deal with the great amorphous mass of unhappiness, anxiety and dejection. That is the role of community psychiatry. Religion once filled this role, then it was tonics, then the barbiturates, then new agents in the 1950s, such as Miltown. The 1960s and 70s brought the benzodiazepines, such as Librium and Valium. Each of these remedies was then defeated by the next new drug set. In the late 1980s, the new drug set was Prozac and its cousins, the so-called SSRIs. Yet the SSRI "antidepressants" turned out to be substantially ineffective. "No more than a third of patients show a response to medication that they would not achieve with placebos," said Roger P. Greenberg, a psychologist at Upstate University Hospital in Syracuse who had studied extensively the trial literature.[5] Unfortunately, the poor efficacy of these drugs, combined with the omnipresence of the new diagnosis "major depression," had the result of trivializing the practice of psychiatry to the point that its great psychopharmacologic arm, once so powerful, dangled uselessly in the byways of commerce.

But did the antidepressants really treat old-fashioned depression? Upjohn sought a depression indication for its new drug Xanax (alprazolam). Paul Leber said in a committee discussion in 1982, "There is probably a point where it is clearly an antidepressant, and it crosses over; it becomes less and less effective in the collection of patients called depressed, where you can't call it an antidepressant anymore. . . . What does it mean to say a patient is severely depressed? Each of us might say terrible anguish, terrible suicidality? If you were doing that, these patients rated very, very low in many scales—that's why they're outpatients."[6] In fact, Xanax ended up being indicated for anxiety and panic disorder, although it was often prescribed for depression as well.

In our search for new antidepressants, one bears in mind that just about any psychoactive drug is an antidepressant, in that it shifts the mood and cognition parameters a couple of notches in some direction. (The problem today in discovering new antidepressants is not a shortage of drugs that act on depression. It is the high placebo responsiveness.) Every drug class in the history of psychiatry has been touted by someone, at some point, as an antidepressant. And there is gold in them thar hills. Acting on the amorphous mass of unhappiness has meant great profits for the pharmaceutical industry. Critic Charles Barber wrote, "Antidepressants have been the most profitable product in the most profitable industry in the most profitable country in the world."[7]

Just How Dangerous Is Depression, Anyway?

In the background was a question about just how dangerous depression was as a disease. And in February 1983, the Psychopharmacologic Drugs Advisory Committee (PDAC) hacked this over. Linda Kessler (a psychopharm group leader at FDA), said that a sponsor brings in a drug as an antidepressant. "Is it sufficient to show that a drug gets the broad spectrum claim of an antidepressant? Do you want to see sicker patients? Do you want to have inpatient studies be a requirement for an antidepressant claim? Do you want to see the HAM-D ratings higher than the HAM-A [anxiety] to make sure that they are depressed?"

Tom Detre, at the University of Pittsburgh, then asked, does it really matter? "95 to 98 percent of all depressed patients are outpatients." [This statistic could be upheld only if huge numbers of outpatients received the diagnosis of depression.]

Paul Leber then said that the FDA had to be very careful. "The risk we run is what happens if you have a drug that is ineffective in a particularly dangerously ill segment of the population? If you put that drug on the market, you have what

I would call dilution of the therapeutic armamentarium. You are displacing individuals from the opportunity of getting treated with an effective drug because you have an ineffective one on the market."[8]

One reads these lines with a shudder, because this is exactly what happened when the SSRIs were introduced 4 years later. The therapeutic armamentarium was diluted when a drug class ineffective in serious, hospitalized, suicidal depression displaced the previous classes of antidepressants that were in fact effective—although not as much as ECT—in the treatment of real depressive illness. Just how the FDA was persuaded to go along with this remains obscure. Leber has now left the FDA, and he has never told us. But it is one of the big questions in the troubled history of psychopharmacology.

Prozac and Its Cousins

> I hope Patrick realizes that Lilly can go down the tubes if we lose Prozac.—Leigh Thompson (1990)[9]

In 1993, the SSRI sales force for SmithKlineBeecham's Paxil was 1,800 representatives, for Lilly's Prozac, 1,600, for Pfizer's Zoloft, 1,250.[10] The SSRIs surfed forward on the greatest promotional tide in the history of American medicine. Effective? Absolutely effective for all depressions! And safe? Much safer than the dangerous old tricyclic antidepressants (TCAs) went the hype. As for the benzodiazepines, prescribing them was characterized as prescribing rat poison. This is an old meme in advertising: detailing your own product by "counter-detailing" the competition, and the TCAs were relentlessly counter-detailed.

The SSRIs became a biochemical carnival. And if we want to know why the science of psychopharmacology died, it was killed off by the most widely prescribed psychiatric drug class in history. By the time the last SSRI went off patent (Lexapro in 2012), the notion that "vitamin serotonin" had anything to do with science was laughable.

Yet in the beginning there was pure science. In 1963, Alec Coppen at the MRC Neuropsychiatry Unit at West Park Hospital proposed an apparent link between serotonin and depression,[11] In a story told elsewhere, investigators at Lilly Research Laboratories then turned the science into the antidepressant drug Prozac.[12] By 1994, Prozac accounted for around a third of Lilly's total sales.[13] The SSRIs were a lifeline for Lilly. Prozac reached the two-billion-dollar level in 1995.[14] Indeed, by the mid-1990s, the SSRIs were demonstrating an "unprecedented [annual] growth" of 56 percent, as *Scrip* put it.[15] This success had a shadow side. It threatened the notion of psychopharmacology as a science. The SSRs were drugs that didn't work for a disease that didn't exist.

246 THE AGE OF PSYCHOPHARMACOLOGY

The 1980s and early 1990s saw the launch of the SSRIs. Astra's zimelidine (Zelmid) was the first, on the market in Europe in 1981—and withdrawn before Merck had a chance to bring it out in the United States. As for other US launches, Lilly brought out fluoxetine (Prozac) in 1988, having received FDA approval in December 1987. (The company had delayed the launch, initially believing the drug ineffective because they had tried it on inpatients; in the later outpatient trials, it worked somewhat better.) Pfizer marketed sertraline (Zoloft) in 1992; SmithKline Beecham launched paroxetine (Paxil) in the United States in 1993; and Forest Labs brought out Lundbeck's citalopram (Cipramil) in 1998, then continued with escitalopram (Lexapro) in 2002.

Commerce, not science, was at stake. One observer lauded "the stroke of marketing genius that led to calling these medications *antidepressants*."[16] The SSRIs were a body blow to the concept of psychopharmacology because they produced such enormous profits that the entire industry focused upon producing more and more SSRIs, so that the endless golden flow would continue. This was deadening to drug discovery. Psychopharmacology was turned into a recipe not for science, but for making more SSRIs.

From the get-go, "SSRI" was a commercial, not a scientific concept. In 1979, a Prozac trialist (whose name was redacted from the source document) filed this rather dubious report about his recent trial: "In review of the eleven patients treated with fluoxetine we were not impressed with the antidepressant activity of the drug. There were two patients that entered remission [but query] whether this was drug related. In the others there was either no change or clinical worsening. Side effects were minimal on any of the dosage regimens."[17] (This would normally be evidence that the compound was inert.)

The SNRIs, or serotonin and norepinephrine reuptake inhibitors, did not fare vastly better. The first was reboxetine (launched as Edronax in Europe and the United Kingdom in 1999); the most important, venlafaxine (Effexor), streeted in the United States in 1994. Much was made of exactly which neurotransmitters these agents acted on,[18] while it is unclear that this has any importance at all. The SNRIs have apparently the same efficacy as the SSRIs[19] and the category exists only for mercantile reasons.

The marketing arm of the British firm SmithKline Beecham (SKB) inserted the SSRI concept into Seroxat ads (Seroxat was the British brand name for Paxil) at the launch in the spring of 1991: "'Seroxat' is more selective and more potent than other available 5-HT [serotonin] re-uptake inhibitors."[20] The acronym SSRI soon sprang into ads on both sides of the Atlantic (see Chapter 16). SmithKline thus hoped to distinguish its antidepressant from Lilly's Prozac and Pfizer's Zoloft, but, as Healy put it, "all three companies used the term to create the appearance of a new class of drugs" and to marginalize the older antidepressants.[21] In a textbook of psychopharmacology edited by Charles Nemeroff and Alan

Schatzberg, both with very close ties to industry, the enthusiastic chapter on SSRIs was written by Gary Tollefson, the vice-president of research at Lilly (Prozac) and Jerrold Rosenbaum, head of psychopharmacology at Mass General Hospital (where Joseph Biederman was allowed to rampage over "pediatric bipolar disorder"). The chapter mirrors the giant wave of academic hype that swept the SSRIs along ("an important advance in pharmacotherapy"). "Sexual dysfunction" is briefly mentioned in a list of six not very important and not very frequent side effects.[22]

The SSRI convulsion transformed psychiatry from being the lowest-prescribing medical specialty to the highest. In 1999, the number of drug mentions per 100 patient visits averaged 150 for all specialties, 170 for family medicine, 180 for psychiatry.[23] Before the launch of Prozac in December 1987, the benzodiazepines had been the mainstay drugs for the vast mass of dysphoria, unhappiness, and fatigue that previously had been called anxiety. Then, with Prozac labeled for depression, the great mass of psychiatric prescribing swung on its axis from the benzodiazepines for anxiety to the SSRIs for depression.

As psychiatry turned toward the SSRIs in the treatment of depression, it swung away from psychotherapy. In 1987, 71.1 percent of depressed patients got psychotherapy from psychiatrists, in 1997, the number was 60.2 percent. By contrast, those receiving antidepressants rose from 37.3 percent to 74.5 percent, and half of the psychopharmacology treatments in 1997 were SSRIs.[24] George Simpson commented of this shift, "For some psychiatrists there had been a little bit of religiosity, a belief in the sanctity of the self which you invade when you give drugs so that you have this notion that the real treatment is the talking. I think that these people began to give drugs with fluoxetine [Prozac]."[25]

This was a shift of historic magnitude. Giovanni Fava, then at the University of Bologna, said in 2016 that, "The shift from benzodiazepines to SSRIs [is] the most successful achievement of pharmaceutical propaganda in psychiatry."[26] Through the skilled use of counter-detailing, the SSRI makers subtly convinced community psychiatrists to switch from Librium and Valium to Prozac and Zoloft. The motto was that the benzos were highly addictive and that the SSRIs, with their "favorable side-effects profile" (nothing was said about impotence or the loss of sexual desire) were the preferable drug class.

The SSRIs, and Prozac in particular, were thus widely celebrated on the grounds that they were "non-addictive," in contrast to the much-cited addictiveness of the benzodiazepines, which the SSRIs largely replaced. By 1989–90, 60.5 percent of drugs prescribed by US psychiatrists were for depression—including 13 percent prescriptions for Prozac. Only 20.8 percent of prescriptions were for anxiety, and all these scrips were for benzodiazepines. (The rest of the prescriptions mainly for antipsychotics.) By that period, sales of Valium (diazepam) had fallen to a mere 3.3 percent of the total.[27]

Shattered Timber

> Clinicians lose sight of the fact that all medicines are poisons (except insulin and vitamins), and the art of medicine lies in knowing when not to treat. We must expect poisons to produce problems and only undertake these risks when there are good grounds to do so, but we have instead drifted into a culture where Prozac has become vitamin serotonin.—David Healy, 2008[28]

A number of disadvantages began to emerge. Fears of addiction had been abolished—or had they? In February 2004, Bob Temple, a man with years of psychopharmaceutical experience behind him (and very much a straight shooter), told the PDAC, "Prozac is a fine drug and everything, but it stays with you more or less permanently, when you stop it, it is very hard to get off, has a very long half-life with active metabolites."[29] This kind of addictiveness doesn't necessarily lead to breaking into old ladies' apartments to steal their televisions, but, for sure, it's addictiveness.

There was more shattered timber. SSRI-related loss of libido is interesting because it shows the gap between what patients and doctors think is important. Max Hamilton, creator of the famous depression scale named after him, said at a conference in 1973 that everyone is interested in suicidality. "But who worries very much about loss of libido? Only the patient or his wife or her husband. Therefore, there are some symptoms which the physician regards as minor ones and ignores, and others which he sees as major ones."[30] Bob Temple said in 2009 that "Sexual dysfunction on SSRIs is in the neighborhood of 50 percent."[31] But the sexual effects story is actually worse than that, because it turns out that men and women can suffer from sexual dysfunction—loss of desire, erectile failure— long after they discontinue the SSRIs. The issue of post-SSRI sexual dysfunction (PSSD) is only now coming to public attention.[32] So, the whole question of side effects was a mosh pit loaded with subjectivity.

But surely the SSRIs have been a public health benefit? One study, based on the United States Survey of Midlife Development for 1995–96 and 2004–2006, followed for 9 years depressed patients who had been treated with medication versus those who had no treatments and no medication. Nine years later, the patients who had received "adequate" treatment for their depression, including medication, were far more symptomatic than the patients who had received no treatment at all; those who had received psychotherapy but no medication fell in the middle. The author said, "This pattern suggests possible long-term iatrogenic effects of antidepressants."[33] Incredibly, these important data appeared in the form of a brief "letter to the editor" in an obscure journal. Jay Amsterdam commented, "This seems to be yet another finding that it is difficult to get published in top-rank journals, as it is almost impossible to get beyond the peer reviewers, who are usually clinical psychopharmacologists who are fixed in their belief that antidepressants couldn't possibly 'poop out' and work less and less well."[34]

A major adverse effect of the new drugs was to smother in their cribs a number of other agents for depression that were probably more promising than the SSRIs. Roche, for example, had under development a monoamine oxidase inhibitor (MAOI) called moclobemide (Aurorix), but Roche withdrew the drug in 1990 from further study in the United States, as *The Pink Sheet* reported, because of "the change in commercial prospects in the antidepressant market in the wake of the Prozac launch and the intense interest in serotonin reuptake inhibitors." Roche went on to market moclobemide successfully in Europe and elsewhere. It was considered by Jules Angst to have imipramine-level effectiveness.[35] At a conference in 1990, Jay Armstrong from the Depression Research Unit at Penn deplored the disappearance of interest in drugs of this class. Earlier, the MAOIs had been plagued by hypertensive crises (the "cheese effect"—the tyramine in cheese and other foods drives up the blood pressure in patients on MAOIs), but Amsterdam said that this problem had been solved with moclobemide and the newer MAOIs.[36] Nobody listened. Prozac was thought to have virtually no side effects.

Wyeth's powerful antidepressant Effexor (venlafaxine) had difficulty making headway against Prozac and its cousins. A Wyeth executive wanted Barney Carroll, then chair of psychiatry at Duke, to come out to California and give some talks on behalf of Effexor. She said Effexor was superior to the TCAs because it caused less sedation and less weight gain, and incurred "no need to do blood levels and no cardiac conduction problems, and in the 14 patients who have attempted suicide with large overdoses—all have recovered without sequel." So what was the problem? Why was Effexor not cleaning up? She told Carroll, "I think I often have more luck selling Effexor against the TCAs than against the SSRIs! However, many psychiatric residents do not have much experience with the TCAs—only SSRIs!"[37] In other words, Prozac and its cousins had blanked from the scene the entire class of TCAs, the effective antidepressants!

The advance of the SSRIs thus left a lot of shattered timber in its wake—psychiatry itself changed from a kind of thoughtful humanism to a prescription machine, with useful drugs destroyed, the side-effects picture seriously distorted, and a sleight-of-hand in which drugs possibly effective for obsessive-compulsive behavior and anxiety turned out to be sure-fire winners for depression. This was progress?

Major Depression

> Antidepressants are generally an order of magnitude overprescribed today, as is depression of the bon-ton ersatz variety. Picking the real McCoy is not so difficult. It is just that it—hiding in prison, on the grate, or in a poorly populated region—is not well represented in meta-analyses. — Mark Kramer, 2017[38]

"Major depression" was the keystone of the vault of uselessness.

Mickey Nardo made clear that, in his backwoods clinic in Georgia's Appalachia, "Most patients I see on 'antidepressants' don't have anything close to major depressive disorder—not by any stretch of the imagination. They're people who are unhappy with their lives, wives, husbands, kids, fate, job, lot in life, friends, lack of friends, etc. They might be helped, but it's sure not with 'antidepressants.'"[39]

Yet DSM's "major depression" conquered the world like Atilla sweeping across the steppes. Previously, psychiatry was alight with rival diagnostic systems and fine psychopathological labels for conditions like "mythomania" (chronic lying). After DSM-III in 1980, only three or four big disease entities were left standing: major depression, bipolar disorder, schizophrenia, and the childhood diagnoses, such as ADHD. All the rest of the historical psychopathology had been eliminated, and one has the feeling that the widely unread DSM team were unfamiliar with much of it.[40] Thomas Ban wrote scathingly of these developments, "By the end of the 1980s, psychopathology and psychiatric nosology, the disciplines which enabled psychiatry to detect the differences in the pathologies of the processing of signals in the brain and in the organization of these pathologies in time, were forgotten languages in psychiatry."[41] But depression's triumphal march did not happen spontaneously, as a result of the power of the concept. It happened because the pharmaceutical industry systematically marketed depression to the medical profession and the public.

Before the advent of Prozac as an antidepressant in 1988, depression was not a widespread diagnosis and remedies for its treatment were not commonly prescribed. "Let's run the numbers," said Mark Kramer. In 1955 in the United States, there were around 80,000 psychiatric inpatients, and 13,000 of them had a diagnosis of depression. If deinstitutionalization had not occurred, inpatient depressives would number about 24,000 today. "This means that drug-appropriate major depressive disorder might merely be [today] an orphan drug development indication—(Yes, you read that correctly!)"[42] An orphan drug, says the former director of psychopharmacology research at Merck, instead of one of the most popular drug classes in the world.

How about medicating those patients with serious (melancholic) depression? The rule of thumb in treating such depressions with the tricyclics was that one third would respond beautifully, one third somewhat, a final third not at all. And the tricyclics sported the standard "anticholinergic" side effects, meaning constipation, blurred vision, dry mouth, and so forth. The National Survey of Psychotherapeutic Drug Use in 1979, supported by the National Institute of Mental Health, found in a nationwide random sample of adults that only 11.0 percent of all men and 20.2 percent of women were on psychotherapeutic medications of any kind. Antianxiety agents were the most commonly prescribed, with 7.5 percent of all men and 14.1 percent of all women on them. As for antidepressants, 1.3 percent of men and 2.8 percent of women took them.[43] These statistics show the extent to which the benzodiazepine drug class and anxiety dominated the psychotropic picture. Depression was scarcely visible in the experience of the average person.

The term "SSRI," almost magical in its incantation of neurochemistry as the solution to your problems, was coined by SmithKline Beecham in 1991 at the time of its launch of Paxil.[44] (Yet only in 1993 did the company begin using it in their US advertising.[45]) Other companies found it impossible to resist the lure of the term and it soon generalized.

And just in time, because suddenly the "worldwide epidemic of depression" was on us. Nardo said, "I never heard about this epidemic until the SSRI drugs came on the market in the late 1980s. And the epidemic is now getting worse as more and more people are taking antidepressants. . . . My personal take is that this whole line of thinking is a market-creation scheme. I don't believe any of it anymore."[46] By 1994, antidepressants had become the fourth best-selling drug class in the US market ($2.89 billion); the number-one sellers were the H_2 antagonists (for ulcers), at $3.95 billion.[47]

The relentless drumbeat about depression and the SSRIs had real-world consequences. In a survey of female outpatients in 1997–98 by the National Center for Health Statistics, 31.3 percent of adult female *outpatients* were currently on antidepressants.[48] In a government-sponsored national survey in 2013 of the population as a whole, 15.9 percent of a*ll* adult women were on antidepressants (compared to 7.7 percent of adult men). In 2013, only 10.3 percent of women were on "anxiolytics, sedatives and hypnotics," and 6.1 percent of men were. (It's important that in 2013 the figures included not just anxiolytics, as in 1979, but hypnotics and sedatives, too.)[49] The take-home message here is that in the three decades between 1979 and 2013, the percent of women on antidepressants had increased almost sixfold!

So much had the diagnosis of depression ballooned that it was inconceivable that all these individuals had a serious mood disorder. But then, what did they have? The argument is not that they had nothing, but rather that other illnesses sheltered under the depression umbrella. One was "demoralization," described by psychotherapist Jerome Frank at Johns Hopkins University in 1974 as "feelings of impotence, isolation, and despair. The person's self-esteem is damaged, and he feels rejected by others because of his failure to meet their expectations."[50] Demoralization is the "helplessness and giving up" syndrome, which is not a mood disorder but a dull resignation to one's fate as something one cannot influence. The treatment is psychotherapy to restore the individual's sense of self-mastery. It differs from depression in the patient's sense of "subjective incompetence," and depression's anhedonia is not found in demoralization. Also, the "hopelessness" of depression is, as Carroll put it, "the cognitive bias that nothing anybody else does will make a difference (as opposed to the helplessness of demoralization: nothing that you do can make a difference)."[51] Misdiagnosis of demoralization as depression led to inappropriate prescribing of antidepressants.

What else other than depression? There was a tradition in biological psychiatry of observing that drugs worked by diminishing nervous "excitability." Leo Alexander, at the Boston State Hospital, said in 1959 that, "The rather broadly effective somatic therapies developed during the past twenty years . . . all worked by rather generally diminishing the excitability of the higher nervous activity of the cortex."[52] Some observers, in an echo of Alexander's analysis, felt that the SSRIs were not really antidepressants at all, but sedated patients rather than undepressing them. David Healy's analysis of the SSRIs was that, "Their primary effect is to emotionally numb."[53] In an online survey of 1,829 New Zealanders who had been taking antidepressants for at least 5 years, "feeling emotionally numb" was reported by 60 percent of the respondents ("feeling not like myself," 52 percent).[54] The authors did not explore the possibility that these "side effects" were precisely the mechanism of the drugs' action.

When Mickey Nardo wound up his practice in Atlanta to go and live in rural Georgia, he reviewed all his previous cases "as sort of an exit exercise, and the surprise to me had to do with SSRIs. . . . Every case I had with significant PTSD was on SSRIs. And I came to think that was because those patients are hypervigilant, have affect storms, and actually do better with the volume turned down. I was surprised that I hadn't noticed that along the way, but I didn't."

There is such a concept as a "serenic," a drug to make people less irritable and aggressive.[55] The SSRIs do this, possibly by influencing cortical levels of the hormone allopregnanolone, the synthetic version of which (brexanolone) was approved by the FDA in 2009 for postpartum depression. Don Klein said, "I don't think the modest antidepressant effects of Prozac, that in my view are limited to mild melancholic states, account for its popularity. It does not make the average citizen happier. My hypothesis is that there is also a fast, general calming anti-irritability effect in the non-depressed. This facilitates subjective peacefulness, positive social feedback, and pleasant socialization."[56] Possibly true, but a serenic is not an antidepressant.

Furthermore, the SSRIs may have an analgesic effect. There is a vast historical literature on the relationship between mood and pain. Belgian alienist Joseph Guislain realized this as early as 1833. "We have always been struck by the appearance of suffering and the convulsive contracture of the face; the sadness, the despondency, their tendency to find mainly themes for self-accusation and complaint." For Guislain, this was the central issue in psychopathology: "Insanity is for us, and in the majority of cases, a pain of the affective sense. We have designated this state under the term 'phrenopathies.'" He continued, "Suffering and lamentation, voilà the primordial symptoms of mental illness. A feeling of oppression is the nature of psychological [morale] pain; a painful sensation is that of physical pain."[57]

There is a huge overlap between depression and pain, which Michael Sullivan, a pain and depression expert at McGill, puts at 50 percent each way. He hypothesizes that each causes the other.[58] Bernard Carroll made central pain dysregulation one of the key features of his depression model.[59] But the literature on SSRIs and pain is sparse.[60] Depression was a much more appealing indication.

What therefore was the big advantage of the SSRIs? Or was there one?[61]

Paxil was not untypical of the SSRIs, and Michael Sugarman's careful meta-analysis of Paxil trial studies in 2014 using efficacy measurements (Cohen's d to check effect size), concluded that "Paroxetine provides only a modest advantage over placebo in treatment of anxiety and depression." (The d values were all less than 0.36, which is the area of "weak effect.")[62]

Was the advantage fighting depression by decreasing the reuptake of serotonin? This sounded like science, but it was the marketing mantra. Neuroscientists had long discounted this, and in any event the reuptake mechanism had been known for decades (see "Chemical Imbalance" in Chapter 8). There was no "revolutionary new principle."

Many investigators had other thoughts. Les Iversen, a psychopharmacologist at Merck, said in an interview that the big advantage of the SSRIs was that "you cannot commit suicide by overdosing because they are not that toxic."[63] Older clinicians, accustomed to fearfulness about suicide on the barbiturates and tricyclics, would have breathed a sigh of relief. (But let's not exaggerate, either: When the body of pediatrician Phoebe Danziger's father was discovered dead of suicide, amid bottles of antidepressants and antihypertensives, on his computer was the recent search, "How to commit suicide with Paxil."[64])

Let's say you recover from Prozac: The longer you are on Prozac, or the greater the number of different antidepressants that you try, the shorter is your time to relapse. Jay Amsterdam, who led a study of Prozac that nailed this, said in an email to colleagues, "The more prior antidepressant-medication trials that a subject has received over the lifetime course of their affective illness, the more likely they are to relapse during antidepressant-medication maintenance therapy, and the more likely they are to remain well on placebo (i.e. no active therapy). These analyses should provide a moment of pause to clinicians."[65]

SSRIs versus Tricyclic Antidepressants

> No man having drunk old wine straightaway desireth new: for he saith, The old is better.—Gospel according to Luke, 5:39

"Occasionally, people will flower on Prozac, [but] not very frequently," said J. Alexander Bodkin at McLean Hospital as the Prozac era was drawing to an end.[66] Why such gloom?

We have here two generations of antidepressant drugs: the tricyclic antidepressants (TCAs), of which Tofranil (imipramine) was the first, launched in Switzerland in 1957, and the SSRIs, of which Prozac (fluoxetine) was the first, launched at the end of 1987. As previously discussed, a good measure of efficacy is not "statistical significance" (a *p*-value) but Number Needed to Treat (NNT): the number of patients you need to treat before getting a response better than the placebo response. A low NNT is good (for severe depression, you have to treat only two or three patients before one responds); a high number is bad (such as, if you have to treat 10 patients before one patient benefits). In neuropathic pain, the NNT for the TCAs is 2–3, for the SSRIs, it's 7.[67] For depression in the elderly, the NNT for TCAs is 5, for the SSRIs, it's 10.[68]

Mark Kramer tabulated the NNT over the years for the different generations of antidepressants: 1954, NNT = 2; 1959–61, NNT = 2; 1975, NNT = 3; post-1980, NNT = 7. Before 1980, the antidepressants were the tricyclics, and one patient in two got better; after 1980, the antidepressants were the SSRIs, and effectiveness had been cut by almost two thirds: only one patient in 7 got better.[69]

In 1994, a trial among melancholic patients at the New York State Psychiatric Institute found that, in patients treated with nortriptyline (a TCA), the intent-to-treat response rate was 67 percent; with fluoxetine (Prozac), it was 23 percent. (Percentages of patients who completed the trial were 83 percent for the melancholics, 10 percent for the fluoxetine group.)[70] One large meta-analysis in 1997 found that, among inpatients (those with serious depression), 51 percent of patients on TCAs responded, compared to 33 percent of those on SSRIs.[71]

Gordon Parker, a Sydney professor of psychiatry who leads the Black Dog Institute, found in a 1999 study of 341 nonpsychotic depressed patients that the "older antidepressants" and MAOIs were more effective than the SSRIs in serious (melancholic) depression.[72] Parker later spoke, on the basis of his enormous experience, of the difference between the TCAs and the SSRIs in treating melancholia: In people under 40, they were equal. In over-40s, TCAs were dramatically superior: "In melancholics, SSRIs equal TCAs in those under 40, TCAs [were] twice better in those 40–60; and TCAs [were] 4 times better in melancholics over 60 (the response to TCAs stayed constant with age increase, the response to SSRIs dropped with age)." He added, "I have long viewed SSRIs as most beneficial for muting emotional dysregulation whether externalized as irritability or internalized as anxious worrying."[73] (On the myth that the SSRIs are "better tolerated and safer than the TCAs," see Michael Alan Taylor's penetrating analysis.[74])

The on-the-ground difference between TCAs and SSRIs is this: "I recently saw a guy in our little clinic," said Mickey Nardo in 2011, "a 50+ year old alcoholic who had been living in a half-way house for six months. He was no derelict, a construction worker whose wife had 'taken it all' in the divorce so he decided to check in and sober up to stop 'wrecking trains.'"

Nardo continued, "I knew that guy was different when I went to the waiting room the first time—different from the garden variety 'I'm depressed' cases that haunt clinics like the one I work in. He was the one that I worried about and would've called if he missed an appointment." How to treat him? "I tried the Celexa trip [an SSRI], going up on the dose when he didn't respond. Still nada."

"So I treated him with Elavil [amitriptyline, a TCA] in a full dose as if it were 1974 when I showed up for my residency. At one month, he walked in and said, 'I think that was it.' He was glad. I was too, but I think I was more mad." Mad because the field had forgotten about the TCAs for patients like this. "So it's not just the fairy tale about SSRIs, it's the DSM-III version of 'MDD' [major depressive disorder] that's awry. He's lumped in there with everyone else."[75]

In 2014, Steve Balt, who had completed a psychiatric residency at Stanford University and a graduate degree in molecular neuroscience at Rockefeller University in New York City, resolved the agonizing over choice of antidepressant that any reader of *Psychiatric Times* might be having with two "stark truths": "First, there seem to be no significant differences among them. . . . Second, and somewhat surprisingly, antidepressant effectiveness is quite low."[76]

The lack of efficacy of the SSRIs in depression meant that therapeutics in psychiatry were going *backward.* The drugs launched in the late 80s and after were less effective in serious depression than previous drug classes. David Healy said, "Modern depression is a creation of the marketing of Prozac. Until recently what is now called depression was called anxiety, nerves or a nervous breakdown, SSRIs can help in some cases of nerves but they are of no use for depression proper—melancholia. But the money for companies lies in treating nerves not melancholia—and as a result any of us with severe depression is likely to get worse treatment now than we once did. We've gone backward."[77]

The Scramble for Indications

> Think of the enormous profit that derives from having vague
> diseases that fit any of the antipsychotics or anticonvulsants . . . and
> makes teaching and treatment easy, but meaningless and usually in-
> effective.—Sam Gershon (2017)[78]

In 2007, one contributor to a psychopharm listserve wrote to another contributor, tongue in cheek, "You are very courageous to treat a suicidal teen with
Prozac." Under ordinary circumstances, Prozac would be the last agent one
would give to a suicidal psychotically depressed teen. Yet the exchange illustrates
how broadly the use of the SSRIs had begun to stretch. Mario Maj, one of the
leaders of European psychiatry and a professor in Naples, suggested in 2002 that
the SSRIs were effective for everything "in the old realm of neuroses."[79] This was
a huge realm. Even though the companies had tried mightily to grow the depression market, other markets lay awaiting. It was not for nothing that David Healy
coined the phrase "Big Panacea," for where "Big Pharma" once stood.[80]

The anxiety market lay ready to grasp, the anxiety indication having been toxic
for a decade after the supposed addictiveness of the benzodiazepines. "From the
beach-head of depression," said Healy, "raids can subsequently be launched on
the hinterlands of anxiety."[81] Lilly began marketing Prozac for "associated anxiety" in Britain in 1994, in the United States in 1996.[82]

In 1990, as Prozac neared a 50 percent share in the "antidepressant" market,
Lilly announced that it intended to market Prozac for obesity.[83] An indication for
obsessive-compulsive disorder was granted to Prozac in 1994.[84] In 1994 as well,
Lilly went after the bulimia indication for Prozac.[85] In 1998, it sought the panic
indication.[86] In 2000, Lilly got permission to market fluoxetine under the brand
name Sarafem for premenstrual dysphoria.[87] In 2002, the company submitted
a New Drug Application (NDA, request for permission) to market a combo
product of Prozac and its antidepressant Zyprexa for "bipolar depression" and
"treatment-resistant depression."[88] The FDA approved this combo as Symbyax in
2009. It is clear by now that Prozac had become a virtual panacea, indicated for
a range of psychiatric indications going far beyond depression, if, in fact, it ever
was a useful antidepressant. Although the NDAs had the ring of science, they
were not based in science. They were motivated by commerce.

For Paxil, it was panic. In 1996, SKB got the panic indication in France and
the United States. Paxil sales soared 59 percent, and SKB's new product group, of
which Paxil was a key member, amounted to a third of the company's total pharmaceutical sales.[89]

Although Lilly had advertised the anxiety indication first, it was actually
Paxil that opened up the anxiety market in 2001 (the year that Lilly's Prozac

patent expired). Jean-Pierre Garnier, the CEO of the company that had become GlaxoSmithKline and that made Paxil, told *The Pink Sheet* in 2001, "The anxiety market holds a bigger growth opportunity for SSRIs than the antidepression market.... There's a lot of runway space there for Paxil." He said that of 90 million antidepressant scrips in the last year, 76 percent were for SSRIs—so that market was about saturated. But for the 72 million antianxiety scrips, only 33 percent were for SSRIs—here was the market of the future! (And in the 12 months ending July 2001, SSRI anxiety scrips had grown 29 percent, SSRI antidepressant scrips only 11 percent.)[90]

Do These Things Actually Work?

> It would not be that bad if the use of these drugs [SSRIs] were diminished, I think, because we don't know whether they actually help most patients.—Thomas Newman, 2004[91]

In the 1970s, Max Fink and Turan Itil were doing research on psychopharmacology using the electroencephalograph (EEG), which gives a picture of the brain's electrical activity (see Chapter 8). This activity is modified by different drugs. Fink later wrote,

> The pharmacologists asked whether we could define EEG profiles of agents that changed serotonin and dopamine. We had defined the CNS effects of cholinergic and anticholinergic drugs in humans, but the SSRI drugs had little effect.
>
> At the same time, we studied clozapine and defined its EEG profile. It was clearly EEG active in humans.
>
> Our failure to define a profile for serotonin agents? We considered them "golden placebos," without confirmed predictable effects on brain chemistry in man. Our work was disregarded, rejected by the marketing folk at various industries and universities and by NIMH.
>
> The failure of fluoxetine to induce characteristic EEG profiles in man predicted the failure of fluoxetine to relieve sick patients. The enthusiasm of Peter Kramer [author of *Listening to Prozac*] was a marketing success, not a demonstrated specific pharmacologic chemical effect.[92]

Many clinicians made this discovery on their own. Carroll's experience: "I have an indelible memory of attending a Lilly satellite meeting at Montecatini Terme outside Florence in 1986. Lilly flew in all their available suits, who almost outnumbered the scientists. The agenda was fluoxetine. The main KOLs for clinical matters were John Feighner and Jay Cohen. After their presentations, there was general unrest, even anger. Ole Rafaelsen in particular erupted like Khrushchev, pounding the desk and accusing Lilly of gilding the lily. A couple of years later, fluoxetine was available in the US. The first patient I treated returned with severe akathisia [restlessness] and dysphoria, something I had not encountered over years of using TCAs. That pretty much sealed the fate of fluoxetine for me."[93]

How much weight should be given such individual expressions of clinical opinion? In my opinion, considerable weight, given that many of the RCTs of the SSRIs, which have constituted the supposed proof of their efficacy, were corrupted by industry and are not valid as scientific evidence. As well, our knowledge of the effectiveness of caffeine, opium, the barbiturates, and the amphetamines was largely derived from clinical opinions, or at best, from open trials, certainly not from RCTs.

But RCTs are indeed valid evidence, if properly conducted, and Prozac flunked trials, too. The early clinical trials were a disaster. In 1996, a Dutch study found Prozac ineffective for the depression of chronic fatigue syndrome.[94] There were few inpatient trials of Prozac, but in the one that Max Fink conducted at Stony Brook, "It didn't work very well," Fink said in an interview in 2008. So they gave ECT or imipramine and the patients got better.[95]

There is an extensive literature,[96] heavily dependent on meta-analyses, comparing antidepressants and reaching various findings, most of which, in my view, are invalid because the literature has been so heavily corrupted with ghosted articles planted by public-relations firms. It would be a vain exercise to compare, let's say, the efficacy or effectiveness of Prozac with those of Zoloft on the basis of the published literature because the data have been so extensively massaged: the conclusion would be fictive. (It was evidently Pfizer's blockbuster Zoloft that got the firm into the KOL sweepstakes. Baum Hedlund, a Los Angeles law firm, argued that in order to "cultivate a body of 'peer-reviewed research' to enhance Zoloft's credibility. . . Pfizer created a large-scale ghostwriting program." A medical communications company would draft the text. "Then, Pfizer would pay 'key opinion leaders'   to put their name on the article and get the article published in specifically targeted medical journals."[97])

One balances the enthusiastic patient anecdotes in media stories and Peter Kramer's book against the statistical finding that fewer than 10 percent of patients taking Prozac "were entirely free of any residual symptomatology," in the words of the study's authors.[98] In a somewhat controversial analysis of data in FDA regulatory submissions, psychologist Irving Kirsch found that the results of antidepressants were scarcely superior to the placebo results, and that the marketed antidepressants may in fact work as placebos.[99] An only slightly less condemnatory judgment was reached by psychologists Brett J. Deacon and Glen I. Spielmans in 2017: "The clinical trials data submitted to the FDA suggest that the efficacy of fluoxetine is small, unreliable, clinically insignificant, and inflated by biased design and reporting practices."[100]

These voices of doubt have not been left unchallenged. Don Klein engaged in an acerbic exchange with Kirsch in *Prevention & Treatment*.[101] Gordon Parker, professor of psychiatry at the University of New South Wales, found Kirsch's conclusions "specious." The problem is that the RCTs submitted to the FDA were for major depression. Parker said that different kinds of depression respond to different agents, and antidepressants like nortriptyline are definitely not placebos in treating melancholic depression.[102]

Robert Whitaker has systematically marshalled the evidence against the effectiveness of the SSRIs, and reference to his work suffices to make the case. Do the SSRIs work? Decidedly no. In fact, they have increased levels of disability as people receive the diagnosis of depression, go on Prozac, and leave the labor force. In the United States, as Whitaker showed, the number of people on government disability due to mood disorders rises in lock step with the percent of the population using antidepressants. In Australia, there is the same parallel upward climb between days on disability and the use of antidepressants.[103] My own impression of these fiercely held opinions is that the question should be, How *ineffective* are the SSRI antidepressants? "Not very effective" or "entirely ineffective and toxic to boot?"

Baron Shopsin, a student of Sam Gershon and chief of the depression unit at Bellevue Hospital in New York, was shocked at what the depression diagnosis had become under the SSRIs. "Children are prescribed drugs as if they were M & M's, whilst more and more adults and children have allegedly become 'treatment resistant', and more children commit suicide. . . . The system is broken. Psychiatrists without an idea about pharmacology bill themselves as psychopharmacologists because they give drugs; they no longer have the time or inclination to listen to or speak to patients. We've created a monster. . . . Diagnostic accuracy and specificity are irrelevant to some of us; it doesn't matter what type of depression— unipolar, bipolar, neurotic, induced or associated with the use of illicit drugs. We are told as long as there are depressive features, the prescribing clinician should give an antidepressant."[104] (Mood disorders in children and adolescents before the onset of puberty are virtually non-existent.[105])

Insiders like Jay Amsterdam at the University of Pennsylvania, with a deep scientific background, felt they were butting their heads against a wall. Here is Amsterdam on the lecture trail before a bug-eyed audience:

> When I would lecture widely about MAOI therapy, most of the psychiatrists in the audience were unbelieving about my bypassing the use of their precious SSRIs. I was always of the opinion that SSRIs only became first-line therapy for depression because of the abject fear of terrible side effects from TCAs

and MAOIs that was put into their heads by Big Pharma. And this marketing ploy worked brilliantly; because all the marketers had to do was get the current generation of medical school educators (at the time) to teach their young psychiatrists-in-training and their medical students that SSRIs were "kinder and gentler" than TCAs and MAOIs (which could kill patients). Once this was taught to that generation of young psychiatrists, it became the educational mantra—to the present day.[106]

(References in the literature to MAOIs decreased from 2008–202 to 2013–2017 by 81.3 percent, to TCAs by 85.0 percent.[107])

Thus, the ineffectiveness of the SSRIs was not something taught to residents. The public story, peddled by the battalion of KOLs in the SSRI file, was that these were wonder drugs. New Zealand journalist Evelyn Pringle wrote in 2009, "Throughout the 1990s, most doctors who attended conferences, medical seminars and other events were not aware that the so-called 'key opinion leaders' encouraging them to prescribe the new generation of antidepressants for everything under the sun, including to children as young as infants, were nothing more than highly paid drug pushers for Big Pharma."[108]

Only insiders like Amsterdam, Carroll, and Fink knew this, so effectively was the literature manipulated by marketing departments. Amsterdam wrote in 2017, "Like it or not, SSRIs are really not that effective (if they are effective at all) and produce substantial side effects, including increased risk for suicidal ideation." None of this, he said, would modify the practice of community psychiatrists of "prescribing SSRIs to the 'walking wounded' (i.e., non-severe, non-melancholic) patients that make up their practice because of unbridled, successful Pharma marketing efforts toward them! Thus, the field is what it is, and this [Peter Gøtzsche[109]] article seems to substantiate what we all know and dislike (i.e., that our most prescribed treatment for depression is crap."[110]

A major review in 2011 of the antidepressant literature (481 references), despite much upbeat rhetoric, conceded that "New pharmacodynamic mechanisms of action [reuptake] have not increased the response rate to a first antidepressant treatment. . . . Moreover, ECT is still the most effective antidepressant treatment."[111]

The SSRIs' lack of effectiveness was long an open secret. At a meeting of the FDA's PDAC on April 8, 2009, Bob Temple had this to say about the antidepressants: "People have been remarking on how small the [treatment] effect of all the antidepressants [is]; it's only 2 or 3 HAMD points and stuff, and that's absolutely true. Tom's [Laughren, director of the Division of Psychiatry Products] been accumulating this stuff over years. Fifty percent of trials can't show anything, like their [Forest Labs] escitalopram study."[112]

It is not widely known that in many of the preliminary trials of Prozac that Lilly organized, another psychoactive drug—usually a benzodiazepine or chloral hydrate—was co-administered. The significance of this is that the positive results of some of these trials may have been owing to the co-administered drug, rather than to Prozac.[113]

Were the patients even real? At a meeting of the PDAC in 1991, Javier Escobar of the University of Connecticut asked Lilly executive Gary Tollefson, "Do you have any idea of what proportion of the individuals who entered those trials were real patients, users of services, and what percentage of them were symptomatic volunteers recruited through newspaper advertisements?"[114] Tollefson waffled and did not answer the question directly.

As David Drachman of the University of Massachusetts told the PDAC in March 1981 on drugs for the elderly, ""Every drug has three actions: the one you want, the one you don't want, and the one you don't know about."[115] When the SSRIs were presented to the FDA for approval the spin was: yes, powerful therapy; no, the side effects are minimal; and there probably won't be any untoward consequences further down the road.

Every point was wrong. David Healy's judgment in 2013 of the SSRIs was severe: "We have ended up in a world in which hints of an effect are used to gain market entry for drugs and when we use these drugs mindlessly on the basis that they are effective, if the RCT evidence is to be believed, we produce greater disability in the long run than if we never had them. The effects may turn out to be worse than if we had encouraged chronic alcohol intake."[116]

To what do psychiatrists owe their clinical success if the medications they hand out are largely useless? For many of them, cultivating the doctor–patient relationship is the therapeutic moment, not the prescription of these largely indifferent drugs. As Benjamin Crocker, a psychiatrist in Portland, Maine, told a listserv in 2008, "It's all motivational interviewing, and the start of that is to get people to tell you and themselves the truth. That's what they pay us for. The meds all work pretty much the same, a hominid could pick em. But we healing artists are supposed to be good at getting people to spill the beans and face the music."[117]

In 2014, Bernard Carroll penned a poignant look back. "In 1961 I was in a pharmacology lab where the hot new drug was imipramine (Tofranil). Across town [in Melbourne], John Cade treated manic patients with lithium, which he discovered in 1948. . . . There was no argument in those early days that the new drugs worked. By 1967 I was a psychiatry resident, and I saw the efficacy of Tofranil and lithium first hand." But then, continued Carroll, the big change came. "Over the past 50 years emphases on increasing sales, on gaming the clinical trials system, on dumbing down the index disorder so as to expand the market, and on voodoo neurochemical explanations of depression supplanted the critical scientific stance in psychopharmacology. That is how we got the plague of KOLs, infomercials, experimercials, CME hijacking, and regulatory capture by Pharma. Our legacy, then, is serious doubt about whether the current antidepressant drugs even work at all."[118]

A Culture of Psychopharmacology Arises

Jamie Reidy, who "carried the bag" for Pfizer, as they say, had a good recipe for gaining entrée to doctors' offices. He gave the staff a case of Zoloft. "Excited, I asked how many samples they'd like. 'As many as you can give us!' they said."[119] This enthusiasm measures how much the SSRIs had become part of the culture. Whether ill or not, the office staff all wanted Zoloft!

A *New York Times* story in 1993 on the rise of "a legal drug culture" began: "Six friends, all highly successful professionals in their mid-30s, met recently for dinner at a restaurant in Washington. The conversation moved quickly from politics to Prozac. It turned out that four people at the table were on the antidepressant." They agreed that they were no longer "seriously depressed." It boggles the mind to think that four of a group of six friends in professional occupations would have been "seriously depressed." The piece featured psychiatrist Peter Kramer and his bestselling book *Listening to Prozac*. "People compare dosages, side effects and results at dinner parties and family gatherings," the piece continued.[120] This was a cultural phenomenon, not a medical one. The belief that one was depressed had become an article of cultural faith, with Prozac as the fairy dust.

Depression changed from being an episodic complaint to a chronic condition. There was no scientific finding involved in this. The growing culture of psychiatric disability inculcated the belief that depression was forever. Of course this belief was not discouraged by industry. "Tom" on the *1BoringOldMan* blog recalled, "I am getting on in years; when I was training in the late 70s and early 80s I was taught that for most people the natural course of a depressive episode was remission even without treatment with a low rate of recurrence.... But then things changed. I remember thinking that it happened almost overnight. All of a sudden, psychiatry married Big Pharma and the message changed. 'Don't EVER stop your meds!' 'You will have to be on them for life or else you will relapse!' "[121] With such a chronic illness, who wouldn't be disabled?

Thus, hand in hand with depression, the SSRIs made their way into the culture. One psychiatrist said in 2008, "I began thinking about the SSRIs about 7 years ago when I asked my internist in passing if he used SSRIs. He said he used them mostly to save marriages. In follow up, he said that he found that husbands became more passive and less angry so the marriage was calmer!"[122]

Calmer to the point of indifference. Journalist Heather Mallick wrote sardonically in 2002, "There are excellent antidepressants now. Doctors call them 'so what drugs' because when you're on them and something bad happens, you just say, 'So what?' "[123]

David Healy said that a culture of "biobabble" had replaced the once ubiquitous culture of "psychobabble" with its complexes and neuroses. "[This] equally vacuous biobabble . . . has consequences for how we view ourselves, how we view the turmoil of adolescence or school underachievement or, finally, moral and criminal culpability. This cannot be blamed on Eli Lilly, but it does stem in great part from the marketing of Prozac and other SSRIs—and it affects the lives even of those who have never heard of Prozac."[124]

The culture of biobabble infected everyone, doctors and patients alike. Whatever the problem, prescribing—or demanding—an SSRI became the solution of choice. Ramin Mojtabai at Johns Hopkins Medical Institutions and Mark Olfson at Columbia University reported in 2011 that among nonpsychiatric physicians, "the proportion of visits at which antidepressants were prescribed but no psychiatric diagnoses were noted" increased from 59.5 percent in 1996 to 72.7 percent in 2007.[125] Thus, in three-quarters of all primary care visits in which Prozac and its cousins were prescribed, the physician did not record a psychiatric issue. It is scarcely an exaggeration to say that the SSRIs were being handed out like candy.

By 1994 Prozac had reached worldwide sales of nearly $1.2 billion a year and merited a breathless *Newsweek* cover.[126] That year it had become the second best-selling drug in the world, behind Glaxo's ulcer drug Zantac.[127] A psychiatric diagnosis was indicated, but it was not depression. It was epidemic hysteria, hardly the best validation for the science of psychopharmacology.

17

Sally

How Sally Laden helped turn the disease of depression into a gold mine.—Mickey Nardo (2011)[1]

In 1997, as part of the FDA Modernization Act, Congress provided that drug makers could get 6 months of patent extension in exchange for conducting trials in the pediatric population. This was called the "pediatric exclusivity provision" and had the laudable purpose of increasing knowledge about drugs in adolescents. So, if a company had a drug earning it $2 billion each year, a 6-month extension on its patent would be worth a billion dollars. The game was worth the candle.

In psychiatry, the depression market had proven so huge that extending it to children would be desirable indeed.[2] In the years 2000 to 2004, four major SSRI makers struggled to get into the pediatric depression market, and the competition was fierce.[3] With the eye of faith, what child or adolescent could not be said to be a bit "depressed"? With all the moodiness, the kicking of the furniture and the dietary whimsies that go with these age groups, "depression" and "bipolar disorder" fairly spring to the lips. Thus, the potential market hung like a piece of ripe fruit.

Hopes were high at GlaxoSmithKline (GSK), as the American branch of the British firm SmithKline Beecham (SKB) was known, headquartered in Philadelphia. GSK made the SSRI antidepressant Paxil (paroxetine), and the firm conceived several trials of Paxil in pediatric depression. Development came along swiftly, and by the end of 1992, GSK had cooked up the protocol for their main RCT of Paxil "in adolescents with unipolar major depression." In house, James McCafferty, a BA from LaSalle University, was to be the coordinator. Martin Keller, professor of psychiatry at Brown University, became the clinician in charge of the trial, together with Neal Ryan at the Western Psychiatric Institute in Pittsburgh as second-in-command. It was to be a six-site study.[4]

Keller was an interesting choice as nominal director. As journalists Dolores Kong and Alison Bass pointed out in the *Boston Globe* in 1999, Keller had been "paid more than $500,000 in consulting fees in 1998, most of it from pharmaceutical companies whose drugs he touted in medical journals and at conferences."[5]

Over time, he received much more than that and evidently belonged to an elite tier of KOLs who cashed out millions of dollars. Indeed, a GSK executive told ghostwriter Sally Laden in 2001 that they were approving Keller's request for 500 gratis copies of the later article in the *Journal of Child and Adolescent Psychiatry* (that she had drafted), "Because Dr. Keller is a member of our advisory board and an influential KOL, we will support his request to purchase 500 reprints." GSK couldn't use the reprints in promotion. "However, we might be able to work with Traci Lee to have reprints sent out as part of our med query on the use of Paxil in children."[6] (If doctors "asked" for information, the company could do off-label promotion.) Keller's ties with industry were so extensive that when the *New England Journal of Medicine* published his article on nefazodone, they didn't list the possible "conflicts of interest" because, as editor Marcia Angell explained, "it would have used too much space to disclose them fully in the *Journal*. We decided merely to summarize them and to provide details on our Web site."[7]

Keller, in any event, was not all that interested in the acute 8-week trial but wanted to conduct a "naturalistic" 2-year follow-up study of the patients, for a large dollar figure,[8] which ultimately the marketing department of SKB agreed to fund, not the research department. The whole thing blew up before the naturalistic study ever got off the ground.

A public relations firm called Scientific Therapeutics Information (STI), led by John Romankiewicz, came on board early. Sally Laden worked for them. The firm evidently had had previous ties to SKB, because in October 1993 Romankiewicz proposed organizing (for $118,000) a 3-day meeting of the "Paxil Advisory Board," which at that point had 10 members, at the Ritz Carlton Hotel in Palm Beach. Charles Nemeroff would chair the meeting and make the main presentations. (Nemeroff was not actually running a trial, but the company wanted his influential imprimatur.)[9]

What kind of trial was Sally asked to write up?

The Trial

By April 1994, the trial of Paxil in adolescent depression, called #329, was up and running at what were to become ten US and two Canadian sites, with a total of 275 adolescent patients (actual patients, not responders to newspaper ads) randomly assigned to Paxil, imipramine, or placebo.[10] The trial concluded in 1997. (The trial was not sufficiently powered to permit a direct comparison of Paxil and imipramine.) Trial designers took to heart Gerald Klerman's advice about incorporating multiple outcome measures in antidepressant studies, regardless of the two designated "primary" goals. You can always claim that the drug does something. In CNS today, he said, almost all trials use such measures.[11]

It was a big problem that the placebo response rate was almost 50 percent,[12] which would have overwhelmed some of the efficacy outcome measurements.

In the early days of the trial, the "primary efficacy variables" were very clear: "change from baseline and the total score on the HAM-D from beginning of treatment to end of the 8-week acute phase," as Sally Laden later put it.[13] Every trial has several of these primary efficacy variables and, if the results were disappointing, departing from them to report secondary variables would be seen as cherry-picking. Very bad form. By September 1995, there was one big secondary variable, the "Schedule for Affective Disorders and Schizophrenia for School-Age Children—Lifetime Version" (abbreviated K-SADS-L). Rachel Klein at Columbia (Don Klein's wife, herself a psychologist, and an important investigator) had drawn it up.[14] Columbia was one of the, at that point, seven trial sites. In addition, "CGI [Clinical Global Impressions] Global Improvement Score and several others also counted as secondary variables.[15] (Changing the outcome variables in a trial is called "outcome switching," or, in a related practice, HARKing: Hypothesizing After the Results are Known.[16])

There were two other Paxil trials, #377 and #701. It was never publicly revealed that both had failed. The Department of Justice (DOJ) later argued that SKB had seriously misled the public about the efficacy of Paxil, a drug the DOJ considered a failure in the management of adolescent depressive illness.[17] (There was a huge subsequent controversy, which is not reviewed here, about the "misbranding" of Paxil, because it was marketed to youth and the elderly. There were also controversies about a tendency to suicide—"suicidality"—among patients who took Paxil and other SSRIs.[18] This whole corner of psychopharmacology was filled with strife.)

Sally

As these developments were brewing, Sally Laden, STI's prime ghostwriter, was underway with a variety of projects. She had graduated in 1981 with a BA in Pharmacy from the University of Connecticut, and in 1983 she received a master's degree in hospital pharmacy from Kansas University. She was employed briefly as a pharmacist, then worked for John Romankiewicz in some capacity beginning in 1985, and she joined him when he founded STI. (She left STI in 2003, but STI's work for GSK continued.[19])

By 1997, the trial was over and the analysis had begun. The results, unfortunately, were not what GSK might have hoped. On the basis of the primary outcome measures, the trial was a failure: In terms of decreasing the HAM-D scores at the endpoint, the Paxil group declined by 10.7 points, the placebo group by 9.1 points. The difference was not statistically significant ($p = 0.133$). For the numerous secondary measures, some results were significant, some not.[20] So hypnotized were people by the concept of statistical significance, that nobody calculated any of the effectiveness measures, such as Number Needed to Treat (NNT). Subsequently, however, Rachel Kline did point out that "effect size" should be discussed as well as "statistical significance."[21] It wasn't.

What to do? Here, Sally raised her hand. In April 1998, she and her boss John Romankiewicz forwarded to GSK a "proposal for a journal article." "The article will be developed for a psychiatry journal. A target journal is recommended, however, the decision on which journal to submit the paper to will be determined after . . . consultation with the primary author [not yet chosen] and the sponsor." They did recommend Marty Keller as the primary author, yet there should not be more than three authors because of "additional charges," meaning they had to pay the "authors" for permission to use their names. STI proposed six drafts. Draft I would be seen only by the sponsor. The primary author would get Draft II, after SmithKlineBeecham's comments had been integrated. Draft III would go to the other two "authors." And so forth. The final draft, Draft VI, would go to the journal that had been selected. Sally made clear that SmithKlineBeecham would be buying a whole package: "STI will provide all necessary resources to complete this manuscript, including writing, editing, library research . . . and the needed coordination with author(s), sponsor, and journal." The total package cost $17,250.[22]

So, Sally went to work, preparing the draft. As raw material she had, as she later said, "data that is given to me."[23] Draft I had 20 "author" names on the title page, led by Keller. Gone were the disappointing primary endpoints! Instead, there were eight "primary efficacy variables," in some of which the Paxil–placebo comparison was significant, in others not. Despite this dog's breakfast of results, Sally concluded, "Paroxetine is [a] safe and effective treatment of depression in the adolescent patient."[24] Paxil in adolescent depression had passed from being a failure to a wonder drug!

There was so much going on! Neal Ryan had to prepare a slide presentation on #329 for the meeting of the European College of Neuropsychopharmacology (ECNP) in Paris in November—the first outing of the #329 results. McCafferty had evidently asked Sally to prepare Ryan's slides, because in May Ryan complained to McCafferty of slides in "his" lecture that he didn't understand. "I don't understand the numbers on the 'Dose Level and Endpoint and Maximum Level' slide. I just don't know what the units are and can't figure it out."[25] Later, McCafferty thanked Ryan for "allowing your name on the ECNP poster."[26]

Back at SKB's head office in London, people were trying to figure out what to do with the failed #329 and the equally failed #377, which had been conducted in Europe, Africa, and South America. As for #377, they would just bury the data (although the data were not concealed from the FDA). Executive Jackie

Westaway wrote staff, "The results of the studies were disappointing in that we did not reach statistical significance on the primary endpoints and thus the data do not support a label claim for the treatment of Adolescent Depression." The best way forward for #329 was, "To effectively manage the dissemination of these data in order to minimize any potential negative commercial impact."[27] In other words, spin!

In line with this suggestion, SKB in London had arranged for another public relations firm, The Medicine Group (TMG), to generate hype for paroxetine. In January 1999, an executive at TMG proposed Jack Gorman and Stan Carson as "authors" for a paper on "Paroxetine—Efficacy Across the Spectrum."[28] TMG, of course, would write the paper. This paper was evidently never published, but Gorman worked extensively for SKB and its British head office.

A total of 10 articles, as well as slide and poster presentations, came out of the #329 trial.[29] As far as can be determined, Sally wrote almost all of them.

What is surprising in all of this is not the behavior of SmithKlineBeecham, which was entirely typical of corporate behavior in these years when hundreds of millions of dollars were at stake. It is the lack of reactivity of the academic authors and trialists to Sally's huge changes. The two primary variables abolished in favor of eight new variables—this might have caused something of a stir. It appears to have caused none. In February 1999, Keller wrote to Sally, "Dear Sally, You did a superb job with this. Thank you very much. It is excellent."[30] Keller later wrote co-authors, "Neal [Ryan] Mike [Strober, at UCLA] and Jim [McCafferty] have edited the first two drafts with me. The initial preparation was done by Sally Laden from STI, who will continue to assist with finalization of the manuscript."[31] Not a hint that something wildly inappropriate had happened in the writing and editing process. Karen Dineen Wagner, at the University of Texas Medical Branch at Galveston, noted that some of the tables were misnumbered and suggested the inclusion of a paper of hers.[32] Keller's own contributions to editing were trivial. Jim McCafferty at GSK was much more worried about the vanished primary endpoints. (McCafferty had a BS in biology from LaSalle University.) He told Sally, "I would state that all endpoints were identified in an analytical plan prepared prior to opening the blind."[33] (This, of course, was a lie.)

Managing the Results

The results were a bit awkward for SmithKlineBeecham. Back in London, a public relations officer at the agency Cohn and Wolfe, which worked for SKB, said there was not going to be a big roll out. "Originally we had planned to do extensive media relations surrounding this study until we actually viewed the results. Essentially the study did not really show Paxil was effective in treating adolescent depression, which is not something we want to publicize."[34]

The paper appeared in a child psychiatry journal in 2001.[35] Three academics in the United Kingdom, led by Raza Silveira, then wrote to the journal a letter mildly critical of the trial.[36] What to respond? Keller, who did not have email (to GSK's irritation), told Ed Zalesky, the administrator of the psychiatry department at Brown, to ask Sally for "a response to this letter to the editor." When she evidently was slow off the mark, Zaleski bugged her: We need the response to JAACAP letter from Silveira et al. in the United Kingdom. "I have to get those materials to Jim McCafferty [at GSK] so he can also work on that response."[37] (This is very cozy for an academic staffer to be so involved in Pharma affairs.) Yet the wait was worth it. Shortly after getting the draft letter, Keller messaged Sally and McCafferty enthusiastically, "This looks great to me. If Sally could prepare a brief cover letter I can send this to the Journal."[38] So, Sally put something together, and JAACAP ran it as a letter,[39] "Drs. Keller and Ryan reply,"[40] just as though Keller and Ryan had written it, and not a public relations firm.

Meanwhile, Sally was tireless in ghosting articles on behalf of Paxil. Later in February 2002, she completed "Draft IV" of an article on "Efficacy and Tolerability of Controlled Release and Immediate Release Paroxetine HCl in the Treatment of Depression, to be authored by Robert N. Golden, MD, Chapel Hill, North Carolina, for submission to *Journal of Clinical Psychiatry*."[41] Charles Nemeroff was enlisted as a "co-author," as were three GSK employees. No reference was made to Sally as the real author or to her company STI. GSK was thanked for "funding."[42] The paper appeared in the *Journal of Clinical Psychiatry* later in 2002.[43] On the title page of the manuscript version, Sally had helpfully written, "STI Cover Page—will be removed upon journal submission."[44] Nemeroff was omnipresent in this work and, according to Mickey Nardo, made "44 paid trips for GSK [in 2001] to give 'talks' as part of their Speakers' Bureau."[45]

Sally stepped away from pediatric depression to ghost, together with C. Gloria Mao at STI, for Kimberly Yonkers, a professor of psychiatry at Yale, an article on paroxetine and premenstrual dysphoria in women.[46] Draft I was completed in March 2003. The piece appeared in a special issue of the *Psychopharmacology Bulletin* in Winter 2003. Sally and Gloria informed Dr. Yonkers that the manuscript title page would "be removed before submission."[47]

And PTSD! Sally and paroxetine were there as well. In 2002, the International Consensus Group on Depression and Anxiety, at a meeting that GSK supported, issued a "consensus statement on Posttraumatic Stress Disorder."[48] In April 2003, Sally produced the first draft of that statement, neatly aligned with GFK's interest in indicating paroxetine for the disorder.[49]

Sally Laden led the indication sprawl for Paxil. To get Paxil into the pregnancy market, D. Jeffrey Newport and Zachary Stowe, both at Emory, were the go-to "authors." In January 2003, Sally prepared an article that appeared under their names in the *Psychopharmacology Bulletin*. The cover page of her draft advised, "To be removed before submission."[50] In the published piece we find: "Disclosure: This work was supported by an unrestricted educational grant from GSK. Dr. Stowe serves as scientific advisor for and receives research grants from Pfizer and GSK."[51]

Again in 2003, Sally got Dwight Evans and Dennis Charney into *Biological Psychiatry* with a piece on Paxil and medical illness.[52] There was, however, one problem with the article: Sally claimed that GSK had not paid her for writing it. "Is there a problem with my invoice for writing Dwight Evans' editorial for the DBSA's [Depression and Bipolar Support Alliance] comorbidity issue to *Biological Psychiatry*? I submitted it over a month ago."[53]

Nardo commented of these antics: "There was a whole issue of *Biological Psychiatry* cheerleading treating depression in physically ill patients introduced by a Sally Laden special. Antidepressants are decidedly unhelpful in medically ill patients, but there are a lot of them so they [GSK] went for the market. Pregnancy is right common too, so off they went. All of this hype solidified the notion that these drugs were 'antidepressants' and any cause of 'depression' required their use."[54]

Even after Sally had left GSK in summer 2003, the company continued to rely on her to ghost such pieces as "The Safety of Antidepressants in Breast Feeding" (Sally's proposed fee was $12,000) and "Safety and Tolerability of Paxil CR" ($17,000).[55] GSK funded a support group, the DBSA, and in August 2003 Lydia Lewis, the president of the DBSA, asked Sally to write up their upcoming consensus meeting in November. The question was: Should Sally bill the DBSA for her services or GSK directly? (Lydia preferred the latter.)[56]

In these years Sally had time to ghost other projects for Charlies Nemeroff as well. But this time it was an entire textbook, to be "authored" by Charles Nemeroff and Alan Schatzberg. By February 1997, her "preliminary draft" was ready for their approval. In a cover letter, Sally said that this was a "sample text for preliminary comment." Draft I, due May 2, would be forwarded to the co-authors and sponsor, as well to the publisher.[57] (So, the American Psychiatric Press was in on the scam from the beginning.) The title page of the preliminary draft said, "Recognition and Treatment of Psychiatric Disorders: A Psychopharmacology Handbook for Primary Care Physicians, Developed by Diane M. Coniglio, PharmD, and Sally K. Laden, MS, at Scientific Therapeutics Information in Springfield. New Jersey." Paxil received prominent play in the "handbook," and competing agents were slaked for their side effects. In the publication, SmithKline was thanked "for providing an unrestricted educational grant to Scientific Therapeutic Information for the development of this handbook."[58] Diane Coniglio was acknowledged for "editorial assistance." Twenty years previously, this kind of wholesale deceit would have been unheard of.[59]

The Sally story does not end with the ghosting of articles on Paxil for adolescents. As the write-up of study #329 was progressing, Sally was working on another GSK study, #352, of Paxil in adult bipolar disorder. It, too, ended in scandal: Jay Amsterdam at the University of Pennsylvania, who contributed the greatest number of patients to the trial, was omitted from the author list because, as his lawyers argued, his "professional ethics would not allow him to lend his name to a ghostwritten work. . . [nor] allow the other 'authors' to turn a failed study into an undisclosed promotional marketing manuscript for the sponsor."[60] The paper was ultimately accepted by the *American Journal of Psychiatry*, "facilitated by the journal editor who also had financial ties to GSK." Trial #352 was, like #329, basically a failed study that the company spun as a resounding success.[61] A much larger story unfolded around the indifference of the University of Pennsylvania to scientific misconduct.[62] But for our purposes, it was Sally who wrote the paper and who recruited Nemeroff to figure among the authors. Mickey Nardo branded #352 as "yet another example of malignant pseudo-science."[63]

Sally Sounds the Alarm About Depression

> Sally Laden is surely one of the most prolific authors in the scientific literature, yet a PubMed search would not reveal this.—Ed Silverman (2012)[64]

As arguably the world's most influential female "psychopharmacologist," Sally sounded the alarm about depression. Each of her creations began with some intonation about the terrible depression epidemic sweeping the globe.

As we have seen, she and Diane Coniglio ghosted the textbook *Recognition and Treatment of Psychiatric Disorders: A Psychopharmacology Handbook for Primary Care* that Nemeroff and Schatzberg were said to have written. GSK subsidized it, and of course it featured Paxil prominently.

And we know that Sally ghosted the article about the big trial #329 of Paxil in adolescents in 2001 that Martin Keller was said to have "authored." "Depressed adolescents grow up to be depressed adults," she stated.[65]

In an editorial in *Biological Psychiatry* that she ghosted for Dwight Evans and Dennis Charney in 2003, she claimed that, "By the year 2030 [depression], will remain a leading cause of disability, second only to cardiovascular disease."[66]

In an article on vagal nerve stimulation therapy that she ghosted in 2006 for Nemeroff and co-authors for *Neuropsychopharmacology*, she asserted that, "Major depression is now recognized as a highly prevalent, chronic, recurrent, and disabling biological disorder."[67]

The above are just a sampling of Sally's many concoctions. It would not be too much to claim that she was the "Typhoid Mary" of the depression world. The recruitment of big names was possible only because GSK was spraying money about the world of upper-level KOLs (see Chapter 9). The #329 trial raised fundamental questions about the nature of "adolescent depression" and whether Paxil was a suitable remedy. One of the reviewers of the first big article on the trial asked if childhood depression was really the same as adult depression. "The field has maintained that the diagnosis of depression in youth is essentially the same as that in adults, yet the treatment literature is strikingly different [meaning very high placebo responses]. Do these findings potentially suggest something about either the method used to diagnose depression, or the validity of the diagnosis itself, in this population? How is it that youth with persistent major depression for a year improve at basically a 50 percent response rate in a placebo arm?" (In the margin, a GSK executive said, "not really addressed.")[68]

So, we find here a fundamental change in the nature of the medical "literature." As one well-informed observer put it, "The medical community is currently trying to come to grips with the idea that much of the clinical trial literature has not been written by the named authors, and, instead, has been written by medical writers employed by pharmaceutical companies who are not listed on the author byline."[69]

The Sally Laden story points like a dagger at the heart of American psychopharmacology, exposing the manipulation of supposedly scientific data for commercial purposes and the extent to which the leaders of the field permitted themselves to be bought off as shills rather than serving, at the summit of their craft, as paladins for the advancement of scientific knowledge. The story of Sally and study #329 became famous only because the accident of litigation made the documents publicly available. But it was in no way egregious. It was typical.

At the end of the day, even Sally's skills at massaging the data could not overcome everything. Apropos a failed trial of Paxil in panic disorder, she told her boss, "There are some data that no amount of spin will fix."[70]

The Paxil Miracle

Paxil was essentially a failed drug. But that did not stop it from becoming, at a certain point, the world's most widely prescribed antidepressant. This was owing to genius marketing.

In 1999, SKG created a 150-person sales force to promote Paxil to psychiatrists. In October 2000, the company organized a Paxil Clinicians Speaker Council ("Psychnet") at the Palace Hotel in San Francisco, to train psychiatrists to be public advocates for the drug. Sally Laden organized the slide presentation, to which participants would be introduced and which would become part of their standard speakers' kit. Participants received an honorarium of $5,000 plus expenses.[71] They were, of course, in every sense shills.

The head office pulled out the promotional stops. In August 2001, a note from Zachary Hawkins, Paxil product management, to "all sales reps selling Paxil" said of the trial's "significance": "This 'cutting-edge,' landmark study is the first to compare efficacy of an SSRI and a TCA with placebo in the treatment of major depression in adolescents. [This was false: the trial was too underpowered to compare imipramine and paroxetine directly.] Paxil demonstrates REMARKABLE Efficacy and Safety in the treatment of adolescent depression." The box was checked saying "The article is for pharma consultants' information only. Do not use it with or distribute to physicians."[72] Yet this was a pro forma disclaimer, along the lines of "wink, wink." Of course the sales reps would mention the trial to clinicians.

Study #329 has been more widely discussed than any other clinical trial in psychiatry, and the impression has arisen that it was largely SKB that was the bad guy in spinning the results. I think this unduly exculpates Sally Laden's work at STI. We don't know if she rearranged the outcome variables on the company's instructions or on her own hook. In a subsequent deposition she blamed McCafferty and that she had worked only with the data the company sent her.[73]

Some people at SKB did try to keep the record straight and to include information unfavorable to Paxil. David Duff at SKB, who reviewed the final draft, noted, for example, that, "There is no mention that insomnia also occurred more frequently on paroxetine than on placebo (15.1% vs 4.6%)."[74] On another occasion, it was Jim McCafferty who had to restrain Sally: "It seems incongruous that we state that paroxetine is safe yet report so many SAEs [serious adverse events]. I know the investigators have not raised an issue, but I fear that the editors will. I am still not sure how to describe these events." He said he would go over the data one more time.[75]

There is plenty of evidence that SmithKline wanted to bend the rules of scientific trials (ghosting!), but the reckless distortion of findings was not in the company's playbook. In view of the meticulousness with which GSK staff conducted the analysis of the data, Bernard Carroll's later judgment, while hitting some central truth, nonetheless seems harsh: "The study has all the hallmarks of an experimercial, a cost-is-no-object exercise driven by a corporate sponsor to create positive publicity for a product in its market niche. This is not clinical science; this is product placement."[76]

18

Atypicals

The treatments we now have are lousy.—Walter Brown, Brown University (2008)[1]

Just as "major depression," a non-existent disease, was the stumbling block to the development of new drugs for mood disorders, "schizophrenia" was the stumbling block for the development of new drugs for disabling disorders of connectivity and mobilization. The parallel is alarming: what were, in both cases, nondiseases became pipelines for billions of dollars in profit for industry. There can be no more striking proof of the failure of psychopharmacology as a scientific paradigm.

Antipsychotics go right back to Smith Kline's chlorpromazine, marketed in the United States in 1954. But, the early antipsychotics had movement disorders as a significant side effect. Thus, the market was ready for a new generation of antipsychotics that did not cause extrapyramidal symptoms (EPS) or tardive dyskinesia (TD). The first antipsychotic with relatively few movement side effects was probably Mellaril (thioridazine), a member of the phenothiazine class (same as chlorpromazine) that Sandoz brought out in 1959. Or, at least, this was Leo Hollister's opinion.[2] Sandoz marketed Mellaril initially as a tranquilizer rather than as an antipsychotic.[3] Yet, among its side effects, it had a tendency to cause sudden death through torsade de pointes (ventricular tachycardia),[4] and after decades of denial, in 2005 the company withdrew it from the market.

The real story of the atypicals[5] shows, once again, how psychopharmacology was downgraded through the conversion of science into commerce.

The market was keen to replace the first-generation antipsychotics (FGAs, typicals) because of their considerable adverse effects on movement: acute EPS and TD. In the mid-1980s, Bob Temple at FDA found the emerging uptick in concern about the FGAs a bit puzzling. In a note in 1983 to a higher-up at FDA, he said: "The association between major tranquilizers and tardive dyskinesia is hardly a new issue and it is difficult to conceive of a practicing psychiatrist who is not well aware of the problem. We are not sure why there has been interest in the problem recently, but there seems to be a relatively small body of physicians who have argued that the [dyskinesia] problem is worse than the disease the drugs are used to treat. It is my impression, and Dr. Leber's, that this reflects a failure to re-member what the treatment of psychosis was like before the major tranquilizers made their appearance."[6] Thus, concern was building. Could this "small body of physicians" be laying the rails for the appearance of the atypicals?

In 1987, on the threshold of the introduction of the second-generation antipsychotics (SGAs, atypicals), Leo Hollister—apparently unaware that the new generation lay just around the corner—complained of the FGAs: "It is more discouraging that more effective pharmacotherapy for schizophrenia has not been developed in the more than three decades since the introduction of the first effective drugs." The current drugs, he said, "are not curative; their ameliorative effects are often limited; many patients remain totally unresponsive; they are un-pleasant to take . . . and they produce major side effects, such as tardive dyski-nesia and tardive psychosis."[7]

For those in the audience at the American College of Neuro-psychopharmacology (ACNP) meeting, the introduction of the first of the SGAs—clozapine—must have seemed Heaven-sent. The Johnson & Johnson publicity machine claimed that all the disadvantages had been overcome.

Yet it was just hype. The SGAs were no more effective than the FGAs. One would never know this from the hopelessly corrupted clinical trial literature.

Clozapine

Clozapine, the first of the true atypical antipsychotics, turned out to be the most effective of them but also the most dangerous. Clozapine, which the US branch of Sandoz marketed as Clozaril, appeared in 1990.

The Wander company in Berne synthesized clozapine in 1963 and put it into animal trials, and then into clinical trials in Berne and in Vienna's Steinhof asylum. The first report appeared in a Viennese medical journal in 1966.[8] The drug did not seem to cause EPS, at least not in short-term use.[9] Wander couldn't believe the results and was "strongly critical" of them, as Jules Angst later said.[10] When Sandoz bought Wander in 1967, they wanted to extract some value from the firm, given all the money they had paid. Clozapine had been launched in Europe in 1969, and Sandoz patented the drug in the United States in 1970. Beginning in 1971, with Angst's randomized controlled trial (RCT) in Zurich, serious investigations commenced.[11]

The easy collaboration between German academics and Swiss drug companies is of considerable interest. Hippius and his "group of five" psychopharmacologists in Berlin began working with the Wander company in Berne over clozapine; they published a brief note in 1966 at an International College of Neuropsychopharmacology (CINP) Congress in Washington DC.[12]

In 1971, Hippius and Günther Stille, pharmacology professor and consultant at Wander, considered the possibility of an antipsychotic without "neuroleptic" (EPS) properties.[13]

But clozapine was bugged by concerns about its toxicity. It had the occasional side effect (in 1.5 percent of patients[14]) of suppressing the production of white cells in the bone marrow, called agranulocytosis. In 1975, Sandoz withdrew the drug from most markets because of the bone marrow problems. Also, because it had so few extrapyramidal effects (side effects that were believed in the day to be a marker of antipsychotic action), Sandoz thought it must be a weak drug. The company was about to ban it entirely when Hippius traveled to Berne and made an impassioned plea for the drug to be kept on the market, at least in Germany.[15]

Clozapine had never been formally admitted to the US market. Sandoz did apply to the FDA in 1971 for permission to put it into trials as an investigational new drug (IND), but clozapine was banned in 1975 and the IND application was withdrawn. Later, Sandoz refused to sell the drug unless clinicians agreed to subject their patients to a weekly monitoring system, which Sandoz originally sold separately. It was cumbersome and off-putting to many, yet it was deemed necessary because in the United States in the first few months of the drug's sales, the monitoring system identified 62 cases of "agranulo," and the company speculated "that at least six deaths could have occurred if the system had not been in place."[16]

Nathan Kline then began treating patients with clozapine, but his IND application was taken away when the drug was banned in 1975, and Kline died before the drug could be developed. In 1975, Sandoz asked John Kane at Hillside Hospital to take over Kline's patients and to wean them off clozapine. Kane began to discontinue clozapine in the patients, and the results were horrible. The patients began importing the drug themselves from Europe and Latin America. Kane said, "I had never heard of anyone doing that with an antipsychotic drug."[17] Furthermore, a small number of psychiatrists, such as George Simpson at Rockland State Hospital, thought clozapine was, as Simpson said, "clearly a unique drug," and they continued to prescribe it.[18]

Herb Meltzer, at Case Western University in Cleveland, was agitating behind the scenes at Sandoz,[19] and in 1983 Sandoz submitted another application to the FDA on behalf of clozapine. Yet it was turned down as too dangerous. Still, the FDA told Sandoz that clozapine might be approvable in a population of treatment-unresponsive patients. So, Sandoz asked John Kane and Meltzer to organize such a trial. This became the famous "study 30." Both researchers were veteran psychopharmacologists and part of the Clozaril Study Group. Sandoz then resubmitted in 1987.

In 1988, Kane and Meltzer confirmed that the drug really did bring about improvements in schizophrenic patients: They tried it on schizophrenics who had failed to respond to three different antipsychotics and were then randomized to a blinded trial of clozapine versus chlorpromazine.[20] (It was somewhat unnerving that clozapine did much better in the trials sponsored by Sandoz then in the non-industry-sponsored trials.[21]) Because of the risk of agranulocytosis, the original indication was for clozapine as a second-line treatment. Clozapine was later considered the first "atypical," or SGA. But when it hit the US market in 1990, it was not marketed as that. Rather, the emphasis was on its use in "latent schizophrenia."[22] Tom Laughren at FDA wrapped up the significance of the Kane-Meltzer trial: "I think that essentially what study 30 shows is that clozapine does for resistant patients what the standard antipsychotic drugs do for the more typical psychotic patients. I personally think that is an important result."[23]

As for neurotransmitters, the clozapine story was not a brilliant affirmation of their centrality. Clozapine was said to have a strong effect on serotonin, quetiapine a weaker one, and so forth. Why any of this mattered is unclear, except to undermine the dopamine theory of psychosis. As Goodman and Gilman's *The Pharmacological Basis of Therapeutics*, the standard pharmacology textbook, observed in 1990, the emergence of clozapine "casts some doubt on the necessity for dopaminergic antagonism in order to produce antipsychotic actions."[24]

And the receptor profile story that gave the drug class its scientific basis? It was mainly just a story. As neuroscience historians Alan Baumeister and Jennifer Francis at Louisiana State University observed in 2002, "Probably the most compelling evidence for the dopamine hypothesis of schizophrenia is the strong correlation between the antipsychotic potency of conventional neuroleptics and the blockage of the D2 dopamine receptor. Even here, however, the evidence is vitiated by the fact that clozapine, an effective atypical [SGA] neuroleptic, is a weak D2 antagonist."[25]

If the dopamine-specificity theory had prevailed, clozapine might never have seen the light of day. As Paul Leber at FDA told Dennis Charney in 1995, "This issue of specific receptor binding affinity might have never developed clozapine, because it seems to be surprisingly weak as a D2 blocker. So the system of classification may not work the way you think, even though it would be another way to put your cookie cutter in the dough of nature.[26]

Clozapine, like so many antipsychotics, also had a history of effectiveness as a serious antidepressant, and were it not for the absurd American insistence on treating antidepressants and antipsychotics as entirely separate drug classes, it might have done good service in the mood area. Early in the development of the drug, Wander brought Frank Ayd over to Berne to talk about a predecessor of clozapine as an antidepressant. Ayd said, "The drug turned out to be a very effective antidepressant in a certain dose range. I had seen no serious adverse effects with it until, ninety percent through the study, 'bingo' a fatal agranulocytosis occurred in an elderly woman."[27] This was an early warning flare.

Thus, a cautionary remark is in order. Clozapine was more dangerous than any other SGAs (if you exempt the weight gains seen with a drug like Lilly's Zyprexa). Pierre Simon, a Parisian psychopharmacologist, participated with Pierre Deniker in one of the earliest clozapine trials. "We treated ten patients. One died from a malignant tumor, one had an agranulocytosis and one had a strange hyperthermia, so the drug was returned to the company, saying that it was too dangerous to develop."[28] In November 1994, Alan Gelenberg at Harvard sounded a warning for the United States: "Clozapine's efficacy in the treatment of chronic psychotic conditions is unquestionable, impressive, and often qualitatively as well as quantitatively different from that of traditional neuroleptics. Nonetheless, it is truly a 'double-edged sword,' as its clinical profile entails many problematic and several life-threatening effects."[29]

The FDA struggled with clozapine, finally approving it in 1989. It was further approved for "recurrent suicidal behavior" in 1992. ("The number [of patients] needed to treat to prevent one suicide attempt was 13," said John Kane in 2003, chief of Hillside Hospital.[30]) In 1995, Paul Leber, at a meeting of the Psychopharmacologic Drugs Advisory Committee (PDAC), called it "a drug which Herb [Meltzer] and others believed must work, and we weren't convinced it worked in circumstances enough to justify the risk."[31] The side effects of clozapine were not limited to agranulocytosis but included cardiomyopathy, cardiomyositis, and diabetes. In a sense, using clozapine was playing with fire, despite the drug's manifest effectiveness. David Healy wrote, "I have had more people die early on clozapine than on all other antipsychotics combined."[32] Clozapine was third on an FDA list of all drugs having fatal outcomes in the years 1998 to 2005 (after oxycodone and fentanyl).[33]

Few thought clozapine ineffective as an antipsychotic, but Paul Janssen, often a contrarian, had contrary views here as well. He said of clozapine, "It sedates. In my opinion this is all. I would very much like to see these fantastic patients that they are always referring to." He mentioned Meltzer: "When Meltzer talks, he pronounces the word clozapine at least once in every sentence if not twice." "Most of the clozapine patients I have seen are very severely sedated. This is not what we want. . . . In my opinion, this whole field of the so-called atypical neuroleptics is a pure invention—doesn't exist."[34] (Of course, Janssen's baby was the rival FGA Haldol.)

The whole clozapine story is a perfect example of a drug creating a disease. Clozapine created "treatment-resistant schizophrenia." When David Healy interviewed Paul Leber, at a time when Leber was still head of neuroscience at the FDA, Healy asked about "the creation of the category of a treatment-resistant indication and [its use] by the industry as a justification for a substantial price hike." Leber: "Absolutely, it is always conceivable when you are trying to do the right thing that you create things that you're not appreciative enough to see what's likely to happen. We are all imperfect. No doubt we may have created an indication that doesn't exist."[35]

At a 1995 meeting of the PDAC on antipsychotics, Carol Tamminga, a leading psychopharmacologist at the University of Maryland, said, "I might suggest that neuroleptic-resistant schizophrenia is a subgroup that was more or less created by the FDA, or at least suggested when clozapine was really approved for this subgroup." She considered the response of schizophrenics to neuroleptic drugs "by and large a continuum, all the way from the very most resistant to the very most responsive to neuroleptic drugs." John Kane seconded the comment: "The concept of treatment refractoriness has sort of taken on a life of its own."[36] Letting drug companies, and their need to find market space, define diagnosis is not really the way we do nosology.

But if treatment-resistant schizophrenia was not a valid subgroup in the amorphous diagnosis of schizophrenia, what were the valid subgroups? Paul Leber asked this question, and it has never really been answered: "The problem is that, given what psychiatric diagnosis is—descriptive, phenotypic, and taxonomic— you really don't have a basis for biologically carving nature at the joints."[37] The comment is interesting because just around the corner lay the question, which he did not ask but might well have, are the "subgroups" in fact separate diseases?

Clozapine occupied, therefore, a kind of twilight status in the rise and fall of psychopharmacology: sounded like a triumph, but maybe not.

What's in a Name?

In the 1970s, the concept of atypical antipsychotics began to emerge with the notion that such agents as pimozide and thioridazine caused fewer EPS. This idea was soon abandoned for those drugs. But with the appearance of such agents as Risperdal (risperidone) in 1993, there was said to be a new and special group of antipsychotics with a distinctive receptor profile that produced fewer dyskinesias.[38] "A new class of antipsychotic" screamed Janssen's first ad for Risperdal in Britain in 1993. Good for positive and negative symptoms and causes fewer EPS than haloperidol.[39] Initially, Janssen called it a serotonin-dopamine antagonist (SDA), as opposed to a "conventional" antipsychotic. Janssen soon ditched the SDA concept, yet it was slow to adopt the term "atypical," and in fact in 2001 Janssen counter-detailed Lilly's "atypical antipsychotic" Zyprexa (without mentioning it by name) as causing hyperglycemia and diabetes. But everybody knew Zyprexa was meant.[40] Finally, in January 2004, Janssen crumbled and began praising its own drug Risperdal as an "oral atypical."[41]

Lilly launched Zyprexa (olanzapine) in 1996, but it wasn't until February 2001 that they discovered the marketing theme of "atypical": "the first and only atypical agent indicated for . . . schizophrenia,"[42] which, as we have just seen, Janssen immediately counter-detailed.

The term "second-generation antipsychotic" seems to have come from the academy rather than industry. It was coined around 2000, possibly by the department of psychiatry of the University of North Carolina (UNC), in a 2001 study led by Miranda Chakos of UNC. Chakos contrasted "second-generation antipsychotics" with "conventional antipsychotics."[43] But it would not have been a stretch to substitute "first-generation" for conventional, and that happened within a year or two. Thus, the second-generation concept comes from the academy rather than industry, yet quickly enough, industry as well was contrasting its second-generation products with Haldol and others from the first generation.

Atypical Antipsychotics

Clozapine had an electrifying effect on the industry. Suddenly, everyone wanted a drug that didn't produce dyskinesias (movement disorders), which were the bugbear of the antipsychotic world. All this would happen within the framework of the dopamine D2 antagonists (drugs that prevented dopaminergic neurons from firing). So, this was the essence of the concept of "atypical": atypicals didn't produce dyskinesias. Although clozapine didn't produce any disordered movements, it was in other respects a dangerous drug. The pharmaceutical chemists went to work, and for them dyskinesia research was an area that was "behaviorally driven," not neurotransmitter or receptor driven. It meant synthesizing compounds, putting them into rats or some other animal, and seeing what the resulting behavior was. There were rat-movement tests that involved climbing, swimming, and so forth, but at the end of the day, keeping track of dyskinesias in the rats was the name of the game. Compounds that produced significant dyskinesias were abandoned.

Janssen's Risperdal was introduced in the United States in 1994 for schizophrenia, Lilly's Zyprexa in 1996, AstraZeneca's Seroquel in 1997, and Bristol-Myers Squibb's Abilify in 2002. There were a dozen other atypicals, but these were the main ones.[44]

The atypicals are powerful drugs, and the original concept was that they should only be used in serious illnesses. So did that meant that in trials half of these seriously ill patients were put on a placebo? No. In 1995, Harvard's Carl Salzman told the PDAC that "placebo control is a fiction; it is not that these patients on placebo didn't get any treatment, they just didn't get any Haldol, but they probably got Ativan and chloral hydrate and maybe some Valium, and who knows what else. It is very rare nowadays for a patient in a placebo control trial to be not allowed to get anything if they are really upset. That is unethical. No informed consent, no IRB [Institutional Review Board] would allow that."[45] So the bar in antipsychotic trials was a bit higher than usually thought: The trial drug didn't have to beat a sugar pill, it had to beat Ativan.

How to Make a Nerve Pill

AstraZeneca's Seroquel had the makings of a nerve pill. The story is this: Ace chemist Edward Warawa was the show-driver. In the mid-1970s, he went to work in the American labs of the British firm ICI, in Wilmington, Delaware. ICI, a chemical company, was new to psychotropics and it took them a while to get the CNS program going, which is why Lilly beat them to the punch with olanzapine (Zyprexa). In 1999, the ICI Pharma Group (now called Zeneca) merged with Astra to form AstraZeneca.

Just as Lilly did, Warawa started out with the three rings of the clozapine molecule, then grabbed a piperazine structure off an older drug called Atarax and attached it to the rings. Then it was a matter of what atoms or molecules ("substituents") to put on the rings to make them as undystonic as clozapine and hopefully more powerful as antipsychotics. There was much experimentation, exchanging sulfur, oxygen, and nitrogen atoms in varying combinations, then putting the compounds into rats to observe the behavioral effects. Seroquel was made in March 1985, and was patented in 1989.[46]

None of this research had anything to do with neurotransmitters, and it was only when presenting a compound for possible patenting that the whole neuro-chemistry of the molecule had to be worked up.

AstraZeneca worked systematically at expanding indications in the Seroquel market, from schizophrenia when it was first marketed in 2002, to "irritability with autism" in 2009, with four other indications in between.

Some thought that, without these expanded indications, Seroquel would have died a quick death, because it was not very powerful as an antipsychotic, and it caused weight gain. But, in the hands of primary care, the indications turned Seroquel into a billion-dollar drug. Thus, Seroquel, which was much more dangerous than Valium, ended up, as a nerve pill, filling the hole left by the "dangerous" benzodiazepines.[47]

But how to spin it? Something was up when, on February 12, 1997, AstraZeneca executive Richard Lawrence messaged a wide distribution[48]: "I am not 100% comfortable with this data [on Seroquel side effects] being made publically [sic] available at the present time—however I understand that we have little choice—Lisa [Arvanitis] has done a great 'smoke-and-mirrors' job!" (a reference to her work in obfuscating the patients' weight gain in one of the trials).[49]

Lisa Arvanitis was a physician and head of the Seroquel team. Nardo said of Dr. Arvanitis's efforts, "I can find no place where it seemed to dawn on her that they had a dog of a drug–a weak antipsychotic that makes patients gain a lot of weight and sometimes develop diabetes. . . . She was as much part of the Sales and Marketing department as anyone else. I doubt this was what the little girl Lisa thought about when she dreamed of being a doctor as a child."[50]

Seven months later, Arvanitis leveled with the rest of the Seroquel team: The big problem was weight gain. "While weight gain slows over the longer term (I only considered to 52 weeks) there still is weight gain. It doesn't stop—the slope just appears to change. The magnitude of weight gain at 52 weeks (regardless of pool or cohort) is about 5 kg. . . . Forty-five percent of all patients showed this kind of "clinically significant weight gain." The problem was what to tell the sales force. Lilly's olanzapine had big weight gain, too. Could they repool some of the studies? "I have to keep asking myself, are we going to go through the motions, using precious resources and not really come up with anything more solid for the sales reps?"[51]

Leaping ahead a few years, Seroquel sales were booming, going from $63 million in 1998 to $2.76 billion in 2005, an increase of 4,280 percent in 7 years. The problem at this point was how to detail the drug to primary care physicians (PCPs). In August 2002, AstraZeneca had arranged for two focus groups with PCPs to talk about their needs. In October, executive Christopher Maurer reported the gist to the team: "Dementia is the most attractive opportunity to expand use of Seroquel with PCPs." (Dementia had not been accepted by the FDA as an indication for Seroquel.) The logic: Family doctors "retain ownership of these patients," and don't refer them to specialists.

How about the accepted indications? Maurer said, "PCPs regard bipolar disorder, like schizophrenia, as beyond their domain and, as a result, they are not eager to treat it."

Treatment-resistant depression? Again, no thanks. "The risk of suicide with these patients makes PCPs nervous."

Maurer concluded that dementia and "treatment-resistant anxiety" were the pathway to the future.[52]

Now key opinion leaders (KOLs) entered the picture to help promote Seroquel. How about bipolar disorder? In June of the following year, 2003, executive William Hess let the team know how the promotional campaign on bipolar disorder called the REACH Program was coming along. In November, there was to be a big launch. "During this meeting, the REACH faculty, comprised of top-tier, internationally esteemed bipolar key opinion leaders (KOLs), will train a subset of national-level KOLs on the program's fundamentals. The goal is that these selected national-level KOLs will subsequently become ambassadors for the program within local markets." There would, for example, be 20 KOLs from

Canada and seven from Austria. Keep in mind that these KOLs were the top psychiatrists in the field. AstraZeneca was going to have a Continuing Medical Education (CME) company "organizing this program."[53]

The term KOL was used entirely without irony. The mind reels. It meant the main international experts on bipolar disorder would be training other experts to spread the AstraZeneca message on Seroquel.

Across the company, "KOL management is one of the hot topics in the organization today," as Johan Hoegstedt told top executives. "We should have a set of core AZ brand slides that we consistently refer to." This would greatly simplify life for the KOLs, because they could just present the company's slides.[54]

AstraZeneca made full use, as did other companies, of medical communications firms to draft papers describing the results of its trials. They had just completed trial "104" and the question was, who should sign on as authors (these "authors," had, of course been completely uninvolved in the study). So, in February 2004, executive John P. Gonzalez wrote the team with troubling news: Nassir Ghaemi, a leading figure in psychiatry at Tufts University, was refusing to play along. Gonzalez said, "As you are aware, trial 104 main paper is authored by Roger MacIntyre and he had requested Nassir Ghaemi be second author. Please note the draft of the paper is well advanced, having already had Roger's comments back. . . . In summary, [Ghaemi] is asking to see the raw data so that he can analyse them himself. All of this . . . is likely to lead to reinterpretation of the study results."

Ed Repp, the Seroquel brand leader, responded, "I vote for 'NOT' giving the raw data. If that's the only path forward, I'd suggest dropping Dr. Ghaemi as an author."[55] Ghaemi was in fact dropped (and for this action, Ghaemi became a hero of Nardo's![56]).

AstraZeneca used medical communications companies to ghostwrite research reports, and the company on the Seroquel file was Parexel Medical Marketing Services. By November 2005, they had completed a titanic assignment: 19 abstracts (that they had written) had been submitted by their Bipolar Execution and Strategy Team for the 2006 meeting of the American Psychiatric Association. For the BOLDER project (Bipolar Execution and Strategy Team) the following abstracts had been submitted: Thase (main results), Macfadden [the AZ physician leader of the Seroquel team] (suicidality), Lydiard (anxiety), Weisler (bipolar I), and Suppes/Hirschfeld (bipolar II).

Lauren Duby at Parexel said, "Thanks to everyone who helped push these through the necessary review procedures."[57]

Wayne Macfadden, the Seroquel medical adviser, left AstraZeneca in 2006 for Janssen. In a deposition in 2007, Macfadden gave insight into the nature of Parexel's assistance.

Q: "And Parexel helped prepare and in fact sometimes prepared entire manuscripts on AstraZeneca's clinical trials. True?"

MACFADDEN: "Parexel would often draft manuscripts for AstraZeneca to complete."

Q: "And Parexel would draft manuscripts and then contact later authors, 'authors,' who would then be listed as the actual author of the paper that was initially drafted by Parexel. True?"

MACFADDEN: "These manuscripts were then circulated to authors for their comments and reviews."

The deposition then drifted to the subject of Seroquel's advantages, if any, over other antipsychotics. Macfadden's true assessment of Seroquel is interesting:

Q: Did Seroquel ever beat any other second-generation antipsychotic in a clinical trial?

MACFADDEN: "My recollection was that there was not a study in which there was a significant advantage in efficacy for Seroquel compared to other atypicals."

Q: "Not only would it be untrue to say that Seroquel was more efficacious than a second-generation antipsychotic, it would be untrue to say that Seroquel was more efficacious than a first-generation antipsychotic, true?"

MACFADDEN: "There was no clinical trial in which Seroquel demonstrated statistically significant superiority over a typical [first-generation] antipsychotic."[58]

The published literature, of course, told a very different story. Isn't the contrast interesting between the principled behavior of the former Astra in Sweden, voluntarily withdrawing zimelidine and remoxipride, and the judgment of US attorneys in 2009, as the Department of Justice sued AstraZeneca for concealing life-threatening conditions like diabetes. "The marketing and promotion efforts of Astra/Zeneca, through its advertisers and sales force, overstated the benefits of Seroquel and minimized, downplayed and concealed the risks associated with this drug. . . . [The company] recklessly, negligently, and with willful wanton indifference to the health and safety of consumers, failed to include any warning regarding hyperglycemia, diabetes mellitus, or related conditions until on or after January 2004."[59]

Turning the Atypicals into Big Bucks

The FDA approved Risperdal for schizophrenia and bipolar mania at the end of 1993. When Janssen launched the drug in the United States in 1994, it was with the idea of replacing Haldol. Risperdal looked to be a "non-lethal Clozaril," in other words, an atypical that was not deadly and did not cause huge weight gains like its competitor Zyprexa (this latter hope was in vain). Yet clozapine sailed under the "treatment-resistant" flag. The article in 1994 that launched Risperdal in the academic press did not assign a new name to this drug class, yet indicated its effectiveness in "treatment-resistant patients."[60] By its fourth birthday in 1998, Risperdal had become "the number one prescribed antipsychotic in the United States," as Johnson & Johnson CEO Alex Gorsky proudly informed company staff.[61] (Gorsky was a J&J lifer, aside from a brief sojourn at Novartis, and had begun with Janssen in 1988 as a sales rep.)

By 2005, Risperdal was an almost $2 billion-a-year drug.

With Zyprexa, Lilly faced the problem of turning a market niche—psychosis—into big bucks. This problem started to be solved for Lilly when Zyprexa was approved for bipolar disorder in 2000. One analyst said, "To get beyond a certain point, companies that manufactured the atypicals needed to expand into the primary-care market." A journalist added, "The big money, in other words, lay in the offices of suburban doctors and family physicians," certainly not populated by chronic schizophrenics. Led by Allan Breier, Lilly planned to move Zyprexa into depression. But it wasn't indicated for depression. The solution: convince the family docs that "what they thought was depression was in fact one half of the mood swings of bipolar disorder."[62]

In 2000, Lilly conceived the "Viva Zyprexa" campaign to persuade PCPs to treat symptoms rather than disorders. The campaign was originally aimed at the "agitation" of dementia. But, in time, schizophrenia became, as Carroll pointed out, "suspiciousness" and mania became "agitation." "In depression, see every sign of agitation as Mania, ergo Bipolar, ergo Zyprexa (approved for 'mixed episodes.')"[63]

So, if you are a sales rep for Zyprexa, how do you handle balky physicians? Here's the guidance from the "objection workshop" for Lilly's sales reps:

Doc: "I do not treat schizophrenia or bipolar disorder."

Sales rep: "Doctor, would you agree that you see patients who present with symptoms of mood, thought, and behavioral disorders who are not responding to your satisfaction?"

[Doc: "Ummmm, yes."]

Sales rep: "For these patients you identify for a psych referral, do you find that there can be delays, insurance coverage issues, or simply patient refusal? How do you approach these patients?'

Lilly instruction: "Bridge into selling at this point."[64]

The bottom line here is that the makers of the second-generation antipsychotics all faced the same problem: How to turn a 1 percent market into a billion dollar drug. So the indications crossed over into the mood disorders, and the clinical audience became the family docs, not psychiatrists. New indications, such as treatment-resistant depression and treatment-resistant schizophrenia, were discovered. But all of these stratagems were driven by marketing, while they were marketed as science.

Are the Second-Generation Antipsychotics Actually Better?

It seems like the conundrum remains, "My patient is sick, they aren't getting much better. I need to do something—if I don't use an atypical, then what do I do?" When backed into a treatment refractory corner, it is always very hard for us physicians not to act.—Matt Keats, Virginia Beach psychiatrist (2009)[65]

Matt Keats captured the therapeutic challenge of dealing with very sick patients who were not responding to first-generation remedies. Maybe the second generation offered more hope? Yet it started to become apparent that, with the exception of two-edged-sword clozapine, the answer to that was No. (Nowhere in this Pharma-dominated discussion was the concept of electroconvulsive therapy ever mentioned.)

The official line was that "newer agents," with presumably superior mechanisms, should replace the "older agents," with their tired old mechanisms. A colleague broached this argument to Jay Amsterdam, who said, "Given that no one presently alive on planet Earth knows the cause of DSM-5 MDD or schizophrenia, etc., what difference does the never-ending onslaught of 'newer' agents mean for the field relative to those that came before—save to sell 'branded' agents for more money? Why not simply have Pharma increase the price of 'older' generic agents (like they have done with MAOIs) to a stratospheric level so that most patients can no longer afford them, either?"[66]

Alarm bells began to ring in 2000 when the National Schizophrenia Guidelines Development Group in England did a meta-regression analysis of 52 RCTs that compared the atypical antipsychotics to the typicals. The result: when the dose of Haldol (the first-generation antipsychotic) was held down to reasonable levels, Haldol did very well. The authors concluded, "There is no clear evidence that atypical antipsychotics are more effective or are better tolerated than conventional antipsychotics."[67] There was a collective dropping of the penny: In the company-sponsored trials, the comparator drug Haldol had been dosed much too high in order to show an unacceptable side-effects profile.

The scientific death knell for the concept of second-generation antipsychotics (SGAs) rang more loudly in 2004 with a government-sponsored trial of over 1,400 patients in 57 centers called CATIE: the Clinical Antipsychotic Trials of Intervention Effectiveness. None of the SGAs except clozapine was proven to be more effective than perphenazine, a first-generation drug. Side-effect profiles were all over the place—with large weight gains troubling such agents as olanzapine (Zyprexa)—and it was unclear which drug was the safest.[68] But, clearly, none was more effective than pokey old perphenazine, patented by Schering in 1958 and marketed as Trilafon. Nobody today has ever heard of it.

CATIE made the year 2004 into a *prise de conscience* about the SGAs. In that year, total expenditure for antipsychotics was $4.1 billion, up from $1.3 billion in 1997.[69] After CATIE, many psychiatrists began shifting back to first-generation antipsychotics. As James Van Norman, a psychiatrist at a community mental health center in Austin, Texas, told a Texas court in 2012, in the course of a lawsuit against the Big Pharma companies for having gulled the Texan mental health authorities, "For a community mental health center strapped for funding, . . . it just made all the sense in the world to really make an effort to shift back over to the first-generation medications where it was clinically appropriate." They were astonished at the weight gains. "Typically, in a maintenance situation, we see somebody about every three months. And people would come in three months later putting on 20, 30 pounds when they're on second-generation medications."[70]

The price for a little efficacy turned out to be a lot of weight gain. Nardo graphed efficacy against weight gain. As efficacy increased, the patients' weight rose.[71] (The one exception to this was iloperidone [Vanda Pharmaceuticals' Fanapt], with which weight gain was toward the max, yet efficacy was low.)

The SGAs were not ineffective. There was general agreement that the atypicals had a sometimes "dramatic" effect on hallucinations and delusions, the so-called positive symptoms. But did they really affect such issues as the ability to think clearly ("cognition"), which were more in the domain of negative symptoms? A study in 2007 of first-episode schizophrenics treated with Zyprexa and Risperdal led by Terry Goldberg at Zucker Hillside Hospital cast doubt on this. The patients improved over time on filling out a questionnaire, to be sure, but no more rapidly than did the normals. And Goldberg and team thought the improvement might be due to increasing practice in filling out questionnaires rather than real cognitive changes.[72] William Carpenter, director of the Maryland Psychiatric Research Center, commented of the study, "It is critical that we not misjudge the efficacy evidence for any drug tested for cognition in schizophrenia. Studies to date show either little or no benefit for cognition with the antipsychotic drugs."[73]

CATIE had demonstrated that the FGAs were equal to the SGAs in such areas as "quality of life." A controlled trial in England in 2006 confirmed this: for schizophrenic patients at baseline, the quality of life with the two drug classes was the same; it was identical at the conclusion of the 52-week trial as well. (In fact, the first-generation drugs were slightly superior. Clozapine was not included in the comparison).[74]

When a panel of specialists held a debate in May 2005 at the annual meeting of the American Psychiatric Association on which was better, the atypicals or the typicals, the advocates of the old-style Haldol-type drugs landed some deadly blows: the trials had been jury-rigged with super-high doses of Haldol; the trials had handled patient dropouts in a highly favorable way for the atypicals; "all of the studies recruited patients," reported one account, "who had failed on FGAs [first-generation antipsychotics], ensuring a bias in the results toward efficacy with SGAs [second-generation antipsychotics]." The room was packed.[75]

Yet the great antipsychotic wheel rolled on. The FGAs fell increasingly into desuetude. George Simpson commented, "I think we are throwing the older typicals out the window very quickly. In the United States, we're soon going to feel that to use typical antipsychotics is malpractice."[76]

The whole "second-generation antipsychotic" wave, with the exception of clozapine, turned out to be mainly commercial hype. There were few differences between them and the chlorpromazine–haloperidol "first" generation. The big selling point of the SGAs had been their low risk of inducing movement disorders. In 2009, investigators at the Connecticut Mental Health Center reported that the risk of tardive dyskinesia in their schizophrenia patients on atypicals was fully two thirds of the risk with FGAs.[77]

Silvio Garattini, director of the Mario Negri Institute in Milan and possibly Europe's foremost psychopharmacologist, said in 1995 in an interview, ""If we look back at the last 40 years, we have not developed any antipsychotics that are clinically more effective than chlorpromazine." He did not even except Clozaril from this statement.[78]

But all the stops had been pulled out for the SGAs. Leo Hollister mused about the success of the SGAs. "There's a big drive to petition the State legislature to appropriate fifty million dollars or whatever to buy atypicals for more patients, and citizens' groups are demonstrating at the Capitol. Now, you know where that orchestration is coming from. It's very well organized by the drug companies, because they would like nothing more than to have these drugs declared first-line treatments." You could get 10-mg tablets of Haldol, a first-generation antipsychotic, for "less than ten cents," said Hollister. But with the SGAs, state health authorities were budgeting tens of millions of dollars. And the receptor profiles, were they really different in the SGAs than in the first generation? Here, Hollister was agnostic. The atypicals all affected serotonin metabolism, but Hollister thought "that serotonin blockade [doesn't have] a damn thing to do with extrapyramidal reactions or schizophrenia." And the blockade of dopamine receptors, was that important? Hollister shrugged. "The new drugs work exactly the same as the old ones, only less."[79]

It is rare that something is published in a mainline medical journal that would cause industry types to actually choke on their coffee. Yet the piece in early 2009 in the *Lancet* by Peter Tyrer, professor of psychological medicine at the Imperial College London, might have achieved that. He said of the so-called second-generation antipsychotics, "As a group they are no more efficacious, do not improve specific symptoms, have no clearly different side-effect profiles than the first-generation antipsychotics, and are less cost effective. The spurious invention of the atypicals can now be regarded as invention only, cleverly manipulated by the drug industry for marketing purposes."[80] He was playing off a meta-analysis of the SGAs by Stefan Leucht at the Technical University in Munich that had just appeared in the *Lancet*: Leucht and colleagues had found the SGAs highly diverse and not at all a unitary group. None was superior to FGAs for negative symptoms.[81]

In 2008, a staff writer from the *St. Pete Times* in St. Petersburg interviewed Allen Jones, who had blown the whistle on the TMAP scam in Texas (see Chapter 19). In 1993, the FDA had forbidden Janssen from promoting Risperdal as superior to other antipsychotics, so, he said, Janssen did an end run by getting academics to make the claim for them. "They got expert opinion," he said, "to be the deciding factor. Essentially the drug companies could pay people to say what the drug companies could not claim themselves," namely that the atypicals were superior to the FGAs. "It was a concentrated, deliberate attempt to substitute illusion for science." Robert Farley, the journalist who did the interview, continued, "The marketing has been a rousing success. Of the prescribed antipsychotics in Florida last year [2007], 86 percent were atypicals."

Farley interviewed Robert Rosenheck at Yale to see if the benefit justified the cost of the SGAs. Rosenheck said, "There was never any evidence that warranted the amount of money we spent on atypicals. If you look at it independently, it is very clear the results [of the CATIE trial] say there is no benefit" to SGAs over FGAs.

Rosenheck said the favorable opinions were purchased. "[The companies] leverage every single angle they can to persuade every person to secure the opinion that their products are superior. Every possible source of opinion. They use money to establish a relationship with them. The issue is not, 'Were these people influenced?' There is nobody who is not influenced."[82]

Schizophrenia?

Let's explicitly avoid the term "psychosis," because, as William T. Carpenter, Jr., professor of psychiatry at the University of Maryland Medical Center in Baltimore, a very senior figure, said in 2002 "To put it bluntly, fifty years of antipsychotic drug development has not resulted in efficacious treatment for the [negative] aspects of schizophrenia that account for poor functional outcomes." He said there would be no progress until the field abandoned its fixation with psychosis.[83]

As discussed in Chapter 5, there could unquestionably be a serious psychic derailment of the lives of young men and women, sometimes temporary, sometimes lifelong. But it was not necessarily psychotic, if psychosis means the loss of contact with reality that delusions and hallucinations entail ("positive symptoms"). Rather, the essence was the "negative symptoms," a portmanteau term for three kinds of core behavior:

First, "emotional blunting" (sometime called "emotional dementia"), meaning the loss of contact with others, retreating into a shell, and deafness to emotional cues.

Second, "executive dysfunction," meaning basically the inability to get anything done, or to hold a job involving any kind of complexity.

Third, "thought disorder," meaning essentially the inability to think in a linear manner.

Schizophrenics do not necessarily have a monopoly on these symptoms, but when they all occur together, and result in disability, the diagnosis is what was once called "hebephrenia," or core schizophrenia.[84] Schizophrenia is not necessarily psychosis (positive symptoms), and nobody has ever developed a drug to treat the negative symptoms. The ongoing inability to do so is one of the reasons for the gathering despair about psychopharmacology.

Atypicals for Everything!

In psychiatry, all treatments are of benefit in all illnesses.—Jay Amsterdam (2017)[85]

For the antidepressants, there was never a shortage of patients. Depression was as common as the common cold, and for anxiety, PTSD, and all the other indications that the SSRIs gained, the supply of patients was endless. The treatment effects were weak, and patients ended up on the drugs for years, but that was scarcely a problem for industry.

With the SGAs, the problem was different. These were powerful drugs, and treatment effects were never an issue. They were effective for psychosis. So, as Nardo said, "[The antipsychotic makers] weren't handed much of a market, unlike the antidepressant makers. They had to create their own. They aimed for a particular set of situations where the drugs were sought by someone other than the patients themselves: mentally impaired children; autistic children;

the kids with 'super angry/grouchy/cranky irritability' that Joseph Biederman called bipolar kids; elderly people in long-term care; psychotics and others in government facilities, including prisons—something like captive audiences."[86] The drug makers were successful: By 2001, more than half (53 percent) of the atypicals were being prescribed "for conditions other than schizophrenia and similar psychotic disorders," as InfoScriber's Clinical Pharmacology Network reported.[87]

The scramble for indications had the result of pushing the atypicals in the direction of panaceas: They were good for everything! In Oregon in 2004, only 15 percent of Medicaid patients on an atypical antipsychotic had a documented diagnosis of schizophrenia. The other 85 percent were receiving an atypical for "sedation" and the like.[88] As Jay Amsterdam, who in his mood disorders clinic at the University of Pennsylvania had a catbird seat, wrote in 2018,

> The field has moved away from identifying and differentiating specific psychiatric disorders (from others) to a less disciplined model of one drug cures all disorders (or, worse yet, Pharma-invented disorders designed for specific drug response—like Prozac for premenstrual dysphoric disorder and Strattera for ADHD). Put simply, no one in the field who is still actively engaged in randomized clinical trials gives a shit anymore about the concept of differential diagnosis. Our field has now been crucified on the cross of special interests and greed, differential diagnosis can be damned—as atypical antipsychotics are able to cure all disorders with virtually no adverse events![89]

This practice gave many senior clinicians the creeps. Ivan Goldberg, a veteran figure in New York who was seen as one of the wise old hands in the field, said in 2007, "As a profession we have been sold a bill of goods by the drug manufacturers regarding the safety of atypical antipsychotics as medications to be used to treat patients with non-psychotic illnesses. There is an old saying, 'Don't swat flies with an elephant gun' and that seems to be exactly what we are doing." Goldberg meant exposing patients to a huge side-effects downside when "MUCH safer alternative treatments" were available. He mentioned tardive dyskinesia, neuroleptic malignant syndrome, and the metabolic syndrome. "Every atypical antipsychotic has the ability to induce [these] side effects."[90]

So successful had Janssen been at expanding the indications for Risperdal that by 2000, 46 percent of all sales were off-label, which is to say, in areas where promotion was forbidden.[91] And by 2012, Bristol-Myers Squibb and Otsuka's Abilify had become the top-selling drug in the United States![92] These figures were a soaring triumph for drugs that had initially been conceived as treating schizophrenia.

The Elder Market

The decision to go after the eldercare market was a particularly cruel one, given that antipsychotics produce a high mortality in patients with dementia.[93] But the elderly were a perfect target. In the nursing homes, unhappiness—manifest as agitation—abounded. Risperdal would be perfect for the agitated elderly, and in 1998 Janssen launched an "Elder Care" sales force to market to physicians who treated the elderly. Risperdal's share of the geriatric market climbed from 21 percent in 1996 to 51 percent in 1999.[94] Mindful of the mortality issue, the FDA admonished Janssen not to promote in that market. Nonetheless, the company barreled right ahead.

In 1998, J&J signed a contract with Omnicare, the huge provider of medication to nursing facilities, to promote Risperdal. Because the FDA had not licensed a geriatric indication for the agent, this promotion would have been off-label and illegal. J&J was never able to convince the FDA to give them the geriatric indication. In 2005, the FDA mandated a black-box warning in the labels of all five atypicals against prescribing them in the elderly. (In any event, such prescriptions would have been off-label.) The death rate of elderly persons on these drugs was about 1.7 times that of patients on placebo.[95]

Finally, the Feds cracked down. In its 2012 Complaint against Janssen, the Department of Justice said, "From the time Risperdal was first approved in 1993, FDA repeatedly advised Janssen not to market the drug as safe and effective for the elderly. Janssen promoted Risperdal to control behavioral disturbances in the elderly until at least 2005."[96] Warning followed warning. All this bureaucratic finger-wagging had little effect on the company's behavior: the elder market was just too tempting. In 2001, for example, the company produced a "Business Plan" for "LTC/Geriatrics" (Long-Term Care). "Many elderly are placed in nursing homes and other extended care facilities due to their psychotic illness . . . so these facilities and the clinicians that deliver care within them remain important targets for RISPERDAL."[97] "Over the years 1999 to 2004, Janssen gave Omnicare tens of millions of dollars in kickbacks to induce Omnicare to purchase and to recommend Risperdal and other J&J drugs," charged the United States in 2010.[98]

By 2001, Risperdal's share of the dementia market was about 54 percent. A billion-dollar drug in the dementia market.[99] The fines for this behavior were enormous, but you can see why Janssen laughed at them.

The Kids' Market

And what more promising market could there be than kids! (See also the Biederman section of Chapter 9.) The use of antipsychotics in children goes way back. Sam Gershon, today one of the very senior figures in psychopharmacology, was trained in Australia and arrived at Bellevue Hospital in New York in 1963, becoming director of the psychopharmacology program at New York University in 1966. Antipsychotics were flooding the market and just starting to be used in children. Gershon was appalled, and he wrote in a later memoir, "We do not know the etiology of the psychotic disorders we are treating. We cannot label them reliably and the treatments are almost certainly harmful to the brain and other organ systems. Yet we blithely persist as if there were no problems." He said, "Increasing proposals to treat younger and younger children should arouse more alarm in our present state of ignorance." He likened the introduction of the antipsychotics to the earlier use of insulin coma (1933). "The similarities between these two historic events, insulin coma and antipsychotic medication, are disturbingly similar: the benefits were overinflated and the risks underestimated. We seem unable to assimilate that lesson and pass it along."[100] The lesson would be that the application of psychopharmacology to the pediatric population has been a false and dangerous trail.

The Sam Gershons of this world were not listened to. Children became the new growth area for second-generation antipsychotics. The drama of the Risperdal story was Janssen's unflagging efforts to expand the indications. After many false starts, it won a coveted pediatric indication in 2006 for "irritability associated with autism," and in 2007 for "adolescents with schizophrenia" and "children and adolescents with bipolar mania." Other pediatric indications then followed, once the door had been battered down.

And Risperdal was a smash in the pediatric market! By 2002, the drug had 54 percent of child and adolescent sales; pediatric use, then off-label, represented 20 percent of all Risperdal sales. The Risperdal people at Janssen vaunted their "Ziprasidone Destruction Plan."[101] (Ziprasidone, or Geodon, was Pfizer's rival drug.)

SGA prescriptions for children rose tenfold between 1994 and 2004: from around 250 per 100,000 doctor visits to 2,500 in 2004. Half of them were prescribed for "disruptive behavior" (including autism and ADHD), 27 percent for pediatric bipolar disorder, 14 percent for depression, and 13 percent for schizophrenia/psychosis. Drugs like Risperdal were supposed to be "antipsychotics," not "a chemical straight jacket," as the FDA warned.[102]

The first big warning light, comparable to the warning that the CATIE trial flashed for adults in 2004, began in 2008 with a NIMH-sponsored study in children and adolescents of two SGAs—Zyprexa and Risperdal—compared to a first-generation antipsychotic, Abbott's Lidone (molindone).[103] All three tied in efficacy, and the SGAs had large side effects: The drugs produced staggering weight gains. "You could stand outside a clinic," said Mickey Nardo, "and pick out the patients on Zyprexa from across the street."[104] Kids in the Zyprexa group gained an average of 13 pounds over the 8 weeks of the trial, and one 18-year-old boy gained 35 pounds on Risperdal. "Kids at school were making fun of me, all that. I knew I had to get rid of it," he told Benedict Carey at the *New York Times*.[105] This was really bad.

Worse than weight gain was the possibility of brain damage in children.

Mark Kramer said that with antipsychotics, there is "the possibility of irreversible neurological sequelae. The verdict is not quite in on 2nd generation antipsychotics, except to say that many who have scrutinized the data, including me, are not impressed. Their neurological adverse effects, now joined by metabolic adverse-effects safety, are an issue. . . . Use in the elderly and children requires extreme evaluation of risk/benefit."[106] The number of children under 5 in the Medicaid system receiving antipsychotics rose from 7,759 in 1999 to 19,045 in 2008.[107] If the therapeutic skies were ever lit up with warning flares, this would be the occasion.

"Treatment-Resistant Depression"

The ingredients are very simple: a false diagnosis (MDD), a false therapy (SSRI) and voilà: un nouveau champs de commerce!—Martin Schumacher (2020)[108]

The concept of "treatment-resistant depression" emerged from the FDA's failed STAR*D study. The SSRIs in STAR*D had performed so poorly in the treatment of depression that the conceit surfaced that some depressions must be "treatment-resistant." It was not that the drugs were inferior, but that the patients' depressions were unresponsive to treatment. As Bernard Carroll put it, "I would say one of Pharma's greatest coups was the invention and adoption of the meme known as TRD or treatment-resistant depression. The entire STAR*D project was built around that, and what did we learn? Bugger all."[109]

Back in the 1960s, the view was that serious depression would be treated with the TCAs or convulsive therapy, less-severe depression with psychotherapy. This changed in 1980 with DSM-III, when the distinction between serious and less-serious was abolished and everything became "major depression." The SSRIs, which debuted in 1988 with Prozac, were billed as suitable for major depression, meaning for everything. Yet a large number of patients didn't respond to Prozac. What to do? The business solution was to call them treatment resistant, and to supplement Prozac with an atypical antipsychotic.

Here was the problem: The schizophrenic market was never more than 1 percent of the population; the depression market, by contrast, was enormous. But none of the SGAs had been indicated as straight-up antidepressants. How could this be sorted out? Indicate the SGAs for depressions that had not responded to "treatment," meaning had not responded to SSRIs! Thus, with atypical antipsychotics in hand, the companies, their KOL linebackers ready to dash, picked it up and ran with it. Treatment-resistant depression, an iatrogenic entity entirely created by treatment with SSRIs, became an important runway for the SGAs.

The term "treatment-resistant depression" went back to 1959 at least, and there were a smattering of references in the 1970s and after.[110] The more recent launch vehicle seems to have been a piece on Risperdal in 1999 by Robert Ostroff, and J. Craig Nelson, both at Yale.[111] (Undoubtedly, the atypicals relieve depressive illnesses of various kinds, as do many other agents; the question is, at what price? The atypicals are full of side effects, such as weight gain, the "metabolic syndrome," and, down the road, diabetes.)

The launching pad for the profitable concept of treatment-resistant depression was a conference that Janssen organized at Emory University in 2003 on "New Therapies for Treatment-Resistant Depression." Charles Nemeroff, still at Emory, gave the main talk, which was then abstracted in 2004[112] and published in 2005.[113] But an embarrassing series of corrigenda then followed in 2006 and 2007, led by Mark Rapaport. It turned out there had been a huge conflict of interest, among other problems.[114] Then, in 2008, Bernard Carroll savaged the whole agenda of nondisclosure of ties to the sponsor, Janssen, and its jury-rigged reporting of the data.[115]

Nemeroff participated in the big Janssen-funded RCT, reported online in 2008, that found Risperdal effective in treatment-resistant depression.[116] Mark Pollack at Harvard suggested that Risperdal seemed effective in PTSD and that the atypicals held promise in the treatment of mixed anxiety-depression.[117] Emory developed a whole program for the supposedly disabling disorder of treatment-resistant depression at its Brain Health Center.

Bernard Carroll commented later, "Ironically, the wide use of [SSRIs] needs to be considered as a cause of the new epidemic of so-called 'treatment resistant depression,' you know, the cases for whom Abilify and Seroquel are being touted. That is a true iatrogenic train wreck, prescribing antipsychotic drugs for nonpsychotic depressed patients because they did not respond to second-rate antidepressants!"[118] (Most antipsychotics have now been approved either for "adjunctive treatment" of depression, or for "treatment-resistant depression," more or less the same thing.)

"Treatment-resistant" became a phrase that made critical spirits squirm. Nardo said, "Every time I hear something like, 'Now approved for augmentation of antidepressant monotherapy in treatment-resistant depression,' I feel ashamed I'm a psychiatrist."[119]

Carroll further questioned the logic of administering an antipsychotic like aripiprazole to massive numbers of patients. "Should we really give this drug to millions of nonpsychotic depressed patients? The marketer's aggressive media advertising appears to have that aim." Carroll noted that the number needed to treat (NNT) for aripiprazole in refractory depression was nine. "The corresponding number needed to treat for lithium is four to five."[120] Carroll found the whole concept of giving antipsychotics to these patients mindboggling. "The very idea of giving antipsychotic drugs to NONPSYCHOTIC depressed patients is so foolish, it can only be explained by academics who should know better buying in to the commercial agenda." He proceeded to name names.[121]

If SGAs had been effective for treatment-resistant depression, that would have been one thing. But they weren't. The KOL-trialists (and the companies) reported only results with "statistical significance." But that wasn't a measure of effectiveness. Nardo went back to the trial data and recalculated the numbers for effectiveness as measured by the Hamilton and MADRS depression scales: They came out between 0.25 and 0.32 (on a scale of a 1.00), which was in the weak to moderate range. But on the patients' self-rated scales, the results were "dramatically near-null," said Nardo (0.14 to 0.20). "Statistically significant, but trivial effect from the subject's perspective."[122] Yet the studies that got into the literature reported all this as wonderful new progress in the treatment of depression.

19

TMAP

A southern extravaganza, the Texas Medication Algorithm Project (TMAP) featured atypical antipsychotics. But it was more a commercial scam than science, cooked up by Johnson & Johnson—with the aid of some helpful academics—to market Risperdal.[1]

TMAP began in 1995 with a grant of $1.7 million from the Robert Wood Johnson Foundation to various officials in Texas and some academics "to develop a model mental health treatment program for incorporation into public mental health and prison systems." This had a feel-good aura. The Foundation was related to the Johnson & Johnson (J&J) company, and what they funded was a "guidelines" project for schizophrenia.[2]

Thus, a group of academics ginned up some guidelines, a term laden with commercial implications. Allen Frances, chair of psychiatry at Duke, was said to have "spearheaded the Expert Consensus Guidelines Project." A. John Rush, professor of psychiatry at the University of Texas Southwestern Medical Center in Dallas, and chair of the DSM-IV Mood Disorders Work Group, led an effort to establish practice "guideline-oriented treatment" in the state of Texas. So, under Rush's supervision, it was in Texas that the guidelines were implemented.

The other four principals in the guidelines project that would become TMAP included Joseph McEvoy, also at Duke, and three psychiatrists from New York institutions: John Docherty, David Kahn, and Peter Weiden. The project was called Expert Knowledge Systems (EKS). Frances and Rush were the drivers of the TMAP project. (As far as is known, the other members of the EKS work group aside from Rush and Frances were not otherwise involved in TMAP. Frances evidently bowed out early.[3]) Frances, Docherty, and Kahn were the steering committee for the Expert Consensus Guidelines.[4]

In November 1995, Frances negotiated an agreement with J&J to develop the "Tri-University guidelines." Questionnaires were sent to experts to establish which antipsychotics were preferable. The experts then came up with a list of agents, all patent protected.

On July 3, 1996, the academics forwarded to Janssen the "Proposal; to Janssen Pharmaceutica" that stated they would help implement the guidelines. There was no doubt where the interest of EKS lay: "We are also committed to helping Janssen succeed in its effort to increase its market share and visibility in the payor, provider and consumer communities." It was signed by Frances, Docherty, Kahn, Daniel Carpenter, and Naakesh Dewan.[5]

J&J cut a check for $450,000 "among the three schools," as David Rothman, a professor of the history of medicine at Columbia who filed a report to the court, wrote. Where this check ultimately landed is unclear. EKS did make it clear that it was committed to helping Janssen promote Risperdal. and to working with Texas "with the assistance of A. John Rush." "All told," wrote Rothman, "J&J paid at least $942,659 [to EKS] on the production and marketing of the Tri-University guidelines."[6] In addition, Frances got $64,000, Docherty, $314,000 [sic], and Carpenter $2,500.[7] This was 100 percent a Janssen show, although EKS courted other companies as well.

Later, all this was reviewed in court. As Rothman continued, "J&J funded a project led by three psychiatrists at three medical centers (Duke, Cornell, and Columbia) to formulate Schizophrenia Practice Guidelines. From the start, the project subverted scientific integrity, appearing to be a purely scientific venture, when it was at its core a marketing venture for Risperdal. In fact, the guidelines produced by this project would become the basis for the TMAP algorithms, giving a market edge to the J&J [Janssen] products in Texas."[8] On the basis of "guidelines," the Texas Department of Mental Health was persuaded to place Risperdal at the top of a treatment algorithm. It was a very expensive guideline, indeed.

But it wasn't just Texas. The organizers of the guidelines, as Janssen's agents, toured the entire country in 1996 "to promote these guidelines, seemingly as an independent third party," said the prosecutor at a later trial. The tour involved free seminars on bipolar disorder and schizophrenia. There were 10 such seminars, in cities from Los Angeles to Boston. The format was schizophrenia on Day 1, bipolar disorder on Day 2. These would have been promotional rallies. "When early versions of these guidelines were published, Risperdal was the only new antipsychotic listed by name." The Tri-University Schizophrenia Treatment Guidelines were, the prosecution argued, one of the main accomplishments in 1996 of the Janssen marketing department. "They took credit for them as a marketing and reimbursement tool, not as a medical breakthrough."[9]

Guidelines? What do we need guidelines for when we've got science?[10] The problem was that science had shown the second-generation antipsychotics (SGAs) to be no more effective than the first-generation, but much more expensive. Only "expert" opinion could contradict these findings. As stated, the guidelines were supposedly established by asking leaders in the field what drugs they recommended. When the authors conducted the poll, it certainly had the appearance of science: dozens of experts were polled, 33 guidelines were established. Their conclusion, "The Experts recommend the newer atypical medications as the treatment of choice for most patients with schizophrenia."[11]

The three were Risperdal, Seroquel, and Zyprexa. (The article appeared only in 1999 and had the appearance of retroactively validating the choice with the "science" of expert opinion.)

TMAP got going in Texas in 1996.[12] When Rush returned to Texas, he laid out that, for the Texas Medication Algorithm Project, Risperdal was the first choice in the treatment algorithm. The algorithm would apply to charity patients in the Texas Mental Health system. The flow chart, or algorithm, that emerged from TMAP was apparently taken "wholesale" from the EKS guidelines (the Tri-University guidelines); it was a thing of beauty.[13] As the final version emerged by 1999, it had six stages, and patients with schizophrenia who had not responded in the previous stage would advance to the next. So, Stage 1 was a trial of Risperdal (which amounted to over 70 percent of all drugs prescribed in the TMAP project), or Zyprexa, or Seroquel.[14]

Patients who failed Stage 1 moved on to Stage 2, where they tried another second-generation product.

Patients who failed Stage 2 went on to Stage 3, where they'd try the third second-generation drug (there were only the three on offer).

Patients who failed Stage 3 were offered a first-generation product (Stage 4), or were moved directly to clozapine. (Clozapine was Stage 5.)

And then, at the end of this martyr's path, patients who failed clozapine would be at Stage 6, where the organizers would throw everything at them, including ECT. It is unknown how many nonresponders made it to Stage 6 and ECT. Very few. The point of the whole exercise was to sell Risperdal.

Janssen greased the skids for Risperdal by bribing everyone in sight. A journalist's phrase was, "Janssen reps went to Texas and trolled for whores."[15] Steven Shon, director of the Texas Department of Mental Health, accepted $47,000 from Janssen and its medical ghostwriter Excerpta Medica; Shon signed an agreement to be a member of J&J's [sic] Speakers' Bureau, reported the *Houston Press*.[16]

Shon was flown all over the country promoting TMAP. Rothman wrote, "When J&J learned in 2001 that competitors 'are NOT happy with Dr. Shon's influence over prescribing behaviors that favor RISPERDAL,' and were mounting 'a full court press' to move him away from J&J, the company responded with alacrity." J&J declared in internal correspondence, "WE WILL NOT LET LILLY OR PFIZER PREVAIL WITH OUR MOST IMPORTRANT PUBLIC SECTOR THOUGHT LEADER."[17] No doubt about it, Shon belonged to J&J.

The Texas officials offered their own sanitized version of the project in 1999, declaring disingenuously that, "The Texas Medication Algorithm Project is a program designed to improve the quality of care of persons with serious mental disorders across sites in the Texas public mental health system." Shon was a co-author, along with several other academics and officials who had received very large amounts of money from Janssen. Janssen's help was buried in a long list of "supporters."[18]

J&J invited the Texas officials to its annual lavish "CNS Summit," in Tempe, Arizona, and typically paid everyone honoraria of $3,000.[19] The meeting was said, in an internal J&J memo, to have been "very well attended, with over 150 of the top US KOLs and 40 international KOLs."

So successful was TMAP in Texas that Janssen tried to export the project to the other 49 states, following the template of giving the chief executives in the mental health authorities of each state generous honoraria for "consulting," or "advising," thus ensuring that Risperdal would be prescribed. Pennsylvania was one of the states experiencing a TMAP expansion.

"What a week! What a week!" exulted Laurie Snyder at Janssen about several recent meetings of mental health professionals in Pennsylvania around June 2002 that Janssen had organized. Snyder was the young woman at Janssen in charge of outreach to state mental health systems. It was her job to line up people for seminars so that Steve Shon could fly up from Texas and explain TMAP to them. The objective was "to establish atypicals as first line, with Risperdal as the standard of care." At one big meeting, "For the first time, the state is taking the initiative to ensure patients have a successful trial on atypicals." There was, regrettably, "still a large amount of conventional usage [first-generation drugs] in the state system."[20] Other Janssen staffers, evidently not Ms. Snyder, rained honoraria all over everybody.

The whole scheme came to light when Allen Jones, an investigator in the Pennsylvania inspector general's office, noticed in 2002 that Janssen was paying $4,000 to fly two state mental health officials to New Orleans, where they were richly wined and dined. Janssen paid additional sums to other officials to organize seminars for doctors and nurses in the state prison system. In February 2004, as the *New York Times* reported, Jones "stumbled upon [the payments] when he was looking into why state officials had set up a bank account to collect grants from pharmaceutical companies."[21]

Jones shared his findings with his superiors, but he was warned off the case. When he persisted, he was fired. In 2004, he filed a whistle-blower's lawsuit in Texas against Janssen, and he was joined in the lawsuit 2 years later by the state of Texas, which by this time was outraged that second-generation antipsychotics were driving the state's mental health budget into bankruptcy. Before TMAP, the Texas Medicaid program spent $250 per patient per year on antipsychotic drugs, such as Haldol; after TMAP, its costs were $3,000 per patient.[22] The State of Texas expended $500 million on Risperdal between 1994 and 2008.[23] Medicaid expenses consumed a quarter of the entire state budget![24]

It was simply too egregious. Texas officials and Janssen protested that it was all above board.[25] Yet TMAP was out by 2006, and a change in leadership at the

Texas Department of Mental Health brought in another algorithm that ranked first- and second-generation drugs equally.[26]

As noted, in 2012 there was a court trial, in the middle of which Janssen folded and paid a fine of $158 million (at the time there were still 400 lawsuits against the company pending over Risperdal.)[27] But it was, in fact, a matter of indifference to the company because they had made so much money from Risperdal that such fines, common across the industry, were just part of the cost of doing business.

Schizophrenia is not a common condition. What was at stake here? In testimony (reviewed in Chapter 13, "Marketing"), Tone Jones, a Janssen sales rep and district manager, explained the imperative for the company to expand the indications and move into the child market, "Can't be a $2 billion product and 1 percent marketing."[28] This was simple arithmetic. No schizophrenia drug was going to make a lot of money, and this was true for all the atypicals and their producers.

Mickey Nardo attended the trial, and when he got back home to Georgia, he wrote,

> I know there are reasons for me to remain stuck on this trial. The kind of pharmaceutical industry misbehavior this story represents changed the field of psychiatry and resulted in a new kind of "drug culture" that rivaled and probably exceeded that of the 1960s. It was a frontal assault on the ethics of psychiatry. It abused the methods and reputation of medical science and made a mockery of large segments of our literature. It corrupted all avenues of disseminating medical information—the literature, academic medicine, Continuing Medical Education, the pharmaceutical "detail men." So I'd like to stay fixated on this trial for a very long time.[29]

The supposed superiority of the second-generation atypicals over the first-generation typicals had been an essential part of the evidence base of psychopharmacology: "We can now cure madness." Within a couple of years, that claim was made to seem garbage. Industry's invasion of clinical psychiatry was corrupting the entire evidence base. Psychopharmacology began to seem increasingly like a branch of industry's marketing department. After the atypicals and TMAP, it would be impossible to hear with a straight face any talk about "science" in psychopharmacology.

20

The Fall of Psychopharmacology

In the course of a few years, their own most favorite theories may be discovered to be as weak and delusive as those which have gone before them.—John Gregory (London, 1770)[1]

In 2012, Mickey Nardo forecast the end of an era. "It was the height of the Age of Psychopharmacology and Clinical Neuroscience (as psychiatry was renamed by NIMH Director Tom Insel in 2005). They set a course in those salad days to sail into a brave new world. Then large cracks began to form in their planet's crust—Senator Grassley's investigations, Chairmen 'stepping down,' large settlements against drug companies with the release of damning documents, an increasingly bad press (well deserved), failed *recent advances* in all directions."[2] This book is about these developments. They marked the end of an era.

At the beginning of the psychopharmacologic era, the excitement was palpable. Psychiatrist Thomas Detre, later a senior figure at the University of Pittsburgh, recalled the enthusiasm of the early meetings of the American College of Neuropsychopharmacology (ACNP). On the beach in San Juan, there would be afternoons of excited conversation with colleagues from all over the neurosciences. "We thought in those days that we have these wonderful new drugs. . . . By using them we will derive some very important information regarding the etiology and the pathogenesis of psychiatry disorders. Well, that hope was not fulfilled; those drugs were dirty drugs which acted on many different systems in the brain."[3] So the pioneers started to become apostate.

The air in Boston was electric in 1965 as Philip Solomon, a professor at Harvard and chief of psychiatry at Boston City Hospital, convened a conference on the new drugs. Opening the conference, Solomon said, "The field is clearly in the midst of a major revolution. The shift is from *diagnosis by description* and treatment-nonspecific to *diagnosis by etiology* and treatment-specific."[4]

No part of this statement turned out to be true. What, in 2021, may we say is the etiology of schizophrenia? What treatments are specific for major depression? The SSRIs? All of the SSRIs are claimed to be effective for every disease in psychiatry except possibly neurosyphilis. It was not without prescience that in 2012 Peter Tyrer, editor of the *British Journal of Psychiatry*, forecast "the end of the psychopharmacological revolution."[5]

Here is a disquieting question. If what psychiatrists do is prescribe ineffective drugs for non-existent conditions, such as major depression, why do we need them at all? This is a Devil's Advocate question. But California's James O'Brien answered it seriously, "What does a psychiatry residency bring to the table that a PhD Program doesn't anymore? Other than eventually having to do the task in 15 minutes instead of 50. No, you don't need three years to learn how to prescribe SSRI/SNRIs, SGAs and mood stabilizers, so let's just stop with the charade."[6] The charade! Really?

Commerce Trumps Science

> The ideal mass market drug is an anxiolytic that kills viruses and is contraceptive in both sexes.—Editorial, *Journal of the Royal College of Physicians* (1977)[7]

From his years at Emory, then in private practice in Atlanta, and then from his mountain perch in Appalachia, Nardo saw it coming: In the 1980s, "We didn't really notice that things were slowly changing, that the firewall between the commercial medical enterprises and academic medicine had eroded a little more with every passing year."[8] "We didn't know anything then. The pharmaceutical invasion of academic psychiatry may have already been well under way, but we didn't know it, at least I didn't. Prozac was still mostly thought of as a wonder drug. Risperdal was the new kid on the block. We had no idea about the conflicts of interest that would later prove to be so extensive and destructive."[9] In 2012, as he wrote those lines, he was describing his lost innocence.

This sense of loss and failure was not confined to the hills of Georgia. In 2014, Susanna Every-Palmer, a psychiatrist at the Otago Medical School in New Zealand, argued that evidence-based medicine (EBM) in general was being discredited by the invasion of industry. "EBM's indiscriminate acceptance of industry-generated 'evidence' is akin to letting politicians count their own votes. . . . Clinical decisions based on such evidence are likely to be misinformed, with patients given less effective, harmful or more expensive treatments."[10] There was a general sense that the whole evidence-based concept, which had been supposedly the battle flag of psychopharmacology, was a snare and a delusion.

What Doomed "Psychopharmacology"?

What doomed psychopharmacology as a scientific concept was its becoming a vehicle for promotion of the industry. Once the "science" of psychopharm became a trope for selling drugs, the scientific concept itself was dead.

The Age of Psychopharmacology had been heavily driven by commercial hype, and the hype ended when the patents expired. With the final expiration of the SSRI patents—escitalopram (Lexapro) in 2012—further commercial enthusiasm was pointless, just easing the way for the generics to cannibalize the market. Mark Kramer, former head of psychopharmacology at Merck, said in 2016, "The days of intense popularity of psychopharmaceuticals had been driven by unparalleled happy-pill marketing of Prozac and its cousins, not the intrinsic value of these agents for whatever it is that ails the masses. The 'feel good fluff' came to an end along with patent exclusivity. Most of the marginally depressed patients and those demoralized by society had been given false hope by all the 4-letter acronym 'mood drugs.'" And once the false hopes were crushed, the disillusionment was great.[11]

It was not that excitement about neuroscience had started to fade. Today, the neurosciences push back the frontiers of knowledge about the brain and central nervous system in ever more thrilling ways. But, as early as the 1980s, it started to become apparent that there was a huge disconnect between the advance of basic neuroscience and the limping pace of drug development. Arvid Carlsson, a leading neuroscientist and Nobel Laureate, noted this in 1987. "In light of the tremendous progress made in basic knowledge, it is remarkable how modest the development in pharmacotherapy has been since the 1950s. . . . The only really striking therapeutic spinoff from basic research," he said, "is the introduction of L-dopa in the treatment of Parkinson's disease."[12] To be sure, 1987 saw the first of the SSRIs, Prozac (fluoxetine). Yet observers did not really regard the SSRIs as new-concept drugs but rather as minor modifications of existing molecules (diphenhydramine, brand-named Benadryl). The SSRI concept was more a marketing trope than a scientific concept, and the "second-generation antipsychotics" (SGAs) had little in common save their recent appearances in the market.

It did not often happen, but it did happen, that clinicians realized the old medications were superior to the new, in other words, that in decades of psychopharmacology, there had been no progress. In 2007, a psychiatrist in Osceola, Wisconsin, told colleagues about recent treatment experiences:

> Four patients, meds driven by penury in my neck of the woods where 3rd party pay is the exception.

(1) Consta [injectable Risperdal]: back in jail, hallucinating (jail staff worried!). I can't continue Consta because of cost, and switch to Haldol dec [decanoate, injectable] (very cheap these days). He improves markedly, no side effects.

(2) Cymbalta [Lilly's duloxetine], after many med trials, pleading for something else. Settle for nortriptyline [a tricyclic antidepressant] (that she pays for herself), with much benefit and mild s/e [side effects].

(3) Clozapine, worse and worse, added haloperidol with great benefit.

(4) Effexor XR [venlafaxine extended release] 300: continuing depression symptoms, backed down to 150 mg and nortriptyline 75 added (patient pay), so far (early) much improvement.

This small-town psychiatrist concluded, "This kind of psychopharm practice is much inhibited by the daily battering of drug reps. Knowing what works here for me included 30 years doing it. The drug reps who want to talk to me know nothing of this, and so are even more useless."[13]

Thus, the failure of 30 years of psychopharmacology in a small town in Wisconsin.

Rats Leaving

There can be no surer sign of the bankruptcy of a field than the rats leaving the sinking ship. Within the past decade, industry has been getting out of psychopharmacology as an expensive and unpromising avenue of drug development. In 2014, it was calculated that the average out-of-pocket cost in developing a drug was $1.4 billion (and another $1.2 billion in foregone revenue from that investment[14]). You couldn't have too many failures in phase III trials before talking real money.

In 2012, Christian Fibiger, a former vice president of neuroscience at Eli Lilly, delivered a shattering judgment of the industry's record of failure: "Psychopharmacology is in crisis. The data are in, and it is clear that a massive experiment has failed: despite decades of research and billions of dollars invested, not a single mechanistically novel drug has reached the psychiatric market in more than 30 years. . . . In recent years, the appreciation of this reality has had profound consequences for innovation in psychopharmacology because nearly every major pharmaceutical company has either reduced greatly or abandoned research and development of mechanistically novel psychiatric drugs."[15]

In 2011, Novartis announced that it was closing its neuroscience division, which included psychiatry, neurology, and pain. Mark Fishman, the director of research at Novartis, told a colleague "[With regard to drug discovery], neurology is too difficult and psychiatry is like alchemy."[16] Astra Zeneca followed, and Pfizer, Sanofi, Janssen, and Merck were said to have "significantly downsized CNS operations."[17] In 2012, Atul Pande, senior vice president of neurosciences at GlaxoSmithKline (GSK), explained why the company had terminated 14 early-stage clinical programs on new psychiatry drugs. "Not a single one of them generated a shred of positive data," he said. Explained a journalist, "Each failure means a multimillion dollar loss for the company. Subsequently, GSK decided to curtail its neuroscience research."[18]

If some promising new drug class comes along, the rats will all climb back on board again: The potential money to be made is staggering. But for the time being, the field lies dormant.

The Failure of Drug Discovery

For the first time in a long time, there are no psychopharmaceuticals in the list of top-20 drugs in the United States. In 2000, the top-20 brand-name drugs included Prozac (ranked #4), Zoloft (#7), Paxil (#8), Zyprexa (#14), and Neurontin (#17). There were five more psychopharmaceuticals ranked at #20 to #30.[19] By contrast, in 2018, *the top 20 did not include a single psychopharmaceutical.*[20] Soon, psychopharmacology will be only a distant memory in people's minds, like the hula hoop or "The Brady Bunch."

After the Golden Age of the 1950s and early 60s, the discovery of drugs with novel mechanisms basically came to an end. One tabulation of "new chemical entities" in psychopharmacology internationally, identified two in 1961–1965, five in 1966–1970, two in 1971–1975, and *none* thereafter (up to 1985).[21] "If all of the medications developed since 1990 disappeared, I believe I could be as effective a psychiatrist as I am today," said one clinician.[22] Barry Blackwell's dismal conclusion was that, "The only truly innovative drug discovered in forty fallow years of research was Viagra." He described the "years of wasted effort on the DSM fantasy that phenotypes, derived by political consensus, might be linked to drug function."[23]

Agents for bipolar disorder boiled down to Depakote (semisodium valproic acid, synthesized in 1882) and lithium, an element, reintroduced to psychiatry in 1949. Again, this was not a stunning choice of treatments—although lithium was effective not just for mania but for the treatment and prophylaxis of mood disorders of all kinds.

For everything else, there remained the SSRIs, the Prozac family. To be sure, there were a couple of outliers, such as amphetamine look-alikes (Ritalin) for the treatment of hyperactivity. But the drugs outlined above are what remained after half a century of psychopharmacology; useful drug categories fell right and left to commercial "counter-detailing," to internal company politics, and to overdrawn concerns about side effects. In story after story, effective drug classes gave way to ineffective drug classes. Bernard Carroll noted the displacement of the effective MAOIs (monoamine oxidase inhibitors) by the ineffective Prozac family. He added, "The story has an eerie parallel with the displacement of lithium by anticonvulsants [called mood stabilizers]—driven by Pharma and by KOLs, of course."[24]

No factor contributed more to ending the Age of Psychopharmacology than its failure to discover new drugs. "Psychopharm" meant drugs, and the last innovative drug class was the benzodiazepines, introduced with Librium in 1960. There were many effective drugs discovered during the rise of psychopharmacology, such as the MAOIs and tricyclic antidepressants, although most of them were blotted out by the SSRIs. What are the chances of reviving them? Zero, said the above-quoted James O'Brien, a psychiatrist in Mira Loma, California, of long experience: "Many pharmacies don't even carry MAOIs in stock and freak out when they see a script for an MAOI. . . . GPs and NPs [nurse-practitioners] will never use MAOIs. Even most psychiatrists are afraid of them. TCAs will continue to be used off label for pain and sleep issues."[25]

This is not supposed to happen in medicine: that therapeutics goes *backward*. Healy commented in the *British Medical Journal* in 2015, "In other areas of life, the products we use, from computers to microwaves, improve year on year, but this is not the case for [psychopharmaceutical] medicines, where this year's treatment may achieve blockbuster status despite being less effective and less safe than yesterday's models."[26]

How could this failure have happened, in an era when neuroscience research was booming? At a very basic level, science became subject to corporate control. Len Cook, a neurochemist looking back over 40-plus years at SmithKline, Hoffmann-La Roche, and Dupont, said that you can't manage science. In the olden days, "We decided what we would do and how we would do it. So the strategy was determined at the bench and we were pretty successful."

But then, continued Cook, the companies, flush with their new success, began to grow. "They started what they called strategic planning groups. They had people come in from Wall Street and Harvard Business School." He said that "Bang for the buck" became the issue. Upper management now determines "what the individual scientist does and how he does it, his time frame of when he's going to do it. . . . So what you have lost in this program of research discovery is the ingenuity of the individual scientist to follow their nose, because it's pretty hard to put a timetable on discovery. In many cases, management will say, 'You now have twenty-two months to prove that the research program is going to work.' After that, that's it."

The restlessly curious neurochemists were called "drughunters." Cook painted an almost romantic picture—although not necessarily a false one—of the pioneering neurochemist out on the frontier. "He's the champion, an intellectual investment, most of the time fighting authority, putting himself on the line, and frequently, against the company. I can think of several instances where the person who made the drug discovery is no longer with the company, because his persistence to get that job done made many enemies. And when their drug came out, [its discoverer was] not there anymore."[27] So management often picked a structure that conduced to failure.

Carroll saw a lurch in the locus of drug discovery from the academy to industry as fatal. "[One perverse shift] was the new conceit that science could be managed and that it was, moreover, too important to be left to the boffin [peculiar but bright] scientists. So the center of gravity in drug development shifted away from academic centers to corporations. Once that happened, then shortsighted short-term objectives elbowed out the commitment to basic science."[28] In other words, the healthy balance between the academy and industry of the 1960s and 1970s basically came to an end. The science of psychopharmacology now meant that industry's commitment was to developing patentable me-too drugs in clinical trials aimed at securing registration rather than new scientific findings. The numerous industry research labs consulted first the marketing departments about what would sell and then, unsurprisingly, were unable to find new drugs.

But there were diagnosis issues, too. The "depression" problem frustrated the development of new drugs. The depression market was so huge that the temptation just to shut one's eyes and barrel after this highly heterogeneous clinical population was overwhelming. But this was the problem: Many of the depressed patients had a number of different conditions, and some had nothing at all. Reflecting on his many years of psychopharmacology at Merck, Mark Kramer noted, "I suspect that drug-responsive real patients constitute an orphan indication: [a new agent] would be plausible for the disabled drug-responsive psychotic endogenous melancholic." It should, he said, be possible to get some underlying biology on this tightly defined, very ill group. "If we cannot get biology in the truly disabled, what are we doing? I figured once that is nailed, then we could . . . go on to chronic dysthymic depression."[29] This would be a rational approach to the depression problem. It would be aided by such approaches as the dexamethasone suppression test (DST), which did isolate a biochemically homogeneous group of patients. Instead, the industry has beat its head against the wall with "antidepressants."

It wasn't just the failure to discover new drugs. Effectiveness was evidently slipping. The new generation of SSRIs seemed to be less effective than previous generations of agents. And the atypical antipsychotics were loaded with side effects. Thus, it cannot be said that, in terms of therapeutics, the psychopharmacology story has had a happy outcome. Surveying this desolate landscape,

Mickey Nardo remarked in 2012 on the "stream of middling drugs like the ones we've had for the last thirty plus years. The pharmaceutical companies seem to know that there's nothing much for them in that kind of situation and are unlikely to stay in the game now that the gold rush is over just to support lonely KOLs and CROs [clinical research organizations]. This says to me that we are at the end of something—an era of sorts."[30]

"The Whole Biobabble About Receptors"

The first big breakthrough of the neurotransmitter doctrine into the clinic was Joseph Schildkraut's 1965 hypothesis that depression was a disorder of norepinephrine metabolism.[31] His article had a huge impact in turning the field toward the study of neurotransmitters as the key to unlocking psychiatric illness, and it was followed closely by Arvid Carlsson's hypotheses about serotonin and dopamine in serious illness. It is thus interesting that Carlsson, in a 2007 interview, turned his back on the neurotransmitter-as-key notion. "I have always been against extrapolating from a drug effect to a hypothesis dealing with pathogenesis." He mentioned his 1963 paper proposing that antipsychotics acted on dopamine and noradrenaline receptors. "But I wouldn't dare from this propose that there would be an aberration in the function of either of these amines as an important pathogenetic factor. These are different things; they should be kept apart."[32]

Among those actually responsible for drug discovery, there was a growing weariness with the whole receptor approach. Alfred Burger, longstanding professor of medicinal chemistry at the University of Virginia and founder in 1959 of the *Journal of Medicinal Chemistry*, said in 1990, "Receptors remained pharmacological rather than biochemical concepts, and [they] did not contribute much to drug design where minor steric or small substituent effects could increase or abolish drug activity without a satisfactory chemical explanation." He mocked the drawing in academic seminars of "circles or rectangles" as the hypothetical shape of the receptor in question.[33] (In FDA submissions, it is still considered obligatory to indicate the "receptor profile" of one's drug as though this explained the mechanism. But it does not, and the "receptor profile" is included mainly because a receptor-conditioned public expects it.)

Other pioneers also began to turn their backs. Frank Berger was the originator of meprobamate (Miltown), the first blockbuster drug in psychiatry. In an interview in 1999, he said, "Research with neurotransmitters is very important, but we're reaching the point where we know as much about neurotransmitters as we need to. . . . We need a new approach. The discoveries of the 1950s have been milked almost to death."[34]

In the late 1990s, David Healy interviewed Solomon Snyder at Johns Hopkins. Snyder, more than anyone, had opened up the whole subject of receptors. Snyder explained that their research into such transmitters as nitric oxide and D-serine had "changed all the rules about neurotransmission": no reuptake, no storage vesicles, no release by exocytosis [discharge into the synapse], no receptor—very, very different."

Healy said, "Things had become very predictable during the 1980s—the monoamines were there and maybe the peptides. Now it's all begun to seem much more mysterious again, would you agree?"

Snyder: "Yes, I'd agree. Interestingly, these weirder neurotransmitters are actually doing more important things than some of the conventional ones."[35]

Any thought that "amine neurotransmitter reuptake" was the basic mechanism of drug action in psychopharm would have been doomed by an exchange that Jay Amsterdam at the University of Pennsylvania and Donald Klein at Columbia had in January 2017. Klein laughed at the claim that Pharma's psych drugs had a "known mechanism" based on the neurotransmitter profile: "It is advertising hype, not science. However, Pharma has spent vast sums on ill-founded stories that this or that agonist or antagonist, based on some action guessed to compensate for some undocumented or irrelevant imbalance, really makes terrific scientific sense." He said this was scientific nonsense.[36]

Amsterdam replied: "When I was a young and less jaded researcher, I sort of bought the pitch that pharmaceutical companies proffered to the medical public on drug mechanism. However, in the early 90s, when I began to wake up from my sleep-walking and realized that the mechanism pitch was simply marketing hype, my views on the antidepressant development field changed drastically." He would tease the residents with a tale of a "new" histamine-active antidepressant generically known as 3-dextro-diphenhydramine. . . . An occasional astute psychiatry resident would pipe up: 'But Jay, this is nothing more than a close congener of Benadryl.' Amsterdam would respond, 'We already showed that our agent beat placebo in two pivotal trials; so don't let facts interfere with a good story! We'll hire a classy medical marketing firm to pitch the histamine basis of antidepressant activity, and the entire field of psychiatry and the NIMH will follow the lead!"[37] This was, of course, a send-up of the Prozac story and the discovery of the SSRIs. Jay Amsterdam's compound had three phenyl groups, Benadryl two. It was, essentially, Benadryl that launched two decades of neurotransmitter "mechanism" hype.

An impatience with the amine neurotransmitters—serotonin, norepinephrine, and dopamine—penetrated even the director's office at NIMH, where the new director, Joshua Gordon, wanted to take NIMH in a different direction from that of his predecessor, Thomas Insel (whose love of research on monoamine neurotransmitters resulted in the waste of hundreds of millions of dollars in public funds). "Enough of monoamines already," said Gordon in 2019, and then pointed the Institute in the direction of ketamine—an anesthetic drug that had started to show usefulness in psychiatry by affecting the non-amine transmitter glutamate (an amino acid acting at the NMDA receptor).[38] (Whether the ketamine gamble will pay off is not clear at this writing.)

At FDA, they were deeply doubtful about postulated "mechanisms." In 1999, Lisa Stockbridge, a regulatory reviewer, told Janssen, "Materials that state or imply that Risperdal has superior safety or efficacy to other antipsychotics due to its receptor antagonist profile are false or misleading because the mechanism of action of Risperdal is unknown, as is the correlation of the specific receptor antagonism to the clinical effectiveness and safety of the drug."[39] Janssen was explicitly enjoined to say in the labeling, "The mechanism of action of RISPERDAL (risperidone), as with other antipsychotic drugs, is unknown."[40] Psychiatrist Eric Turner shared with colleagues in January 2017, "Regarding mechanism, at the FDA, Paul Leber used to say, 'We don't care if it's horse manure as long as it works.' "[41]

As George Beaumont, Geigy's medical director (and a psychiatrist), remarked in 1998 about antidepressant research, "All this emphasis on separating neurotransmitter systems and identifying receptors seems really to have got us nowhere and we have gone back full circle more or less to where we started in the 1950s." He said, "It's even worse in the field of anxiety," where none of the research on the "5-HT [serotonin] receptors . . . suggesting that here was a new group of drugs which would be immensely valuable, none of these observations have proved to be of much use clinically."[42] This was a reference to the SSRIs not from some marginal maverick but from a deep insider.

In schizophrenia as well, the amine neurotransmitters had dominated the picture. In the early 1970s, Sol Snyder at Johns Hopkins and Philip Seeman at the University of Toronto opened up the "dopamine model" of schizophrenia, believing that the disease was geared by the dopamine D1 receptor, and then attention turned to the D2 receptor. It was therefore believed that the schizophrenia puzzle was basically solved as a disorder of dopamine metabolism. It does not trivialize the first-class science that led to the discovery of these receptors to note that they are not really the heart of the schizophrenia story.

And there are lots of neurotransmitters. Those that had the greatest impact on psychiatry were the amine transmitters, such as dopamine and serotonin, because they quickly became commercial marketing devices. In Leo Hollister's interview of Yale psychopharmacologist George Aghajanian about the latter's work on ketamine, Aghajanian told Hollister that the ketamine research was exciting because it had gotten them into research on glutamate. Hollister said, "This is exciting, because we've been desperately trying to get off the dopamine hypothesis."[43] Hollister, a former president of the ACNP, was merely expressing the impatience of much of the field with what had become a marketing trope.

Decreasing serotonin reuptake? Is that the story? The group of the London-based neurochemist Gerald Curzon found that the quite effective antidepressant tianeptine (Servier's Stablon) *increased* serotonin reuptake rather than inhibiting it.[44] Although inhibiting the reuptake of various neurotransmitters was a real phenomenon, it was only a piece of some larger yet unclarified mechanism of drug action.

The problem was that drug development had been hijacked by the neurotransmitters. Martin Schumacher, a Novartis scientist, commented skeptically, "The whole disease model based on neurotransmitters . . . reminds one of Galen's humoral pathology. His four temperaments [sanguine, choleric, phlegmatic, melancholic] correspond schematically to the most important neurotransmitters: dopamine, serotonin, noradrenaline, and maybe acetylcholine or glutamate. But just as Galen's humoral pathology was replaced by Rudolf Virchow's doctrine of cellular pathology, psychopharmacology today needs a very different new departure."[45]

The great volumes of neurotransmitter research had yielded no new drugs. Yet subsuming neurotransmitter research to the marketing needs of industry had a pernicious effect on research in neurochemistry. Researchers could get funding only for neurotransmitter and receptor studies, and this was the case long after advances in such research ceased to lead to the discovery of new drugs. Tom Ban commented, "In trying to prevent the falling apart of the neuroleptic market, industry is lavishly supporting and propagating neuropharmacologic research on receptor changes in schizophrenic brains or linkages through the D4 receptor to genetics. This kind of research is based on the assumption that schizophrenia, a concept, is one disease." By contrast, Ban continued, industry had little interest in supporting research that might "disentangle the biologic heterogeneity of schizophrenia."[46]

Sam Gershon explained sardonically in 2017 how the neurotransmitter game was played. "A did not work, let's tweak A and try that —or be really scientific: add a second purported mechanism, like norepinephrine to serotonin, and we will definitely have a super compound. We had these experiences [at New York University] when we showed that blocking the manufacture of norepinephrine with AMPT [alpha-methyl-para-tyrosine] did not prevent the antidepressant effect. We confirmed these findings in studies with Leo Hollister. The norepinephrine group were shocked and suspicious and we received some very unhappy phone calls."[47] So much for the norepinephrine model of depression, in other words. It is not hard to understand why exciting new drugs failed to come out of this scientific mishmash.

But there are alternatives to following the amine neurotransmitter pathway. Recent investigators have started pursuing the trail of dysregulation in the opioid system as a means of finding new therapeutic approaches in depression.[48] This picks up a thread that is millennia old: using opiates to treat serious (melancholic) depression, an approach begun by the ancients and reactivated with success in the nineteenth century. Opioid therapy is not something that we as a society, in the midst of an opioid epidemic, are thrilled at hearing about. But the science is what it is.

On balance, the relevance of basic science to clinical psychiatry has been way overhyped. In the psychiatry residency program of a major North American medical school, the mantra is "science." But in 2016 the British neuroscientist blogger "Neuroskeptic" had a different take on this: "The whole of the past decade in psychiatry might be called the Decade of Jumping the Gun. The fact is that we simply don't have good enough neuroscience tools yet to allow us to answer the clinically important questions. We just don't. We might get there eventually, but at the moment we are not there."[49]

Biological Tests Lie Fallow

In 1954, Charles Shagass at McGill University proposed the "sedation threshold" test with barbiturates to differentiate different kinds of illnesses. Relying on the onset of slurred speech or nystagmus to mark the threshold, this was an early diagnostic "marker" or "test" (see Chapter 8). Shagass found that patients with "neurotic depression" needed larger amounts of amobarbital for sedation than did patients with psychotic depression and organic brain disease.[50]

In the 1970s, the endocrine system popped up on psychiatry's horizon. In 1968, Bernard Carroll, still in Australia, explained in the *British Medical Journal* how a test used in endocrinology to check levels of cortisol could be applied in psychiatry. The test, called the dexamethasone suppression test (DST), showed that in melancholic depression, an injection of the artificial hormone dexamethasone would maintain serum cortisol at high levels. This was a paradoxical effect, because in normal people an injection would cause a fall in (suppression of) cortisol, as the adrenal glands (which produce cortisol) get the message they can turn off for a while. Dexamethasone "nonsuppression" thus became a biological marker of melancholia.

But in the 1980s, the DST went out of fashion. Jay Amsterdam tried to figure out why. It was because you couldn't study serious depression in fake patients. "We all know the real problem—and that's with the inappropriate application of the current diagnostic system, as well as the 'dummying down' of symptom severity [to enable] enrolling 'symptomatic volunteers' into RCTs—which are now our vaunted 'evidence base' for treating depression, and the Pharma colonization of treatment of all types of depressions of all severities—because insurers long ago established the 'standard of care' as a 15-minute 'med check' for depression. For greed and filthy lucre, psychiatry sold its soul to Pharma and big insurers. Thus, the DST went the way of the Dodo bird."[51]

As described in Chapter 8, in the 1960s Max Fink and Turan Itil, then at the Missouri Institute of Psychiatry, began to work out procedures for pharmaco-EEG, using the EEG to identify different brain patterns of drug response (so that the manufacturer could tell if its drug was an antidepressant or an antipsychotic). As a scientific innovation, this seemed a deeply promising way of hooking psychiatry up with basic science.

All three tests—sedation threshold, DST, and pharmaco-EEG—were important, not because they would tell you whether your patient had depression or schizophrenia (you could probably figure that out clinically) but because *they identified biologically homogeneous groups of patients who evidently had a similar biochemistry.* Yet none of these tests was followed up, and by the end of the 1980s psychiatry had, incredibly, lost sight of all three.

They had been elbowed aside by an almost hypnotic fascination with the neurotransmitters.

Academics Begin Bailing Out

> A drug is a chemical substance which, when brought into contact with a living organism, produces a paper.—Nathan Kline (1971)[52]

For 30 years, the collaboration between scientists and industry had been fruitful. Then, for many, it ceased to be. Jay Amsterdam had a major lab at the University of Pennsylvania for the investigation of mood disorders. Then he bailed. "I ceased doing this sort of consulting work when I realized that the Pharma companies really did NOT want my opinion on scientific matters. What they really wanted was 'my name'. At the end of my tenure with Pharma, I came to realize what the medical affairs or market folks meant when they would smile at you and say: 'Of course we want your opinion, Jay—no, really we do.' That was actually code for: Dr. Amsterdam, when we want your opinion we'll give it to you (along with enough money for me not to tell them to f.o.). But all of this Pharma ill-will was late in the game (say the late 1990s to early 2000s)—when I severed all ties of any sort with Pharma."[53]

Barry Blackwell, the discoverer of the "cheese effect" with the MAOIs, bailed around the same time as Amsterdam. Speaking of the ACNP, he said, "[The founders] recognized, from the start [1961], the need for close collaboration and communication with basic scientists in an extended environment conducive to translational dialogue. This is how the ACNP was born in 1961. For the first decade (1962–72) this was a fruitful enterprise driven by intellectual curiosity and a profound desire to help people with severe mental illness. . . . [Then] this atmosphere, its motivations, and rewards were quickly and progressively eroded and no longer exist."[54] (This was written in 2011.)

Or, it might be fair to say that the KOLs were hailed by their own devising. Industry critic and blogger Roy Poses commented in 2013 of the companies that were ending CNS programs, "For 50 years, no fundamentally incisive innovations have occurred, so the defectors [companies] are telling the academics to get their act together in respect of better understanding disease mechanisms. Trouble is, too many academic clinical investigators have devolved into key opinion leaders promoting corporate marketing messages at the expense of generating original clinical science."[55] The KOLs had emphasized lucre to the detriment of science, and now that science was needed, the money flow stopped.

Psychiatry's Marquee Disorders Begin to Run Out of Gas

Psychopharmacology rested on two big diagnoses, schizophrenia and major depression, and treatments for the two disorders constituted the core of the discipline. But in the later years, warning flags started to be raised.[56] Progress in treatment of the two diseases had dropped off sharply.

As early as 1958, Manfred Bleuler, professor of psychiatry in Zurich—the very birthplace of schizophrenia, the diagnosis itself conceived by his father Eugen— rang the alarm about psychopharmacology. He said at the first meeting of the CINP in Rome, "Modern neuropharmacology has hitherto contributed nothing to the understanding of the pathogenesis of schizophrenia. . . . The clinician's task today is to show the basic researcher on what dangerous and precarious ground he is moving if he wishes to build up a doctrine on schizophrenia based on his latest discoveries."[57] Here, at the very beginning of psychopharmacology, was a counsel of despair about its utility in the study of schizophrenia.

In 1987, Gerald Klerman at Harvard, the guiding figure of psychiatric diagnostics, noted that very little progress was being made with this troublesome diagnosis. "We must acknowledge," he told the ACNP, "that the past decade has not been one of great optimism and triumph in the field of schizophrenia and the field has not flourished." There had been no treatment advances beyond the neuroleptics. "The patients are improved, but not well enough to be socially independent." Given the lack of progress, "interest in schizophrenia research seemed to decrease."[58]

Nancy Andreasen at the University of Iowa, who revived the distinction between positive and negative symptoms, mused in 1990 about the great diversity in patients with schizophrenia. "They may experience intense emotions . . . or seem completely impoverished of emotion. Their speech may be normal and log-ical, disorganized and confused, or empty and laconic. In motoric activity they may be agitated and restless, manifest stereotypies or repetitive behavior, or sit inactively or even in a stupor. [These symptoms have since been hived off as a separate disease, catatonia.] Their personal relationships may be marred by in-tense jealousy and suspicion and fear, or disinterest and apathy."[59] These are all the same disease?

Events since the late 1980s have done little to show that these critics were wrong. Even though the volume of schizophrenia research today is huge, since Klerman's time there have been no advances in the basic biology, diagnostics, or therapeutics of schizophrenia. And now there is widespread doubt about whether the disease even exists as a single entity, comparable to tuberculosis. Conan Kornetsky, a member of the departments of psychiatry and pharma-cology at Boston University Medical School, told an interviewer in 1995, "We are dealing probably with more than one disease."[60]

The whole dopamine-neurotransmitter story was called into question. Amphetamine, a dopamine releaser, was supposed to worsen the condition in schizophrenia, supposedly a dopamine-driven disease relieved by dopamine blockers. But a number of Kornetsky's patients improved on amphetamine. The findings caused Kornetsky to think that maybe the dopamine hypothesis of schizophrenia needed to be re-evaluated.[61]

Another old-timer with vast clinical experience, George Simpson, who had worked with Nate Kline at Rockland State Hospital, told Thomas Ban in 2001, "I can see where [DSM-style] nosology might get in our way because we can see in schizophrenia a group of illnesses; it creates problems if we treat them as one en-tity and lump them together in imaging or genetic studies."[62]

And the spavined old nag major depression made it into DSM-5 despite three decades of furious criticism. How did that happen? As Jan Fawcett, head of the mood workgroup in DSM-5, said, "Examination of existing genetic, imaging, and clinical data led to the realization that we on the DSM-5 mood workgroup had been born 20–30 years too early and that the current data available were not adequate [to make this distinction about melancholia]." The data just weren't there! (The claim is ludicrous.) After a century's torrent of clinical and biochem-ical evidence on melancholia, he shook his head sadly and said, "Maybe thirty years from now."[63]

Dusk

They say that the "Owl of Minerva flies at dusk," meaning that wisdom is achieved only as night falls. For Thomas Insel, director of NIMH, dusk was

2011. An interview in the *British Medical Journal* quoted him as saying, "The field of mental health is on the cusp of a revolution, which is set to transform the diagnosis and treatment of mental illness and reverse the lack of major progress . . . over the past 100 years."[64] And then it *was* dusk. None of this turned out to be true. There were no revolutionary breakthroughs in knowledge, and DSM-5 in 2013, if anything, set the field back, rather than accelerating the rush toward singing tomorrows. There were no new meds, and the two existing drug sets—atypicals and SSRIs—were, if anything, inferior to their predecessors. Neurotransmitters, imaging, genetics: no practical new knowledge emerged from any of this. The woods were now dark and silent.

By the year 2000, many long-time industry insiders had the feeling that something fundamental had shifted. Thomas Ban spoke of "the post-neuropsychopharmacology era."[65] Others had a sense of "paradigm exhaustion."[66]

Looking back fondly on the past is typical "golden age thinking." But this was not that. It was the dim but real apprehension that the ground was shifting under them, and under the entire field. Jay Amsterdam, writing in 2019, said: "In a sense, entering the field of psychiatric research in 1976, at the sunset of those halcyon days of modern psychiatry, I was able to witness, first hand, the slow creep of the academic–industrial complex (AIC) (also as Barney [Carroll] once said) into the framework of scholarly activities. By the late 1990s, the dark curtain of the AIC had descended, and much that was vital in the process of academic research was henceforth a simple matter of the accumulation of *filthy lucre*."[67]

What were the signs that the era of psychopharmacology was fading? One was that grasp of the knowledge base was slipping—because the "base" had become commercialized. And rather than remembering the names of the cranial nerves (science), the field had been reduced to remembering the names of competitive drug products—and that poorly. At a meeting of the Psychopharmacologic Drugs Advisory Committee (PDAC) in 1995, John Davis, a major expert in psychopharmacology at the University of Illinois Medical School in Chicago, rose to make a point about obsessive-compulsive disorder: "Both clozapine and chlorpromazine were available in Europe for many years." He has confused clomipramine (Anafranil), an anti-obsessional drug with chlorpromazine (Thorazine, the first antipsychotic).

Paul Leber, the head of psychiatric drugs at FDA, continued the confusion. He declared, full of umbrage, "I don't even think your facts are fully accurate. Chlorpromazine was introduced in England as an antidepressant, widely used, has one of the biggest death rates in overdose that you will ever run into, and is seizurogenic as heck." He had clearly confused chlorpromazine with clomipramine (which is "seizurogenic").

Nobody noticed the confusion.

Then, Denis Charney, another huge psychopharmacology expert, rose to speak: "I don't think you are completely accurate about chlorpromazine in terms of OCD, because there was substantial data prior to the large Ciba-Geigy study suggesting its efficacy." (Clomipramine was a Ciba-Geigy drug; chlorpromazine, of course, came from Smith, Kline & French.)

The authorities huffed and puffed at one another for a while about chlorprom-azine, hopelessly tangled in confusion.[68] We'll grant them their momentary lapses; some of the drug names are confusing. But still, what was once hard and fast knowledge was somehow all running together.

And the meds were increasingly products of the profit motive rather than the public interest. Israeli public health scholar Mayer Brezis wrote, "Public health now emerges as a grave example of conflict of interests with private enterprise." He indicted in particular the SSRIs. "These medications may in fact have no clin-ically meaningful advantage over placebos, and antidepressants have not been convincingly shown to affect the long-term outcome of depression."[69] The con-flict between industry and public health is, in other words, irremediable and intrinsic.

It was no accident that an SSRI producer led the charge away from corpo-rate responsibility and into profit. Mark Kramer at Merck pointed his finger di-rectly at Pfizer (and its drug Zoloft). "While [I was] at Merck and Co, it seemed that Pfizer had been the first of Big Pharma to align its governance accordingly. Hordes of financial engineers were recruited to put profit first. Corporate social responsibility (CSR) had been marginalized. As Pfizer began to overtake each pharma company on the 'Forbes Best' list, pharma followed Pfizer's lead."[70]

There once was once a time when the efforts of industry were indisputably of benefit to public health, and collaboration with the academy was not mercenary but scientific. There is no reason why these times should not come again, and, once the corrupting concept of psychopharmacology has expired, in the area of psychiatric drugs, progress might resume.

21
Conclusion

At the end of the nineteenth century, if a man was fat, balding, impotent and shy, his best course of action would have been to keep his chin up and muddle through. Today, he has the pharmaceutical industry.—*Scrip* (2000)[1]

In this dismaying story of rise and fall, what can we cling to? What actually works? The late Ivan Goldberg, a New York psychiatrist of vast experience, will help us. He told correspondents in 2008, apropos "disclosures":

Maybe we need to have a new sort of disclosure, i.e., disclosing our prejudices. My chief ones are:
- TCAs and MAOIs are superior to SSRIs and SNRIs;
- First-generation antipsychotics are as effective, if not more effective than the newer ones;
- Antipsychotics of all classes should be reserved for patients with psychotic symptoms;
- Lithium is more often than not the "mood stabilizer" of choice.[2]

In other words, in psychopharm, old is better than new. We have done better on the upswing than on the down.

The psychopharmacologic model has led to the prescription of the wrong drugs for the wrong indications. In Max Fink's judgment, "Clinical psychiatry is an extraordinarily weak discipline, split from clinical medicine, with its roots in unfounded psychological fantasies that disregard effective diagnostic and treatment practices. Floundering by confusing syndromes for studies of causes, the profession is unable to identify and treat most of the complaints of patients coming to the psychiatric clinics."[3]

A model that started out with such a promising future has become little more than ad copy for the pharmaceutical industry. The failure of drug discovery is not a cause, but a consequence, of this larger failure. The diseases that we now have are the wrong diseases because the diseases that the system offers are artifacts—you can't discover drugs for diseases that don't exist. And the drugs that we now have are the wrong drugs: a commercialized infatuation with the amine neurotransmitters has blocked the imaginative exploration of the vast world of neural connectivity that might have produced new drug entities. So that is the problem.

Nowhere has the air leaked more audibly out of the tire than in the exhausted DSM series. DSM-5, launched in 2013, was supposed to incorporate all the revolutionary new discoveries psychiatry was making into its nosology. In 2002, David Kupfer, the dynamic head of psychiatry at the University of Pittsburgh and co-chair of the later DSM-5 Task Force, looked to a glowing DSM future with the confident expectation that anticipated discoveries in neuroscience would make a new nosology necessary. But the promised breakthroughs never occurred. In 2006, Ross Baldessarini said in an interview, "Sometimes I feel as if I'm waiting for Godot. We keep being told about all these wonderful breakthroughs that are just around the corner, and they never seem to quite pay off."[4] Sometime later, Kupfer and Daryl Regier, the other co-chair of DSM-5 Task Force, rowed back from the coming breakthroughs, noting that the revolutionary new discoveries had stayed in the wings.[5]

Then there was the melancholia morass. DSM-5 adopted what Gordon Parker called the *Totschweigtaktik* (killing something by ignoring it) in dealing with melancholia.[6] The diagnosis didn't even make it into the index. Instead, the drafters burbled, "Major depressive disorder represents the classic condition in this group of disorders."[7] All the cheery upspeak coming from the DSM-5 organizers ignored that one huge issue had not been solved. As Ivan Goldberg commented in 2012, "It is interesting that none of the [organizers'] planning conferences drilled down into the major depression problem. That is such a lame mess, but the DSM-5 people are acting like there are no problems. Duh."[8]

DSM-5 delegitimized the whole psychopharmacology enterprise even further by extending the range of what was considered "mental illness"—all of it, as Kupfer and Regier asserted—"on a solid biological footing."[9] Psychiatrist James O'Brien was scathing on this subject. "Where APA screwed up from the beginning was making every problem in life a mental illness. Had they stayed with the Feighner/St. Louis diagnoses (excluding homosexuality), we would have been taken seriously by the mangled [managed] care executives. But you can't expect them to take us seriously when psychiatry claims that Mood Disorder NOS [not otherwise specified] is a disease 'just like neuroblastoma.' It's not just insurance companies that can't abide that, but the public [—and] anyone with common sense won't either." This smells like a big discrediting of psychopharmacology

What Is to Be Done?

On the basis of this analysis, what needs to be done to restore science to psychiatry and to enable the discovery and development of effective new drugs?

One approach is that some kind of government-run trial service, comparable to the Jon Cole's Psychopharmacology Service Center (PSC), with its Early Clinical Drug Evaluation Units, needs to be restored. These units tested drugs reliably and without self-interest, unlike the industry-sponsored trials, the only purpose of which was registration of the drug. The cancellation of the PSC was an act of colossal shortsightedness that led to, and opened the way to, the disaster that psychopharmacology has become.

Second, reliable "phenotypic" diagnoses must be developed, which means diagnoses that correspond to diseases as they exist in Nature, not as they exist in the minds of a group of academic psychiatrists seated around a table. There will be no progress until drugs are tested for convincing phenotypes.

Three, responsibility for nosology needs to be taken away from the American Psychiatric Association, which is a trade organization with a heavy commitment to industry to keep the status quo, and responsibility must be given to a scientific organization, such as the Karolinska Institute in Stockholm or the National Institute of Mental Health in Bethesda. The Scandinavians have a long history of judiciousness in specifying diagnoses, and they cannot possibly fail to improve on our own dismal performance. As DSM-5 was being drafted, Allen Frances, who had helmed DSM-IV, sprang onto the other side of the barrier and became one of DSM-5's fiercest critics. In October 2012 he told *Psychology Today* that, "APA has lost its competence and credibility as a custodian for DSM. A diagnostic system that affects so many crucial decisions in our society cannot be left to a small professional association whose work is profit driven, lacking in scientific integrity, and insensitive to the public weal."[10]

Finally, the debasement of psychiatric science is a public-health issue. Psychiatric disease is very common. The public has a right to be diagnosed and treated on the basis of science. In 2016, Donald Klein saw industry's corruption of psychiatry as a matter of public health. "Much different [from the low-scale corruption of academics] is the corruption of truth-telling by industry's business-minded leadership—because it sabotages our medical practice's supposed reliance on an evidential basis. That's directly relevant to our patients' vital concern about getting the right pills. So far they don't get that because of their trusting relationship with their own doctor." Klein continued, "So the point is that Pharma corruption far exceeds academia. We won't get necessary public support—for any correction—until the public feels, correctly, that they are personally endangered. How to bring that danger to their sustained attention is our premier problem."[11] Klein and others cited in these pages are the canaries in the coal mine. The drugs don't work, and the public is clueless.

In this record of postmodern misadventure in pharmacology, psychotherapy doesn't look so bad after all. Freud has taken a beating, but that doesn't mean that psychotherapy is invalid or inferior to drugs. There are many psychotherapies, and each time a doctor sees a patient in a consultation, a form of psychotherapy is performed. It's called using the doctor–patient relationship therapeutically. Joel Paris, former head of psychiatry at McGill, wrote in 2019, "In an era dominated by neuroscience, diagnostic checklists, and overly aggressive pharmacology, patients are not getting the care and understanding they need."[12] This is absolutely true.

Acknowledgments

I am indebted to Max Fink, Martin Schumacher, and Peter Tyrer for comments on an earlier draft. Mary van Beuren was a formidable copyeditor.

As often in the past, I express here once again my gratitude to Susan Bélanger, the administrator of the History of Medicine Program at the University of Toronto, for her help. Katherine Wilson has also done yeoman service.

And, once again, I have the pleasure of working with Andrea Knobloch at Oxford University Press.

Notes

Preface

1. On irritability as a separate category not necessarily connected to mood, see Gin S. Malhi and Erica Bell, "Fake Views: Irritable Mood or Moody Irritability or Simply Being Irritable *and* Moody?" *Australia & New Zealand Journal of Psychiatry*, 53 (2019), 1126–1129. doi:10.1177/0004867419885017
2. Alec Coppen, interview, in David Healy, ed., *The Psychopharmacologists* (London: Chapman and Hall, 1998), I, 285. Hereafter cited as Healy, ed., *Psychopharmacologists*.

Chapter 1

1. Joel Elkes, "Psychoactive Drugs: Some Problems and Approaches," in Philip Solomon, ed., *Psychiatric Drugs: Proceedings of a Research Conference Held in Boston* (New York: Grune & Stratton, 1966), 4–21, 18. The conference was held in 1965.
2. Nardo, "One Boring Old Man" (hereafter *1BOM*), January 31, 2012, 2.
3. Nardo, *1BOM*, January 31, 2012, 2–3.
4. C. M. Hales et al., "Prescription Drug Use Among Adults Aged 40–79 in the United States and Canada," *NCHS Data Brief,* no. 347 (Hyattsville MD: NCHS, 2019).
5. Thomas J. Moore et al., letter: "Adult Utilization of Psychiatric Drugs and Differences by Sex, Age, and Race," *JAMA Internal Medicine*, 177 (2017), 274–275.
6. Nardo, *1BOM*, January 2, 2017, 3.
7. Mark Kramer, to correspondents, March 28, 2017.
8. Barry Blackwell, *Treating the Brain: An Odyssey* (INHN Press: Philadelphia, 2019).
9. Michael Balint, *The Doctor, His Patient and the Illness* (1952; reprint, New York: International Universities Press, 1972).
10. See, for example, Kevin M. McKay et al., "Psychiatrist Effects in the Psychopharmacological Treatment of Depression," *Journal of Affective Disorders*, 92 (2006), 287–290.
11. Nardo, *1BOM*, August 11, 2013, 1.
12. Roger P. Greenberg, "Reflections on the Emperor's New Drugs," *Prevention & Treatment*, article 27, vol 5, posted July 15, 2002. http://journals.apa.org/prevention/volume5/pre0050027c.html
13. Heinz Lehmann, interview, in Healy, *Psychopharmacologists*, I, 181–182.
14. United States Senate, Labor-Health, Education, and Welfare Appropriations, 1958, session of April 8, 1957; *Hearings Before the Subcommittee of the Committee on Appropriations, United States Senate, Eighty-Fifth Congress, First session, on H.R. 6287* (Washington DC: United States Government Printing Office, 1957), 1382.

15. Robert Cancro, "The Uncompleted Task of Psychiatry," in Thomas A. Ban et al., eds., *From Psychopharmacology to Neuropsychopharmacology in the 1980s and the Story of CINP, As Told in Autobiography* (Budapest: Animula, 2002), 237–241, 239.

16. Nardo, *1BOM*, October 4, 2014, 1.

17. Samuel B. Woodward, "Observations on the Medical Treatment of Insanity," *American Journal of Insanity [Am J Psych]*, 7 (1850), 1–34, 34.

18. Ralph Gerard, "An Analysis of the Program," in Jonathan O. Cole and Ralph W. Gerard, eds., *Psychopharmacology: Problems in Evaluation. Proceedings of a Conference on the Evaluation of Pharmacotherapy in Mental Illness* (Washington DC: National Academy of Sciences, 1959), 9–10. The conference was held in 1956.

19. George H. Simmons, "The Commercial Domination of Therapeutics and the Movement for Reform," *JAMA*, 48 (May 18, 1907), 1645–1653, 1645.

20. William Osler, "The Treatment of Disease," *Canada Lancet*, 42 (1909), 899–912, 905–906.

21. Paul Nicholas Leech, discussion, Chauncey D. Leake, "The Pharmacologic Evaluation of New Drugs," *JAMA*, 93 (November 23, 1929), 1636.

22. Ernest E. Irons, "The Clinical Evaluation of Drugs," *JAMA*, 93 (November 16, 1929), 1523–1524.

23. Mindel C. Sheps, "The Clinical Value of Drugs: Sources of Evidence," *American Journal of Public Health*, 51 (1961), 647–654, 651.

24. On the AMA's various committees in this area, see John P. Swann, "Sure Cure: Public Policy on Drug Efficacy Before 1962," in Gregory J. Higby et al., eds., *The Inside Story of Medicines: A Symposium* (Madison WI: American Institute of the History of Pharmacy, 1997), 223–261, 233.

25. Arthur J. Cramp, *Nostrums and Quackery* (Chicago: American Medical Association, vol. 2, 1921), 160–162.

26. George H. Simmons, "The Commercial Domination of Therapeutics and the Movement for Reform," *JAMA*, 48 (May 18, 1907), 1645–1653, 1649.

27. Rhonda S. Karg et al., "Past Year Mental Disorders among Adults in the United States: Results from the 2008–2012 Mental Health Surveillance Study," SAMHSA, Center for Behavioral Health Statistics and Quality, *CBHSQ Data Review* (October 2014), 5. http://www.samhsa.gov/data/sites/default/files/NSDUH-DR-N2MentalDis-2014-1/Web/NSDUH-DR-N2MentalDis-2014.htm

28. Ida Macalpine and Richard Hunter, "The Pathography of the Past," *Times Literary Supplement*, March 15, 1974, 256–257.

29. Nardo, *1BOM*, March 11, 2014, 2.

30. Nardo, *1BOM*, September 30, 2010, 2.

31. Joseph Zubin, discussion, Lee N. Robins and James E. Barrett, eds., *The Validity of Psychiatric Diagnosis* (New York: Raven Press, 1989), 244.

32. Frank M. Berger, interview, in Thomas A. Ban, ed., *An Oral History of Neuropsychopharmacology, The First Fifty Years: Peer Interviews* (Brentwood TN: ACNP, 2011), III, 92. Hereafter cited as Ban, ed., *Oral History of Neuropsychopharmacology*.

Chapter 2

1. Robert Rubin, to correspondents, September 13, 2017.
2. Ida Macalpine and Richard Hunter, "The Pathography of the Past," *Times Literary Supplement*, March 15, 1974, 256–257.
3. World Health Organization, *Ataractic and Hallucinogenic Drugs in Psychiatry: Report of a Study Group* (Geneva: WHO, 1958), 4–5. WHO Technical Report Series, no. 152.
4. Torald Sollmann, "Experimental Therapeutics," *JAMA*, 58 (January 27, 1912), 242–244, 243.
5. Heinrich Laehr, *Ueber Irrsein und Irrenanstalten* [On Insanity and Insane Asy;ums] (Halle: Pfeffer, 1852), ix, 10.
6. Henry Maudsley, *Responsibility in Mental Disease* (New York: Appleton, 1874), 17.
7. E. W. Anderson, "Foreword," in F. J. Fish, *Schizophrenia* (Bristol: Wright, 1962), ix.
8. Malcolm Lader, interview, in Healy, ed., *Psychopharmacologists*, I, 470.
9. U.S. National Library of Medicine, *Index-Catalogue of the Surgeon General's Office, United States Army*, 4th series (Washington DC: GPO, 1942), VII, 958–960.
10. Nardo, *1BOM*, April 20, 2012, 2.
11. Frederick K. Goodwin and Peter P. Roy-Byrne, "Future Directions in Biological Psychiatry," in Herbert Y. Meltzer, ed., *Psychopharmacology: The Third Generation of Progress* (New York: Raven Press, 1987), 1691–1698, 1698.
12. Santiago Ramón y Cajal, *Advice for a Young Investigator* (1897), English translation by Neely Swanson (Cambridge MA: MIT Press, 1999), 47.
13. Walter Jacobi and Helmut Winkler, "Encephalographische Studien an Schizophrenen" ["Encephalographic Studies in Schizophrenics"], *Arch f Psych*, 84 (1928), 208–226.
14. Daniel R. Weinberger et al., "Lateral Cerebral Ventricular Enlargement in Chronic Schizophrenia," *AGP*, 36 (1979), 735–739.
15. Johannes Vorster, "Ueber das Verhalten des specifischen Gewichtes des Blutes bei Geisteskranken" ["On Specific Blood Values in Patients with Mental Illnesses"], *Allgemeine Zeitschrift für Psychiatrie* [General Journal of Psychiatry], 50 (1894), 1081–1082. This meeting of the "Südwestdeutsche Irrenärzte" [Southwest German Psychiatrists]. took place in 1892.
16. For a cool-headed assessment, see D. Louis Steinberg, "Hematoporphyrin Treatment of Severe Depressions," *AJP*, 92 (1936), 901–913.
17. Claude Bernard, "Des effets physiologiques de la morphine et de leur combinaison avec ceux du chloroforme" ["Physiological effects of morphione and of its combination with chloroform"], *Bull. Thérapeutique* [Therapeutic Bulletin], 77 (1869), 241–256.
18. G. B. Verga, "Contribuzione allo studio della circolazione cerebrale" ["Contributions to the Study of the Cerebral Circulation"], *Archivio Italiano per le Malattie Nervose* [Italian Archives of Nervous Illness], nos. 3-4 (1884), 282–283.
19. Jean-Pierre Couerbe, "Du cerveau, considéré sous le point de vue chimique et physiologique" ["On the brain, considered from a chemical and physiological point

of view"], *Annales de Chimie et de Physique* [Annales of Chemistry and Physics], 56 (1834), 160–193, 192.

20. Jacques-Joseph Moreau de Tours, *Du hachisch et de l'aliénation mentale* [On hashish in mental illness] (Paris: Masson, 1845) . The Société Moreau de Tours was founded by Henri Baruk and associates in 1958. See H. Baruk et al., "Préface," *Annales Moreau de Tours,* 1 (1962), vii–xv, ix.

21. Alfred T. Poffenberger, " General Reviews and Summaries: Drugs," *Psychol Bull,* 16 (1919), 291–292.

22. Walter Freeman, "Psychochemistry," *JAMA,* 97 (August 1, 1931), 293–296.

23. William R. Houston, *The Art of Treatment* (New York: Macmillan, 1936), 78.

24. Joel Elkes, "Psychopharmacology: Finding One's Way," in Ingrid G. Farreras et al., eds., *Mind, Brain, Body and Behavior: Foundations of Neuroscience and Behavioral Research at the National Institutes of Health* (Amsterdam: IOS Press, 2004), 201–220, 201.

25. Eliot Slater, "Psychiatry in the Thirties," *Contemporary Review,* 226 (1975), 70–75, 70.

26. Henry M. Hurd, *The Institutional Care of the Insane in the United States and Canada* (Baltimore: Johns Hopkins Press, 1916), II, 668.

27. Ian Tait, discussion, in E. M. Tansey et al., eds., *Wellcome Witnesses to Twentieth Century Medicine,* vol. 2 (London: Wellcome Trust, 1998), 169.

28. Daniel W. Cathell, *Book on The Physician Himself,* 10th ed. (Philadelphia: David, 1893), 150–151.

29. See "Deaths Due to Barbituric Acid and Amphetamines, US, 1959, Memorandum for the File," August 3, 1961; US National Archives, RG88, 1961, box 3078, 502. Number of suicide deaths total from US Vital Statistics, 1959, 132. At the same time, it is true that barbiturates were involved in suicide far more frequently than any other drug class. See Annakatri Ohberg et al., "Antidepressants and Suicide Mortality," *J Affect Disord,* 50 (1998), 225–233. Whereas in Finland in 1987–88, the number of suicides per Defined Daily Dose (DDD) for individuals using barbiturates was 105.3, imipramine 17.7, benzodiazepines 0.3.

30. Max Hamilton, discussion, in M. Hamilton, "Mixed Anxiety-Depressive States," in W. Linford Rees, ed., *Anxiety Factors in Comprehensive Patient Care* (Amsterdam: Elsevier, 1973), 18–26, 26.

31. A. G. Young, discussion, in Chauncey D. Leake, "The Pharmacologic Evaluation of New Drugs," *JAMA,* 93 (November 23, 1929), 1635.

32. Louis Lewin, *Phantastica: Die betäubenden und erregenden Genussmittel* [Hallucinatory Drugs: The Sedative and Stimulative Pharmaceuticals of Pleasure] (Berlin: Stilke, 1924), 1–2.

33. For an overview, see John P. Swann, "Sure Cure: Public Policy on Drug Efficacy Before 1962," in Gregory J. Higby et al., eds., *The Inside Story of Medicines: A Symposium* (Madison WI: American Institute of the History of Pharmacy, 1997), 223–261.

34. Suzanne White Junod, *FDA and Clinical Drug Trials: A Short History*, US Food and Drug Administration. www.fda.gov

35. W. A. Puckner and Paul Nicholas Leech, "The Introduction of New Drugs," *JAMA,* 93 (November 23, 1929), 1627–1630.

36. "An Interview with Morris Fishbein, M.D.," 10–11; History of the U.S. Food and Drug Administration, transcript in the NLM, History of Medicine Division, FDA Oral History Collection, interview of March 12, 1968.

37. Robert P. Fischelis, interview, 158; History of the U. S. Food and Drug Administration, transcript in the NLM, History of Medicine Division, FDA Oral History Collection.

38. Leonard A. Dub and Louis A. Lurie, "Use of Benzedrine in the Depressed Phase of the Psychotic State," *Ohio Med J*, 35 (1939), 39–46.

39. Constantine Pascal, "Le Dynamisme de la Démence Précoce," ["Dynamics in Schizophrenia"] *Presse Médicale*, 40 (April 13, 1932), 568–572.

40. Wallace F. Janssen, interview (1984), 109–110; History of the U. S. Food and Drug Administration, transcript in the NLM, History of Medicine Division, FDA Oral History Collection.

41. Torald Sollmann, "The Evaluation of Therapeutic Remedies in the Hospital," *JAMA*, 94 (April 26, 1930), 1279–1281.

42. Torald Sollmann, "The Evaluation of Therapeutic Remedies in the Hospital," *JAMA*, 94 (April 26, 1930), 1280.

43. Emil Kraepelin, Psychiatrie: Ein Lehrbuch für Studierende und Aerzte, 8th ed (Leipzig: Barth, 1913), III, 1392–1394.

Chapter 3

1. Henri Ey, ed., *Premier Congrès Mondial de Psychiatrie* [Firset World Congress of Psychiatry], Paris, 1950 (Paris: Hermann, 1952), IV, 494.

2. See Cohen, in Ingrid G. Farreras et al., eds., *Mind, Brain, Body, and Behavior: Foundations of Neuroscience and Behavioral Research at the National Institutes of Health* (Amsterdam: IOS Press, 2004), 198, n. 4. Johns Hopkins was unaccountably left off this list—its program was based in the Phipps Clinic, which opened in 1913 as a section of the Johns Hopkins Hospital.

3. *Hearings Before the Subcommittee on Antitrust and Monopoly of the Committee on the Judiciary, United States Senate, Eighty-Sixth Congress, Second Session, part 16: "Administered Prices in the Drug Industry (Tranquilizers)," January 21–29, 1960* (Washington DC: Government Printing Office, 1960), 9035.

4. Reinhard Lorich, *Psychopharmakon, Hoc est Medicina Animae* (1548); see O. K. Linde, "Historischer Abriss: Geschichte der Psychopharmaka" [Historical Atls of the History of Psychopharmaceuticals], in P. Riederer et al., eds., *Neuro-Psychopharmaka* (Vienna: Springer, 1992), I, 41–65..

5. David I. Macht, "Contributions to Psychopharmacology," *Johns Hopkins Hospital Bulletin*, 31 (1920), 167–173.

6. Melvin Wilfred Thorner, "The Psycho-pharmacology of Sodium Amytal," *Journal of Nervous and Mental Diseases*, 81 (1935), 161–167.

7. Len Cook, interview, in Healy, ed., *Psychopharmacologists*, II, 22–23.

8. Jacques S. Gottlieb et al., "Psychopharmacologic Study of Schizophrenia and Depressions," *Psychosomatic Medicine*, 14 (1952), 104–114.

9. Jean Thuillier, interview, in Healy, ed., *Psychopharmacologists*, III, 543.

10. Jean Delay and Jean Thuillier, "Psychiatrie expérimentale et psychopharmacologie" ["Experimental Psychiatry and Psychopharmacology"], *Semaine des Hôpitaux de Paris* [Parisian Hospital Bulletin], 32 (October 22, 1956), 3187–3193.

11. Henri Baruk, and J. Launay, "Aperçu historique sur la psychopharmacologie" ["Historical Overview of Psychopharmacology"], *Ann Moreau de Tours* [Annals of Moreau de Tours], 2 (1965), 3–29, 5. P. Chanoit gave 1934 as the founding date and the title. http://ancien.serpsy.org/histoire/adeline_8.html

12. http://ancien.serpsy.org/histoire/adeline_8.html

13. Jean Thuillier, *Ten Years that Changed the Face of Mental Illness* (1981), English translation by Gordon Hickish (London: Dunitz, 1999), 137–138.

14. Thuillier, *Ten Years*, 138–139. Thuillier told David Healy that he was director of "the first department of neuropsychopharmacology in the world" from 1955 to 1976. Healy, ed., *Psychopharmacologists*, III, 546.

15. Anthony Clare, personal statement, in Michael Shepherd, ed., *Psychiatrists on Psychiatry* (Cambridge: Cambridge University Press, 1982), 23.

16. Joel Elkes, "Psychoactive Drugs: Some Problems and Approaches," in Philip Solomon, ed., *Psychiatric Drugs: Proceedings of a Research Conference Held in Boston* (New York: Grune & Stratton, 1966), 4–21, 5. The conference was in 1965.

17. Leo Hollister et al., "Meprobamate in Chronic Psychiatric Patients," in Frank M. Berger, ed., *Meprobamate and Other Agents Used in Mental Disturbances* (New York: Academy of Sciences, 1956), 789–800, 797.

18. Jean Delay, discussion, in P. B. Bradley et al., eds., *Neuro-Psychopharmacology: Proceedings of the First International Congress of Neuro-Pharmacology,* Rome, September 1958 (Amsterdam: Elsevier, 1959), 205.

19. Heinz Lehmann, discussion, in Nathan S. Kline, ed., *Psychopharmacology Frontiers: Proceedings of the Psychopharmacology Symposium* (Boston: Little Brown, 1959), 422–423. Hereafter cited as Kline, ed., *Psychopharmacology Frontiers.* That these proceedings were brought out by a major commercial publisher testifies to the public interest the issues aroused.

20. Alfred Pope, discussion, in Jordi Folch-Pi, ed., *Chemical Pathology of the Nervous System: Proceedings of the Third International Neurochemical Symposium, Strasbourg 1958* (Oxford: Pergamon Press, 1961), 709.

21. Irvine H. Page, "Neurochemistry and Serotonin: A Chemical Fugue," in Seymour S. Kety, ed., "The Pharmacology of Psychotomimetic and Psychotherapeutic Drugs," *Annals of the New York Academy of Sciences*, 66 (1957), 592–601, 592.

22. Irvine H. Page, *Chemistry of the Brain* (Springfield, IL: Charles C Thomas, 1937).

23. Linford Rees, interview, in Healy, ed., *Psychopharmacologists*, II, 177.

24. Mayer-Gross, op cit., 8–9. Willi Mayer-Gross, "A survey of the pharmacological possibilities in psychiatry," in Jean Delay, ed., Colloque International sur la Chlorpromazine et les Médicaments Neuroleptiques en Thérapeutique Psychiatrique [International Colloquium on Chlorpromazine and Neuroleptic Medications in Psychiatric Therapeutics] [1955] (Paris: Doin1956), 7.

25. M. D. Armstrong, A. McMillan, and K. N. F. Shaw, "3-Methoxy-4-Hydroxy-*O*-Mandelic Acid: A Urinary Metabolite of Norepinephrine," *Biochem Biophys Acta*, 25 (1957), 422–423.

26. Merton Sandler, interview, in Ban, ed., *Oral History of Neuropsychopharmacology*, III, 463–464.

27. Benjamin Brodie, discussion, in Kline, ed., *Psychopharmacology Frontiers*, 463.

28. Jonathan Cole, discussion, in Jonathan O. Cole and Ralph W. Gerard, eds., *Psychopharmacology: Problems in Evaluation* (Washington DC: National Academy of Science—National Research Council, 1959), 615. The conference was in 1956.

29. David Healy makes this point in Healy, ed., *Psychopharmacologists*, II, 204.

30. Gordon Claridge and David Healy, "The Psychopharmacology of Individual Differences" [an interview of Claridge by Healy], *Human Psychopharmacology*, 9 (1994), 285–298, 296.

31. Theodore L. Sourkes, "A Biochemist in Psychiatry: Dropping in on the Psychopharmacology Era," in Thomas Ban et al., eds., *Reflections on Twentieth-Century Psychopharmacology*, vol. IV of the series *The History of Psychopharmacology and the CINP, As Told in Autobiography* (Budapest: Animula, 2004), IV, 291.

32. For a year-by-year chronicle of events in psychopharmacology, see Ross J. Baldessarini, "American Biological Psychiatry and Psychopharmacology, 1944–1994," in Roy W. Menninger et al., eds., *American Psychiatry After World War II (1944-1994)* (Washington DC: American Psychiatric Press, 2000), 371–412. The "highlights" chronicle is at pp. 374–375.

33. Ralph W. Gerard, "The Biological Roots of Psychiatry," *AJP*, 112 (1955), 81–90, 82.

34. "In Conversation with Max Hamilton," *Royal College of Psych Bull*, 7 (1983), 42–45, 62–66, 63.

35. See, for example, Joel Elkes, "Psychopharmacology: Finding One's Way," *Neuro-psychopharmacology*, 12 (1995), 93–111, 96.

36. Joel Elkes and Charmian Elkes, "Effect of Chlorpromazine on the Behaviour of Chronically Overactive Psychotic Patients," *British Medical Journal*, 2 (September 4, 1954), 560–576.

37. Michael Alan Taylor, *Hippocrates Cried: The Decline of American Psychiatry* (New York: Oxford University Press, 2013), 46.

38. Frank Ayd interview, Healy, ed., *Psychopharmacologists*, I, 88.

39. Paul McHiugh, *Perspectives of Psychiatry*, 2nd ed. (1998), 12–13. Baltimore: Johns Hopkins University Press.

40. News story, *F-D-C Reports ("The Pink Sheet")*, July 22, 1957, 6.

41. B. Carroll, post, *1BOM*, May 31, 2011, 2.

42. Michael Shepherd, "An English View of American Psychiatry," *AJP*, 114 (1957), 417–420, 419.

43. Tim Bergling, *Sissyphobia: Gay Men and Effeminate Behavior* (New York: Harrington Park Press, 2001), 41.

44. Max Fink, interview, in Ban, ed., *Oral History of Neuropsychopharmacology*, IX, 76.

45. Klein interview, in Healy, ed., *Psychopharmacologists*, I, 330.

46. B. Carroll, comment, in *1BOM*, December 17, 2016, 3.

47. David Healy [interview with] "Mandel Cohen and the Origins of the *Diagnostic and Statistical Manual of Mental Disorders, Third Edition: DSM-III*," *History of Psychiatry*, 13 (2002), 209–230, 210.

48. Jan Fawcett, interview, in Ban, ed., *Oral History of Neuropsychopharmacology*, V, 132.

49. Melvin Sabshin and Joshua Ramot, "Pharmacotherapeutic Evaluation and the Psychiatric Setting," *AMA Archives of Neurology and Psychiatry*, 75 (1956), 362–370, 365, 367.

50. Roy R. Grinker, Sr., "The Phenomena of Depression," in Thomas A. Williams et al., eds., *Recent Advances in the Psychobiology of the Depressive Illnesses: Proceedings of a Workshop Sponsored by the Clinical Research Branch, Division of Extramural Research Programs, National Institute of Mental Health, April 30 through May 2, 1969* (Washington DC: Superintendent of Documents, Government Printing Office, 1972), 295–297, 296.

51. Jonathan Cole, discussion, in Kline, ed., *Psychopharmacology Frontiers*, 439. The congress was held in 1957.

52. Ralph W. Gerard, "Orientation," in Jonathan O. Cole and Ralph W. Gerard, eds., *Psychopharmacology: Problems in Evaluation* (Washington DC: National Academy of Sciences—National Research Council, 1959), 9–19, 10. The conference was in September 1956.

53. Samuel H. Barondes, interview, in Ban, ed., *Oral History of Neuropsychopharmacology*, III, 69–70.

54. Fritz Freyhan, "General Problems of Psychopharmacology," in Kline, ed., *Psychopharmacology Frontiers*, 8–9.

55. Eric Strömgren, essay, in Michael Shepherd, ed., *Psychiatrists on Psychiatry* (Cambridge: Cambridge University Press, 1982), 152–169, 159.

56. Robert A. Cohen interview, in Ban, ed., *Oral History of Neuropsychopharmacology*, I, 200.

57. Burton Angrist, comment, in Samuel Gershon, "Events and Memories," 30; *INHN*. http://inhn.org/fileadmin/user_upload/User_Uploads/INHN/EBOOKS/Samuel_Gereson_s_Events_and_Memories.pdf

58. Ralph W. Gerard, "Drugs for the Soul: The Rise of Psychopharmacology," *Science*, 125 (1957), 201–203.

59. Eugène Asse, ed., *Lettres de Mlle de Lespinasse* (Paris: Charpentier, 1876). The letter in question was dated November 8, 1775.

60. Robert Spitzer, interview, in Healy, ed., *Psychopharmacologists*, III, 427.

61. Gina Bellafante, "Big City," *New York Times*, April 20, 2020, 38.

62. Librium ad, "Wellsprings of Anxiety: The Search for Identity," *Dis Nerv Syst*, 31 (1970)

63. Jean Thuillier, *La Folie: Histoire et Dictionnaire* (Paris: Laffont, 1996), 6. "Le fou n'était plus un aliéné."

64. World Health Organization, *Ataractic and Hallucinogenic Drugs in Psychiatry: Report of a Study Group* (Geneva: WHO, 1958), 10–11, 43. WHO Technical Report Series, no. 152.

65. Nathan S. Kline, "Presidential Address," in Daniel H. Efron, ed., *Psychopharmacology: A Review of Progress, 1957–1967: The Proceedings of the Sixth Annual Meeting of the American College of Neuropsychopharmacology, San Juan, Puerto Rico, December 12–15, 1967* (Washington DC: Government Printing Office, 1968, PHS Pub. No. 1836), 1–3, 3.

66. Nardo, *1BOM*, March 1, 2014, 3.

67. *Hearings Before the Subcommittee on Reorganization and International Organizations of the Committee on Government Operations, United States Senate, 88th Congress, First Session*, "Agency Coordination Study," part IV, 1288–1289.

68. News story, *F-D-C Reports ("The Pink Sheet")*, March 16, 1959, 6.

69. On reserpine and the tranquilizers, see Edward Shorter, *Before Prozac: The Troubled History of Mood Disorders in Psychiatry* (New York: Oxford University Press), 37–38.

70. Max Fink to correspondents, March 15, 2017.

71. Malcolm Lader, interview, in Healy, ed., *Psychopharmacologists*, I, 467.

72. Jonathan Cole, interview, in Healy, ed., *Psychopharmacologists*, I, 241. See Albert Kurland, "Chlorpromazine in the Treatment of Schizophrenia: A Study of 75 Cases," *JNMD*, 121 (1955), 321–329.

73. Donald Klein to correspondents, January 18, 2017.

Chapter 4

1. Nathan S. Kline, ed., *Psychopharmacology* (Washington DC: American Association for the Advancement of Science, 1956), v.

2. Gerald J. Sarwer-Foner, interview, in Ban, ed., *Oral History of Neuropsychopharmacology*, IX, 280.

3. T. Sourkes, in Ban, ed., *Oral History of Psychopharmacology*, IV, 293.

4. George Simpson, interview, in Healy, ed., *Psychopharmacologists*, II, 297.

5. Mogens Schou, "The Theoretical Basis of Psychiatric Pharmacotherapy," *Report on the Twelfth Congress of Scandinavian Psychiatrists in Copenhagen, Denmark, 1958* (Copenhagen: Munksgaard, 1959), 12–15, 14. This is *Acta Psych et Neurol Scand*, Suppl. 136, vol. 34 (1959).

6. See Irwin Kopin, "Psychopharmacological Research in the 1950s," in Ingrid F. G. Farreras et al., eds., *Mind, Brain, Body, and Behavior: Foundations of Neuroscience and Behavioral Research at the National Institutes of Health* (Amsterdam: IOS, 2004), 267–280, 271. Hereafter, Farreras, ed., *Mind, Brain, Body*.

7. Jonathan O. Cole and Ralph W. Gerard, eds., *Psychopharmacology: Problems in Evaluation* (Washington DC: National Academy of Sciences—National Research Council, 1959), 9–19, 10. The conference was in September 1956. On these events, see Robert A. Cohen, "The Early Years of the NIMH Intramural Clinical Research Program," in Farreras, ed., *Mind, Brain, Body*, 183–200, 192.

8. On this, see Stephen Bernstein, "A Ten-Year History of the Early Clinical Drug Evaluation Unit (ECDEU) Program," *Psychopharmacology Bulletin*, 6 (2) (April 1970), 1–21, 3.

9. See news stories, *F-D-C Reports ("The Pink Sheet")*, August 11, 1958, 17; and *F-D-C Reports ("The Pink Sheet")*, October 20, 1958, 15.

10. See Max Fink, memoir, in Thomas Ban et al., eds., *The Triumph of Psychopharmacology and the Story of CINP* (Budapest: Animula, 2000), 85–86.

11. News story, *F-D-C Reports ("The Pink Sheet")*, April 8, 1957, back cover.

12. [Jonathan Cole, The National Institute of Mental Health Psychopharmacology Service Center Collaborative Study Group, "Phenothiazine Treatment in Acute Schizophrenia," *AGP*, 10 (1964), 246–261.

13. Leo E. Hollister, "The ECDEU Program: A View From the Field," *Psychopharmacology Bulletin*, 6 (2) (April 1970), 82–85, 84. For statistics, see Roland R. Bonato et al., "BLIPS: The Information Processing System for the ECDEU Program," ibid, *Psychopharmacology Bulletin*, 1970, 22–47.

14. Frances O. Kelsey to Roger L. Black, November 18, 1964; National Archives, UD - WW, E 35, 88-72-4049, 505.51, box 280.

15. William E. Bunney, Jr., and John M. Davis, "Norepinephrine in Depressive Reactions: A Review," *AGP*, 13 (1965), 483–494, 492.

16. John M. Davis, interview, in Ban, ed., *Oral History of Neuropsychopharmacology*, V, 115.

17. Heinrich Waelsch, ed., *Biochemistry of the Developing Nervous System. Proceedings of the First International Neurochemical Symposium held at Magdalen College, Oxford, July 13–17, 1954* (New York: Academic Press, 1955). See also Elkes, in Farreras, ed., *Mind, Brain, Body*, 211.

18. See New York State Psychiatric Institute, *Annual Reports*, 1948–1961.

19. Sidney Malitz et al., "Preliminary Evaluation of Tofranil in a Combined In-Patient and Out-Patient Setting," [Proceedings] McGill University Conference on Depression and Allied States, Montreal," *Canadian Psychiatric Association Journal*, Suppl. 4 (1959), S152–S159, S152.

20. Harold A. Abramson, ed., *Neuropharmacology: Transactions of the First Conference, May 26, 27 and 28, 1954, Princeton, NJ* (New York: Macy Foundation, 1955).

21. Karl Rickels, *A Serendipitous Life: From German POW to American Psychiatrist* (Evergreen CO: Notting Hill Press, 2011), 156–158, 171.

22. Jean Delay, "Introduction au Colloque International," in Delay, ed., *Colloque International sur la Chlorpromazine et les Médicaments Neuroleptiques en Thérapeutique Psychiatrique* (Paris: Doin, 1956), 5.

23. Fritz Flügel, "Thérapeutique par Médication Neuroleptique Obtenue en Réalisant Systématiquement des États Parkinsoniformes," ibid., 790–792.

24. Hans-Joachim Haase, "Über Vorkommen und Deutung des psychomotorischen Parkinsonsyndroms bei Megaphen—bzw. Largactil-Dauerbehandlung," *Nervenarzt*, 25 (1954), 486–492.

25. Nathan S. Kline, ed., *Psychopharmacology Frontiers: Proceedings of the Psychopharmacology Symposium of the Second International Congress of Psychiatry* (Boston: Little Brown, 1959), 61.

26. Silvio Garattini, interview, in Healy, ed., *Psychopharmacologists*, I, 135.

27. Wolfgang de Boor, *Pharmakopsychologie und Psychopathologie* (Berlin: Springer, 1956).

28. Thomas A. Ban, interview, Healy, ed., *Psychopharmacologists*, I, 588.

29. Oldrich Vinar, interview, in Healy, ed., *Psychopharmacologists*, III, 68–69.

30. On these events see Thomas A. Ban, "Preface," in Ban, ed., *Oral History of Neuropsychopharmacology*, X, x–xi.

31. Joseph J. Schildkraut, John M. Davis, and Gerald L. Klerrman, "Biochemistry of Depressions," in Daniel H. Efron, ed., *Psychopharmacology: A Review of Progress, 1957-1967: The Proceedings of the Sixth Annual Meeting of the American College of Neuropsychopharmacology, San Juan, Puerto Rico, December 12-15, 1967* (Washington DC: Government Printing Office, 1968, PHS Pub. No. 1836), 625–648.

32. Max Fink, "Neurophysiological Response Strategies in the Classification of Mental Illness," in Martin Katz et al., eds., *Classification in Psychiatry and Psychopathology* (Washington DC: USDHEW-PHS, 1965, PHS Pub. No. 1584), 535–540, 537. Hamilton's comment is on p. 542.

33. Thomas A. Ban, interview, in Ban, ed., *Oral History of Neuropsychopharmacology*, IV, 24.

34. Undated note from Bernard Carroll to [IJ?] Oberman, in Carroll Papers, Neuroscience History Archives, Brain Research Institute, UCLA.

35. Steven Marc Paul, interview, in Ban, ed., *Oral History of Neuropsychopharmacology*, III, 389.

36. Elkes, in Farreras, ed., *Mind, Brain, Body*, 214.

37. Nathan S. Kline and Heinz E. Lehmann, eds., *Psychopharmacology* (Boston: Little Brown, 1965), ix. *International Psychiatry Clinics*, Oct 1965, vol. 2, no. 4.

38. Harry F. Dowling, "Twixt the Cup and the Lip," *JAMA*, 165 (October 12, 1957), 657–661, 657.

39. On these events, see Max Rinkel, "The Psychological Aspects of the LSD Psychosis," in M. Rinkel, ed., *Chemical Concepts of Psychosis: Proceedings of the Symposium on Chemical Concepts of Psychosis Held at the Second International Congress of Psychiatry in Zurich, Switzerland, September 1 to 7, 1957* (New York: McDowell, 1958), 75–84.

40. See A. R. Green, "Gaddum and LSD: The Birth and Growth of Experimental and Clinical Neuropharmacology Research on 5-HT in the UK," *British Journal of Pharmacology*, 154 (2008), 1583–1599. 5-HT is serotonin. doi:10.1038/bjp.2008.207

41. Joel Elkes in Farreras, ed., *Mind, Brain, and Behavior*, 206.

42. [Philip R. Lee, ed., *The Drug Makers and The Drug Distributors* (USDHEW—Office of the Secretary, December 1968), 19.

43. Jean Thuillier, *La Folie: Histoire et Dictionnaire* (Paris: Laffont, 1996), 184.

44. On these developments, see Edward Shorter, *A History of Psychiatry* (New York: Wiley, 1997), 264–266.

45. Fritz A. Freyhan, "Vier Jahrzehnte klinischer Psychiatrie—aus persönlicher Sicht," *Fortschr Neurol Psychiat*, 47 (1979), 436–441, 438.

46. Arthur J. Prang, Jr., interview, in Ban, ed, *Oral History of Neuropsychopharmacology*, V, 274.

47. A convenient overview of the drugs discussed in this section may be found in Edward Shorter, *Before Prozac: The Troubled History of Mood Disorders in Psychiatry* (New York: Oxford University Press, 2009), xi–xvi.

48. Many observers are dubious about the whole concept of "treatment-resistant depression" (TRD), which usually means nonresponse to the SSRIs. Jay Amsterdam said that, in his mood disorders clinic at the University of Pennsylvania, he "learned a hell of a lot about MAOI therapy in TRD and the abject fear of the field to use MAOIs for TRD—despite the fact that they (and ECT alone) demonstrated the best promise for response." Jay Amsterdam to correspondents, January 5, 2017.

49. Jay Amsterdam to correspondents, April 8, 2016.

50. Jonathan O. Cole, Gerald L. Klerman, and Reese T. Jones, "Drug Therapy," in *Progress in Neurology and Psychiatry,* 15 (1960), 540–576, 542–543.

51. See Establishment Inspection Endorsement, A/S Syntetic, June 3, 1971; Federal Archives, RG88, General Subject Files 1971, box 4531.

52. Sidney Cohen, "TP-21, A New Phenothiazine," *AJP,* 115 (1958), 358. TP-21 was thioridazine.

53. Donald F. Klein and Max Fink, "Behavioral Reaction Patterns with Phenothiazines," *AGP,* 7 (1962), 449–459, 454.

54. Donald Klein, interview, in Healy, ed., *Psychopharmacologists,* I, 348.

55. Rinaldo De Nuzzo, "1972 Prescription Survey by the Albany College of Pharmacy," *Medical Marketing & Media,* 8 (4) (1973), 3–26, 28, tab. 2.

56. "Record 63 New Therapeutic Chemicals Marketed in 1959," *F-D-C Reports ("The Pink Sheet"),* January 11, 1960, 19–21.

57. These examples are from Librium ads in *JAMA,* 220 (4) (April 24, 1972), 512–514; *JAMA,* 225 (9) (August 27, 1973), 1125–1126; and *JAMA,* 228 (11) (June 10, 1974), 1388–1391.

58. Elavil ad, *JAMA,* 188 (3) (April 20, 1964), 92–93.

59. Triavil ad, *JAMA,* 206 (11) (December 9, 1968), 2426–2428.

60. See, for example, Nick Craddock and Michael J. Owen, "The Kraepelinian Dichotomy—Going, Going—But Still Not Gone," *BJP,* 196 (2010), 92–95. doi:10.1192/bjp.bp.109.073429

61. David Drachman, discussion, Psychopharmacologic Drugs Advisory Committee (PDAC), March 13, 1981, II-77. Obtained from the FDA through the Freedom of Information Act.

62. George Gardos, interview, in Ban, ed., *Oral History of Neuropsychopharmacology,* IV, 127.

63. Nathan S. Kline, testimony, "False and Misleading Advertising (Prescription Tranquilizing Drugs)," *Hearings Before a Subcommittee of the Committee on Government Operations, House of Representatives, Eighty-Fifth Congress, Second Session, February 11–26, 1958* (Washington DC: Government Printing Office, 1958), 6–14.

64. Nardo, *1BOM,* August 25, 2011, 3.

65. Nardo, *1BOM,* August 12, 2015, 12.

66. Paul Leber, discussion, PDAC, February 24, 1983, I-155-156. Obtained through the Freedom of Information Act.

67. Robert Whitaker, *Anatomy of an Epidemic: Magic Bullets, Psychiatric Drugs, and the Astonishing Rise of Mental Illness in America,* 2nd ed (New York: Broadway Books, 2015), 7.

Chapter 5

1. John Ferriar, *Medical Histories and Reflections* (London: Cadell, 1810), II. 1.
2. Max Fink, Donald F. Klein, and John C. Kramer, "Clinical Efficacy of Chlorpromazine-Procyclidine Combination, Imipramine and Placebo in Depressive Disorders," *Psychopharmacologia*, 7 (1965), 27–36, 34.
3. Ludiomil ad, *JAMA*, 247 (10) (March 12, 1982), 1417.
4. Allan V. Horwitz, "How an Age of Anxiety Became an Age of Depression," *Milbank Q*, 88 (2010), 112–138. https://www.ncbi.nlm.nih.gov/pmc/articles/PMC2888013/
5. Morton Kramer, discussion, in Joseph Zubin, ed., *Field Studies in the Mental Disorders* (New York: Grune & Stratton, 1961), 115. The conference was in 1959.
6. Benjamin Pasamanick, in Zubin, ed., Field Studies, ., 118. Morton Kramer, discussion, in Zubin, ed., *Field Studies*.
7. Karl Jaspers, *Allgemeine Psychopathologie* [General Psychopathology], 4th ed. (Berlin: Springer, 1946), 4.
8. These events are described in Edward Shorter, *History of Psychiatry* (New York: Wiley, 1997), and Edward Shorter, *What Psychiatry Left Out of the DSM-5: Historical Mental Disorders Today* (New York: Routledge, 2015).
9. Richard Hunter, "Psychiatry and Neurology: Psychosyndrome or Brain Disease," *Proceedings of the Royal Societty of Medicine*, 66 (1973), 359.
10. B. Carroll, comment, in *1BOM*, March 28, 2014, 4.
11. Brainstorm Consortium, "Analysis of Shared Heritability in Common Disorders of the Brain," *Science*, 360 (June 22, 2018).
12. Thomas Willis, *Two Discourses Concerning the Soul of Brutes,* Latin ed. 1672, English ed. 1683 (Gainesville FL: Scholars' Facsimiles, 1971), 211.
13. Frank Fish, discussion, in E. Beresford Davies, ed., *Depression: Proceedings of the Symposium Held at Cambridge 22 to 26 September 1959* (Cambridge: University Press, 1964), 349.
14. On this, see Edward Shorter, *What Psychiatry Left Out of the DSM-5: Historical Mental Disorders Today* (New York: Routledge, 2015), 99–129.
15. Paul Janssen, interview, in Healy, ed., *Psychopharmacologists*, II, 60.
16. See Max Fink and Michael Alan Taylor, *Catatonia: A Clinician's Guide to Diagnosis and Treatment* (New York: Cambridge University Press, 2003); Edward Shorter and Max Fink, *The Madness of Fear: A History of Catatonia* (New York: Oxford University Press, 2018).
17. Oswald Bumke, *Lehrbuch der Geisteskrankheiten* [Textbook of the Mental Illnesses] (1919), 2nd ed. (Munich: Bergmann, 1924), 866.
18. See the Leber-Laughren exchange in Psychopharmacologic Drugs Advisory Committee (PDAC), November 4, 2002, 192.
19. Paul Leber, discussion, PDAC, July 24, 1995, 45–46. Obtained through the Freedom of Information Act.
20. News story, *Scrip*, September 10, 1996, 19.
21. Thomas P. Rees, "A Note on the Indications for Shock Therapy," *Journal of Mental Science*, 97 (1951), 144–145, 145.

22. Leo Alexander, *Objective Approaches to Treatment in Psychiatry* (Springfield IL: Charles C Thomas, 1958), 4–5.

23. Eliot Slater, *Man, Mind, and Heredity: Selected Papers of Eliot Slater on Psychiatry and Genetics*, eds. James Shields and Irving I Gottesman (Baltimore: Johns Hopkins Press, 1971), 8–9.

24. Raymond Battegay, "Forty-four Years of Psychiatry and Psychopharmacology," in Healy, ed., *Psychopharmacologists*, III, 387.

25. Laszlo J. Meduna, *Oneirophrenia: The Confusional State* (Urbana: University of Illinois Press, 1950), 62.

26. Emmanuel Régis, "Les psychoses d'auto-intoxication: Considérations générales" ["The autointoxication psychoses: general considerations"], *Archives de Neurologie*, (1899), 278–303.

27. Ralph W. Gerard, "The Nosology of Schizophrenia," *AJP*, 120 (1963), 16–29, 17, 29.

28. Courtenay Harding, George W. Brooks et al., "The Vermont Longitudinal Study of Persons With Severe Mental Illness: Long-Term Outcome of Subjects Who Retrospectively Met *DSM-III* Criteria for Schizophrenia," *AJP*, 144 (1987), 727–735.

29. W. Mayer-Gross, Eliot Slater, and Martin Roth, *Clinical Psychiatry* (London: Cassell, 1954), 296.

30. W. Jacobi and H. Winkler, "Encephalographische Studien an chronisch Schizophrenen" ["Encephalographic Studies of Chronic Schizophrenia"], *Archiv für Psychiatrie*, 81 (1927), 299–332; Jacobi and Winkler, "Encephalographische Studien an Schizophrenen" ["Encephalographic. Studies of Schizophrenia"], *Archiv für Psychiatrie*, 84 (1928), 208–226.

31. Daniel R. Weinberger et al. "Lateral Cerebral Ventricular Enlargement in Chronic Schizophrenia," *AGP*, 36 (1979), 735–739.

32. On this distinction, see Norman Sartorius et al., "Two-Year Follow-Up of the Patients Included in the WHO International Pilot Study of Schizophrenia," *Psychol Med, 7* (1977), 529–541.

33. See Gerald Goldstein et al., "High-functioning Autism and Schizophrenia: A Comparison of Early and Late Onset Neurodevelopmental Disorder," *Arch Clin Neuropsychol,* 17 (2002), 461–475. https://www.sciencedirect.com/science/article/pii/S0887617701001299

34. Thomas A. Ban, interview, in Healy, ed., *Psychopharmacologists*, I, 619.

35. John S. Strauss, William T. Carpenter et al., "Speculations on the Processes That Underlie Schizophrenic Symptoms and Signs: III," *Schizophrenia Bulletin*, 1 (1974), 61–69.

36. Leo Hollister, interview, in Ban, ed., *Oral History of Neuropsychopharmacology*, I, 54; IX, 146–147.

37. R. S. Kahn and R. S. Keefe, "Schizophrenia Is a Cognitive Illness: Time for a Change in Focus," *JAMA Psychiatry*, 70 (2013), 1107–1112, 1107.

38. See Michael Alan Taylor and Nutan Atre Vaidya, *Descriptive Psychopathology: The Signs and Symptoms of Behavioral Disorders* (New York: Cambridge University Press, 2009), 384–385.

39. Daniel R. Weinberger, interview, in Ban, ed., *Oral History of Neuropsychopharmacology*, II, 294.

40. Ewald Hecker, "Die Hebephrenie: ein Beitrag zur klinischen Psychiatrie," *Archiv für pathologische Anatomie und Physiologie und für klinische Medicin* [Archives of Pathological Anatomy and Physiology and od Clinical Medicine], 52 (1871), 394–429.

41. Michael Alan Taylor, *Hippocrates Cried: The Decline of American Psychiatry* (New York: Oxford University Press, 2013), 174.

42. Eli Robins and Samuel B. Guze, "Establishment of Diagnostic Validity in Psychiatric Illness: Its Application to Schizophrenia," *American Journal of Psychiatry*, 126 (1970), 983–987.

43. Donald W. Goodwin to Harrison G. Pope, Jr., and Joseph F. Lipinski, October 30, 1978; in Paula Clayton Papers, Neuroscience History Archives, UCLA, box 31.

44. Seymour Kety, discussion, in Robert L. Spitzer and Donald F. Klein, eds., *Critical Issues in Psychiatric Diagnosis* (New York: Raven Press, 1978), 250. This exchange took place at a meeting of the American Psychopathological Association in 1977.

45. M. Harrow et al., "Do All Schizophrenia Patients Need Antipsychotic Treatment Continuously Throughout Their Lifetime? A 20-Year Longitudinal Study," *Psychol Med*, 42 (2012), 45–55. doi:10.1017/S0033291712000220

46. Benjamin Wiesel, interview, August 16, 1990; Hamilton Archives at Hartford Hospital, 21.

47. Louis A. Gottschalk, interview, in Ban, ed., *Oral History of Neuropsychopharmacology*, IX, 124.

48. Robert M. Kessler, interview, Ban, ed., *Oral History of Neuropsychopharmacology*, II, 287–288.

49. See, for example, Jim Van Os, editorial, "The Dynamics of Subthreshold Psychopathology: Implications for Diagnosis and Treatment," *AJP*, 170 (2013), 695–698; H. Häfner et al., "ABC Schizophrenia Study: An Overview of Results since 1996," *Soc Psychiatry Psychiatr Epidemiol*, 48 (2013), 1021–1031.

50. Joseph J. Schildkraut and Donald F. Klein, "The Classification and Treatment of Depressive Disorders," in R. I. Shader ed., *Manual of Psychiatric Therapeutics* (Boston: Little Brown, 1975), 39–61, 42–43.

51. Donald Klein to correspondents, July 17, 2012

52. Karl Leonhard, *Die Aufteilung der endogenen Psychosen* [The Classification of the Endogenous Psychoses] (East-Berlin: Akademie-Verlag, 1957). n response to medication, see Frank Fish, "The Influence of the Tranquillisers on the Leonhard Schizophrenic Syndromes," *L'Encéphale*, 53 (1964), pp. 245–249, tab. 1, p. 248.

53. C. M. Banki et al., "Neuroendocrine Differences among Subtypes of Schizophrenic Disorder?" *Neuropsychobiology*, 11 (1984), 174–177.

54. Charles L. Bowden, interview, in Ban, ed., *Oral History of Neuropsychopharmacology*, IV, 57.

55. Robert A. McCutcheon et al., "Schizophrenia: An Overview," *JAMA Psychiatry*, published online October 30, 2019. jamapsychiatry.com

56. Barry Blackwell, *Bits and Pieces of a Psychiatrist's Life* (Philadelphia: Xlibris Corp, 2012), 150.

57. News story, *F-D-C Reports (The Pink Sheet")*, March 16, 1959, 6–10.

58. Herman van Praag et al., "The Vital Syndrome Interview," *Psychiatria, Neurologia, Neurochirurgia*, 68 (1965), 329–346. Herman van Praag, interview, in Healy, ed., *Psychopharmacologists*, I, 360–361. Kurt Schneider, "Die Schichtung des emotionalen Lebens und der Aufbau der Depressionszustände" ["The layering of emotional life and the structure of depressive conditions"], *Zeitschrift für die gesamte Neurologie und Psychiatrie* [Journal of Global Neurology and Psychiatry], 59 (1920), 281–286. He revived it in Schneider, *Beiträge zur Psychiatrie* [Contributions to Psychiatry] (Wiesbaden: Thieme, 1946), 8–9.

59. Gordon Parker and Dusan Hadzi-Pavlovic, *Melancholia: A Disorder of Movement and Mood* (Cambridge: Cambridge University Press, 1996).

60. Michael Alan Taylor and Max Fink, *Melancholia: The Diagnosis, Pathophysiology, and Treatment of Depressive Illness* (Cambridge:: Cambridge University Press, 2006).

61. Thomas A. Ban, *From Melancholia to Depression: A History of Diagnosis and Treatment* (2014). http://inhn.org/ebooks/thomas-a-ban-from-melancholia-to-de-pression-a-history-of-diagnosis-and-treatment.html

62. Merton Sandler et al., "Is There an Increase in Monoamine-oxidase Activity in Depressive Illness?" *Lancet*, 1 (May 10, 1975), 1045–1049. A. S. Hale et al., "Tyramine-Conjugation Deficit as a Trait-marker in Endogenous Depressive Illness," *J Psychiatr Res*, 20 (1986), 251–261. A. S. Hale et al., "Tyramine Conjugation Test for Prediction of Treatment Response in Depressed Patients," *Lancet*, 1 (February 4, 1989), 234–236. There has been a lively academic discussion about first use of the term "antidepressant," but Smith, Kline & French Laboratories, as it then was, claimed in 1950 of its new drug Dexamyl (a combo of amphetamine and barbiturate) that "The 'Dexedrine,' because of its 'smooth' and profound antidepressant action, restores mental alertness and optimism and dispels psychogenic fatigue." The Amytal treated other symptoms. There almost certainly were earlier uses. *New York State Journal of Medicine*, 50 (1950), 511.

63. W. M. Harrison et al., "The Tyramine Challenge Test as a Marker for Melancholia," *Archives of General Psychiatry*, 41 (1984), 681–685.

64. Merton Sandler, interview, in Ban, ed., *Oral History of Neuropsychopharmacology*, III, 464.

65. Israel Strauss, discussion of Peter G. Denker, "Results of Treatment of Psychoneuroses by the General Practitioner: A Follow-Up Study of 500 Patients," *AMA Archives of Neurology and Psychiatry*, 57 (1947), 504–512, 511.

66. Mark S. Kramer, "Commentary" on Barry Blackwell: Corporate Corruption in the Psychopharmaceutical Industry, October 13, 2016, 29. https://inhn.org/fileadmin/user_upload/User_Uploads/INHN/FILES/Kramers-__LM_Revised_commentary_-_October_13__2016.pdf

67. J. W. Stewart, P. J. McGrath, F. M. Quitkin, and D. F. Klein, "Atypical Depression: Current Status and Relevance to Melancholia," *Acta Psych Scand,* Suppl., 433 (2007), 58–71. J. W. Stewart, P. J. McGrath, F. M. Quitkin, and D. F. Klein, "DSM-IV Depression with Atypical Features: Is It Valid?" *Neuropsychopharmacology*, 34 (2009), 2625–2632.

68. Bernard Carroll to Shorter, March 6, 2010.

69. Thomas A. Ban, "From Melancholia to Depression: A History of Diagnosis and Treatment" ms., tab. 10, p. 34. A revised version of this paper was subsequently published online (https://pdfs.semanticscholar.org/42b0/9e82bb9f61b4416e00d0aa4cf27dc16d54b2.pdf) yet without tab. 10.
70. DSM-III, 215.
71. DSM-5, 185.
72. Bernard Carroll, "Dexamethasone Suppression Test in Depression," *Lancet*, 2 (December 6, 1980), 1249. https://doi.org/10.1016/S0140-6736(80)92507-6
73. Henri Ellenberger, "Comparison of European and American Psychiatry," *Bull Menninger Clinic*, 19 (1955), 43–52, 49. Ellenberger's book, a must-read for any student of the history of psychiatry, is *The Discovery of the Unconscious* (New York: Basic Books, 1970).
74. Emil Kraepelin, *Psychiatrie: ein kurzes Lehrbuch für Studirende und Aerzte* [Psychiatry: A Short Textbook for Students and Physicians], 4th ed. (Leipzig: Abel, 1893), 435–445. Spelling was later changed to "Studierende."
75. Nardo, *1BOM*, February 7, 2016, 2.

Chapter 6

1. Barry Blackwell, *Bits and Pieces of a Psychiatrist's Life* (Philadelphia: Xlibris, 2012), 191.
2. G. W. B. James, discussion, "Hypnotic Drugs: Uses and Dangers," *BMJ*, 2 (December 30, 1933), 1213–1214.
3. On this, see William C. Bogner, *Drugs to Market: Creating Value and Advantage in the Pharmaceutical Industry* (Tarrytown NY: Pergamon/Elsevier Science, 1996), 62–64.
4. [Philip R. Lee, ed., *Task Force on Prescription Drugs, Background Papers: The Drug Makers and the Drug Distributors* (Washington DC: US DHEW, December 1968), 4.
5. Erik Verg et al., *Milestones: The Bayer Story in 130 Chapters* (Leverkusen: Bayer, 1988), 136.
6. Robert P. Fischelis, interview, September 17–19, 1968, 75; "History of the U. S. Food and Drug Administration," transcript in NLM, History of Medicine Division, FDA Oral History Collection.
7. C. Rufus Rorem et al., *The Costs of Medicine: The Manufacture and Distribution of Drugs and Medicines in the United States and the Services of Pharmacy in Medical Care* (Chicago: University of Chicago Press, 1932), 119.
8. Thomas Ban, interview, in Healy, ed., *Psychopharmacologists*, I, 607.
9. Frank Ayd interview, in Healy, ed., *Psychopharmacologists*, I, 82. Ayd was often criticized for his close relations with industry. Yet he was at pains to tell Congress in 1958 that he had profited very little from the ties. "Half the compounds I have screened, I have screened for nothing." Frank Ayd, Jr., testimony, "False and Misleading Advertising (Prescription Tranquilizing Drugs)," *Hearings Before a Subcommittee of the Committee on Government Operations, House of Representatives, Eighty-Fifth*

Congress, Second Session February 11 ... 1958 (Washington DC: GPO, 1958), 56). Ayd was a very observant Catholic, and his big ambition in life was closer relations with the Pope, not with the pharmaceutical industry.

10. Ayd, in Healy, ed., *Psychopharmacologists*, I, 86.

11. Max Fink, "Clinical Evaluation of Psychoactive Drugs in the 21st Century," in Thomas A. Ban et al., eds., *From Psychopharmacology to Neuropsychopharmacology in the 1980s and the Story of CINP, As Told in Autobiography* (Budapest: Animula, 2002), 21–26, 24. Vol. 3 of the series *The History of Psychopharmacology and the CINP*.

12. T. Ban, interview, in Healy, ed., *Psychopharmacologists*, I, 619.

13. "Administered Prices: Drugs." *Report of the Committee on the Judiciary, United States Senate, Made by its Subcommittee on Antitrust and Monopoly ["Kefauver Committee"], Eighty-Seventh Congress, June 27, 1961* (Washington DC: GPO, 1961), 130.

14. P. Roy Vagelos and Louis Galambos, *Medicine, Science, and Merck* (New York: Cambridge University Press, 2004), 71.

15. Philip R. Lee, *Task Force on Prescription Drugs, The Drug Makers and the Drug Distributors* (USDHEW: Office of the Secretary, December 1968), 9. The 2019 figure is from the website of the Pharmaceutical Research and Manufacturers of America.

16. David Taylor, "The Pharmaceutical Industry and the Future of Drug Development," *Pharmaceuticals in the Environment* (2015), 1–33, 27. doi:10.1039/9781782622345-00001

17. Ernst Rothlin, "Opening Address," in P. B. Bradley et al., eds., *Neuro-Psychopharmacology: Proceedings of the First International Congress of Neuro-Pharmacology* (Rome, September 1958) (Amsterdam: Elsevier, 1959), 6.

18. Ralph Landau et al., eds., *Pharmaceutical Innovation: Revolutionizing Human Health* (Philadelphia: Chemical Heritage Press, 1999), 36–37.

19. Barrie G. James, *The Future of the Multinational Pharmaceutical Industry to 1990* (London: Associated Business Programmes, 1977), 75, tab. 4.7.

20. News story, *Scrip*, July 15, 1994, 8.

21. Nicolas Rasmussen, "The Drug Industry and Clinical Research in Interwar America: Three Types of Physician Collaborator," *Bull Hist Med*, 79 (2005), 50–80, 57.

22. Material in these two paragraphs is mainly from John E. Lesch, "Sulfapyridine," in Gregory J. Higby and Elaine C. Stroud, eds., *The Inside Story of Medicines: A Symposium* (Madison WI: American Institute of the History of Pharmacy, 1997), 101–138, 123–124.

23. Gardiner Harris, "With Big Drugs Dying, Merck Didn't Merge—It Found New Ones," *Wall Street Journal*, January 10, 2001, 1.

24. P. Roy Vagelos and Louis Galambos, *Medicine, Science, and Merck* (New York: Cambridge University Press, 2004), 181.

25. P. Roy Vagelos and Louis Galambos, *Medicine, Science, and Merck* (New York: Cambridge University Press, 2004), 161.

26. William Potter, discussion, in Food and Drug Administration, Psychopharmacologic Drugs Advisory Committee (PDAC), February 6, 2008, 299. Obtained through the Freedom of Information Act.

27. Roy Vagelos and Louis Galambos, *Medicine, Science, and Merck* (New York: Cambridge University Press, 2004), 226.

28. Mark Kramer to Edward Shorter, January 30, 2019.

29. Mark S. Kramer, "Commentary" on Barry Blackwell: Corporate Corruption in the Psychopharmaceutical Industry, October 13, 2016, 29. https://inhn.org/fileadmin/ user_upload/User_Uploads/INHN/FILES/Kramers-__LM_Revised_commentary_ -_October_13__2016.pdf

30. News story, *Scrip*, February 21, 2001, 9. The molecule, EMD 68843, was never marketed.

31. Paul J. Fouts, O. M. Helmer et al., "Treatment of Human Pellagra with Nicotinic Acid," *Proceedings of the Society of Experimental Biology and Medicine,* 37 (1937), 405–407.

32. See Robert H. Furman, "A Brief History of the Lilly Laboratory for Clinical Research," in *Clinical Investigation in the 1980s: Needs and Opportunities: Report of a Conference* (Washington DC: Institute of Medicine, Divisions of Health Sciences Policy and Health Promotion and Disease Prevention, National Academy Press, June 1981), Appendix E-1 to E-3.

33. Jay Amsterdam to correspondents, September 18, 2017.

34. News story, *Scrip*, April 24, 1998, 7.

35. LexisNexis Academic, Lilly v. Zenith Goldline, US District Court for the Southern District of Indiana, Indianapolis Division, 2005 US Dist. LEXIS 6448, decided April 14, 2005, p. 21.

36. Quoted in Glen I. Spielmans and Peter I. Parry, "From Evidence-based Medicine to Marketing-based Medicine: Evidence from Internal Industry Documents," *Bioethical Inquiry*, 7 (2010), 13–29, 20.

37. News story, *Financial Times*, November 20, 2019, 11.

38. Paul Janssen, interview, in Healy, ed., *Psychopharmacologists,* II, 56.

39. News story, *Scrip*, February 16, 1990, 16.

40. Leo Hollister, interview, in Ban, ed., *Oral History of Neuropsychopharmacology*, I, 57–58.

41. Leo Hollister, interview, in Ban, ed., *Oral History of Neuropsychopharmacology*, I, 65.

42. On these events, see Steven Brill, "America's Most Admired Lawbreaker," *Huffington Post* (2015, 5–6). http://highline.huffingtonpost.com/miracleindustry/ americas-most-admired-lawbreaker/

43. Hanns Hippius, interview, in Healy, ed., *Psychopharmacologists*, I, 201–202.

44. G. Stille and H. Hippius, " Kritische Stellungnahme zum Begriff der Neuroleptika (anhand von pharmakologischen und klinischen Befunden mit Clozapin)," *Pharmaco- psychiatry*, 4 (1971), 182–191.

45. Ivan Östholm, *Drug Discovery: A Pharmacist's Story* (Stockholm: Swedish Pharmaceutical Press, 1995), 33–34.

46. News story, *Scrip*, May 9, 1995, 11.

47. News story, *Scrip*, February 25, 1997, 9.

48. News story, *Scrip*, February 4, 2005, 12.

49. Sam Gershon to correspondents, June 23, 2016.

50. B. Carroll to correspondents, June 24, 2016, attached to Amsterdam thread of August 24, 2016.

51. B. Carroll to correspondents, September 18, 2017

52. B. Carroll, comment, *IBOM*, May 5, 2015, 3.
53. On Dexamyl, see Edward Shorter, *Before Prozac: The Troubled History of Mood Disorders in Psychiatry* (New York: Oxford University Press, 2009), 33.
54. http://inhn.org/biographies/eulogies/alfred-pletscher-1917-2006.html
55. See Thomas A. Ban and Hanns Hippius, *Thirty Years CINP* (Berlin: Springer, 1988), 5–6. The founding figures of CINP traveled extensively between industry and academe.
56. Gerald F. Meyer, interview, May 24, 1995, 40; "History of the U. S. Food and Drug Administration," transcript in NLM, History of Medicine Division, FDA Oral History Collection.
57. See Alex Gorsky, deposition, September 5, 2012, 8–9. https://highline.huffingtonpost.com/miracleindustry/americas-most-admired-lawbreaker/assets/documents/1/gorsky-deposition-2012.pdf?build=02281049
58. Fran Hawthorne, "Merck's Fall from Grace," *The Scientist*, May 1, 2006. https://www.the-scientist.com/uncategorized/mercks-fall-from-grace-47598
59. William Lazonick et al., "US Pharma's Financialized Business Model," Institute for New Economic Thinking, *Working paper* no. 60 (July 13, 2017), 17. https://www.ineteconomics.org/uploads/papers/WP_60-Lazonick-et-al-US-Pharma-Business-Model.pdf
60. Mark Kramer to correspondents, September 18, 2017.
61. Klaus Bogeso and Vagn Pedersen, interview, in Healy, ed., *Psychopharmacologists*, II, 566.
62. David Healy, *Pharmageddon* (Berkeley: University of California Press, 2012), 54.
63. Wallace F. Janssen, interview, January 30–31, 1984, 78; "History of the U. S. Food and Drug Administration," transcript in NLM, History of Medicine Division, FDA Oral History Collection.
64. "Administered Prices: Drugs." *Report of the Committee on the Judiciary, United States Senate, Made by its Subcommittee on Antitrust and Monopoly ["Kefauver Committee"], Eighty-Seventh Congress, June 27, 1961* (Washington DC: GPO, 1961), 145.
65. Steven Shapin, *A Social History of Truth: Civility and Science in Seventeenth-Century England* (Chicago: University of Chicago Press, 1994), 410.
66. Janssen, FDA Oral History Collection, 109.
67. Joel Elkes, "Psychopharrmacology: Finding One's Way," in Farreras., ed., *Mind, Brain, Body*, 201–220, 209.
68. James H. Kocsis, interview, in Ban ed., *Oral History of Neuropsychopharmacology*, IV, 223.
69. Thomas Ban to Edward Shorter, November 18, 2007.
70. Owen L. Wade, discussion, in Joseph D. Cooper ed., *Decision-Making on the Efficacy and Safety of Drugs* (Washington DC: Interdisciplinary Communication Associates, 1971), 167.
71. Len Cook, interview, Healy, ed., *Psychopharmacologists*, II, 18.
72. Thomas Ban to Edward Shorter, November 18, 2007.
73. Donald S. Robinson, interview, in Ban, ed., *Oral History of Neuropsychopharmacology*, V, 309.

74. Leslie L. Iversen, interview, in Ban, ed., *Oral History of Neuropsychopharmacology*, III, 240–241.

75. Shorter and Healy, interview with Arvid Carlsson, February 27, 2007, 90.

76. Food and Drug Administration, Bureau of Drugs, Minutes, Psychopharmacologic Drugs Advisory Committee (PDAC), January 23, 1978, pp. 5–6; Federal Archives, US-WW, E20, 88-85-32 (Advisory Committee Minutes, 1978). At this point, only summaries of the PDAC meetings were available, not transcripts.

77. Mark Kramer to correspondents, June 21, 2016.

78. Mark S. Kramer, "Commentary" on Barry Blackwell: Corporate Corruption in the Psychopharmaceutical Industry, October 13, 2016, 3. http://inhn.org/fileadmin/user_upload/User_Uploads/INHN/FILES/Kramers-__LM_Revised_commentary_-_October_13__2016.pdf

79. Jay Amsterdam to colleagues, April 17, 2017.

80. Michael Alan Taylor, *Hippocrates Cried: The Decline of American Psychiatry* (New York: Oxford University Press, 2013),67.

81. Taylor, *Hippocrates Cried*, 67–68.

82. Donald F. Klein, "Commentary by a Clinical Scientist in Psychopharmacological Research," *J Acad Child Adol Psychopharmacol*, 17 (2007), 284–287, 284–285. For an early report, see Donald F. Klein and Max Fink, "Psychiatric Reaction Patterns to Imipramine," *AJP*, 119 (1962), 432–438.

83. Marcia Angell, editorial, "Is Academic Medicine for Sale?" *New England Journal of Medicine,* 342 (May 18, 2000), 1517. See also Angell's exchange with various psychiatrists in *The New York Review of Books*, June 23, July 14, and August 18, 2011. https://www.nybooks.com/articles/2011/08/18/illusions-psychiatry-exchange/

84. Nardo, *1BOM*, December 2, 2014, 1.

85. Leo Hollister, interview, in Ban, ed., *Oral History of Neuropsychopharmacology*, IX, 146.

86. Nardo, *1BOM*, November 13, 2011, 2.

87. Comptroller General of the United States, Report to the Congress: Problem Areas Affecting Usefulness of Results of Government-Sponsored Research in Medicinal Chemistry, ms. (August 12, 1968), 14–15. In Pharmacy Library, University of Wisconsin.

88. Jonathan Cole interview with Edward Shorter, July 17, 2002, 22–23.

89. The proceedings cited in this section are at: http://1boringoldman.com/index.php/2012/01/26/the-trial/

90. Texas v. Janssen, January 18, 2012, 214, 220; Texas v. Janssen, January 9, 2012, 215. The TMAP proceedings cited in this section are at: http://1boringoldman.com/index.php/2012/01/26/the-trial/

91. Texas v. Janssen, January 18, 2012, 221–223.

92. Texas v. Janssen, January 18, 2012, 225–228.

93. Texas v. Janssen, January 18, 2012, 229–230.

94. The discussion of the three unreported trials is at Texas v. Janssen, January 18, 2012, 234–253. Weight increase–decrease discussion is at 247–248.

Chapter 7

1. Audrey Newell, February 11, 2008, to psycho-pharm@psycom.net
2. Paula Clayton, interview, in Ban, ed., *Oral History of Neuropsychopharmacology*, VII, 99.
3. Fritz A. Henn, interview, in Ban, ed., *Oral History of Neuropsychopharmacology*, VIII, 154.
4. See David Healy, "Mandel Cohen and the Origins of the *Diagnostic and Statistical Manual of Mental Disorders, Third Edition: DSM-III*," *History of Psychiatry*,13 (2002), 209–230, 210–211.
5. John P. Feighner, Eli Robins, Samuel B. Guze, Robert A. Woodruff, Jr., George Winokur, and Rodrigo Muñoz, "Diagnostic Criteria for Use in Psychiatric Research," *Archives of General Psychiatry*, 26 (1972), 57–63.
6. Hannah S. Decker, *The Making of DSM-III* (New York: Oxford University Press, 2013), 56. Decker's account is highly sympathetic to the APA and the DSM Task Force. For another account, see Edward Shorter, "The History of DSM," in Joel Paris and James Phillips, eds., *Making the DSM-5: Concepts and Controversies* (New York: Springer, 2013), 3–20.
7. Samuel B. Guze, "Biological Psychiatry: Is There Any Other Kind?" Psychol Med, 19 (1989), 315–323. https://www.cambridge.org/core/journals/psychological-medi-cine/article/biological-psychiatry-is-there-any-other-kind/319025FCF7A19410E18 C4DB67201562F
8. Donald W. Goodwin and Samuel B. Guze, *Psychiatric Diagnosis*, 4th ed. (New York: Oxford University Press, 1989), iii.
9. Eli Robins and Samuel B. Guze, "Establishment of Diagnostic Validity in Psychiatric Illness: Its Application to Schizophrenia," *AJP*, 126 (1970), 983–987.
10. "The disease of medical 'model.'" In the preface to the first edition, reprinted in the sixth edition, Carol S. North et al., eds., *Goodwin and Guze's Psychiatric Diagnosis*, 6th ed. (New York: Oxford, 2010), xvii. The authors of the first edition were Robert A. Woodruff, Jr., Eli Robins, and Samuel B. Guze.
11. Samuel Guze, comment, in Roger K. Blashfield, "Feighner et al., Invisible Colleges, and the Matthew Effect," *Schizophrenia Bulletin*, 8 (1982), 1–12, 6–7.
12. Blashfield, "Feighner et al.," 3–4. *Schizophrenia Bulletin* (1982).
13. See Edward Shorter, *What Psychiatry Left Out of the DSM-5: Historical Mental Disorders Today* (New York: Routledge, 2015), 68–98.
14. Karl Leonhard, *Aufteilung der endogenen Psychosen* [The Classification of the Endogenous Psychoses] (Berlin: Akademie-Verlag, 1957).
15. "Altostrada," in *IBOM*, February 15, 2014, 6.
16. Nassir Ghaemi, May 15, 2017, to colleagues.
17. R. E. Kendell, comment, in Blashfield, "Feighner et al.," 11–12.
18. Robert Spitzer, in "Affective Meeting," April 20, 1984; APA Archives, Williams Papers, Research—DSM-III-R, box 4, folder "Affective (Mood) Meeting."
19. Transcript of Proceedings, DHEW, Psychopharmacological Agents Advisory Committee, March 21–22, 1977, 234–235, 248–249; National Archives, UD-WW, E18, 88-85-27, box 16.

20. Michael Alan Taylor, *Hippocrates Cried: The Decline of American Psychiatry* (New York: Oxford University Press, 2013), 205.
21. Nardo, *1BOM*, May 17, 2012, 1.
22. Joseph J. Schildkraut, "The Catecholamine Hypothesis of Affective Disorders: A Review of Supporting Evidence," *AJP*, 122 (1965), 509–522.
23. Joseph J. Schildkraut, interview, in Ban, ed., *Oral History of Neuropsychopharmacology*, V, 326–328.
24. B. Carroll review of *Comprehensive Textbook of Psychiatry*, *AJP*, 138 (1981), 705.
25. Interview of Robert Spitzer by Max Fink and Edward Shorter, March 14, 2007. Thomas A. Williams, Martin M. Katz, and James Asa Shield, Jr., eds., *Recent Advances in the Psychobiology of the Depressive Illnesses: Proceedings of a Workshop Sponsored by the Clinical Research Branch, Division of Extramural Research Programs, National Institute of Mental Health, Hosted by the College of William and Mary in Virginia, April 30 through May 2, 1969* (Washington DC: GPO, 1972); DHEW Pub No. (HSM) 70-9053. On Klerman's role in the genesis of DSM, see also Myrna Weisman, interview, in Healy, ed., *Psychopharmacologists*, II, 521–542. Weisman was married to Klerman.
26. Martin Katz, interview, in Ban, ed., *Oral History of Neuropsychopharmacology*, IX, 199–200.
27. Donald F. Klein, interview, in Ban, ed., *Oral History of Neuropsychopharmacology*, IX, 214–215.
28. Julius Hoenig, "Nosology and Statistical Classification," *Canadian Journal of Psychiatry*, 26 (1981), 240–243, 240–241.
29. Robert L. Spitzer, Jean Endicott, and Eli Robins, "Research Diagnostic Criteria: Rationale and Reliability," *AGP*, 35 (1978), 773–782. For a helpful overview of national systems for classifying psychiatric illness, see Erwin Stengel, "Classification of Mental Disorders," *WHO Bulletin*, 21 (1959), 601–883.
30. See Walter Barton to Sidney Malitz, March 20, 1973; American Psychiatric Association, Archives, box 17, folder 188.
31. Boyd L. Burris to Jules Masserman, April 18, 1979; in Paula Clayton Papers, Neuroscience History Archive, UCLA, box 31.
32. Nardo, *1BOM*, May 17, 2011, 3.
33. Jean Endicott attributes the phrase to Zubin. See her interview in Ban, ed., *Oral History of Neuropsychopharmacology*, VII, 203.
34. Donald F. Klein and John M. Davis: *Diagnosis and Drug Treatment of Psychiatric Disorders* (Baltimore: Williams & Wilkins, 1969), 2, 9.
35. Shorter-Fink interview with Spitzer, March 14, 2007, 1.
36. See American Psychiatric Association, Archives, box 17, folder 188. "Task Force on Nomenclature and Statistics, Meeting of September 4, 5, 1974." Spitzer clearly dominated the proceedings. Helen Decker also studied these events, but, as a partisan of psychoanalysis, she downplayed the ideological conflict between Spitzer's Task Force and the Board. H. Decker, *The Making of DSM-III* (New York: Oxford University Press, 2013), 141–142.
37. Samuel Guze, interview, in Healy, ed., *Psychopharmacologists*, III, 408–409.
38. Nardo, *1BOM,* August 30, 2011, 1–2
39. Exchange in *1BOM*, January 9, 2016, 3–4.

40. See, for example, Spitzer to the Task Force, October 11, 1977. Source: Paula Clayton Papers, Neuroscience History Archive, UCLA, box 31.

41. The four documents quoted in these paragraphs be found in the Paula Clayton Papers, Neuroscience History Archive, UCLA, box 31.

42. Nardo, *1BOM*, November 2, 2011, 3.

43. Thomas A. Ban, interview, in Ban., ed., *Oral History of Neuropsychopharmacology*, IV, 19.

44. Robert Temple, discussion, Psychopharmacologic Drugs Advisory Committee (PDAC) meeting of March 12, 1981, 234. Obtained through the Freedom of Information Act.

45. Hostility to psychoanalysis was definitely on Spitzer's mind, as he stated in interviews. Yet Don Klein said there was "no specific anti-psychoanalytic animus" on the DSM-III Task Force. Klein, *1BOM*, November 2, 2011, 6–7. Two analysts did join it, but only later in the process. Nardo noted that "The St. Louis group had Dr. Spitzer's ear, and they were taking no prisoners [on psychoanalysis]." *1BOM*, May 12, 2011, 3.

46. Michael Shepherd, "Evaluation of Drugs in the Treatment of Depression," in "McGill University Conference on Depression and Allied States," *Canadian Psychiatric Association Journal*, 4 (Suppl.) (1959), S120–S128, S124.

47. American Psychiatric Association, *Diagnostic and Statistical Manual of Mental Disorders*, 2nd ed. (DSM-II) (Washington DC: APA, 1968), 35.

48. Robert L. Spitzer, Jean Endicott, Eli Robins, Judith Kuriansky, and Barry Gurland, "Preliminary Report of the Reliability of Research Diagnostic Criteria Applied to Psychiatric Case Records," in Abraham Sudilovsky et al., eds., *Predictability in Psychopharmacology* (New York: Raven Press, 1975), 1–47.

49. Robert L. Spitzer, Jean Endicott, Eli Robins, "Research Diagnostic Criteria," *AGP*, 35 (1978), 773–782.

50. Hagop S. Akiskal and William T. McKinney, Jr., "Depressive Disorders: Toward a Unified Hypothesis," *Science*, 182 (October 5, 1973), 20–29, 21. It was, moreover, a point the authors made just in passing.

51. Nardo, *1BOM*, January 14, 2015, 3.

52. Edward Shorter, "The History of DSM," in Joel Paris and James Phillips, eds., *Making the DSM-5: Concepts and Controversies* (New York: Springer, 2013), 3–20.

53. Paula Clayton, "Cassette 5—Making a Diagnosis: Definition of Affective Disorders," Paula Clayton Papers, Neuroscience History Archive, UCLA, box 30, folder 16 ("DSM III—Affective Disorders and Schizophrenia)," 11–12.

54. Nardo, *1BOM*, March 26, 2015, 2.

55. Nardo, *1BOM*, May 16, 2011, 2.

56. Bernard Carroll to Spitzer, February 19, 1979; APA Archives, Williams Papers, DSM-III-R, box 1, DSM-III Files "Major Depressive DO."

57. Donald Klein, "Endogenomorphic Depression: A Conceptual and Terminological Revision," *AGP*, 31 (1974), 447–452.

58. B. Carroll, comment, *1BOM*, December 5, 2011, 3.

59. B. Carroll, comment, *1BOM*, May 17, 2011, 3.

60. See Spitzer to "Affective Disorder Mavens," July 10, 1978; APA, Williams Papers, Research—DSM-III-R, DSM-III Files, "misc affective."

61. Spitzer to "Dear Colleague," April 30, 1979; APA, Williams Papers, DSM-III-R, loose DSM-III files, "neurosis" folder.
62. Donald F. Klein to "Members of DSM-III Task Force," March 30, 1979; APA, Williams Papers, Research—DSM-III-R, box 2, "Glossary folder selections." Klein was responding to an earlier note from Spitzer about the "Neurotic Peace Treaty" with the psychoanalysts.
63. Henry Pinsker to Robert Spitzer, March 8, 1982; APA Archives, Research—DSM-IIIR, box 1; DSM-III Proposed Revisions.
64. Max Fink, discussion, in Robert L. Spitzer and Donald F. Klein, eds., *Critical Issues in Psychiatric Diagnosis* (New York: Raven, 1978), 332–333.
65. Max Fink, discussion, in Robert L. Spitzer and Donald F. Klein, eds., *Critical Issues in Psychiatric Diagnosis* (New York: Raven, 1978), 334.
66. Bernard Carroll, "Beyond Symptom Counts to Case-wise Probabilities," *Bipolar Disorders* (2017). doi:10.1111/bdi.12525
67. Bernard Carroll, comment, *1BOM*, May 12, 2012, 5.
68. George Arana, interview with Max Fink, January 4, 2006, 12. In Fink Papers, Stony Brook University Archives.
69. Werner H. Mombout (?) to Spitzer, June 9, 1983; APA, Medical Director's Office, Range 37, box C-1, "DSM-III Conference."
70. See Robert Spitzer to Donald Klein, September 17, 1984, and associated letters. APA Archives, Research—DSM-III-R, box 2, "loose DSM-III-R papers."
71. Donald Klein to Robert Spitzer, August 31, 1984; APA Archives, Research—DSM-III-R, box 2, "loose DSM-III-R papers."
72. See Robert Spitzer to "Dear Colleagues," March 13, 1986; APA Archives, Williams Papers, Research—DSM-III-R, box 4, folder "Mood."
73. "Tom," *1BOM*, April 29, 2011, 4. The discussant was a psychiatrist.
74. Laura Batstra and Allen Frances, "Holding the Line Against Diagnostic Inflation in Psychiatry," Psychotherapy and Psychosomatics, 81 (2012), 5–10, 6.
75. Mark Kramer to correspondents, May 15, 2017
76. Nassir Ghaemi, "Letter to a Foreign Psychiatrist," *Psychiatric Times*, April 11, 2013, 1.
77. On this, see Edward Shorter, *What Psychiatry Left Out of the DSM-5: Historical Mental Disorders Today* (New York: Routledge, 2015).
78. Thomas A. Ban, "RDoC in Historical Perspective," February 19, 2015. http://inhn. org/perspectives/thomas-a-ban-the-rdoc-in-historical-perspective.html
79. Martin Roth, "Phobic Anxiety-depersonalization Syndrome," *Proceedings of the Royal Society of Medicine*, 52 (1959), 587–595.
80. Peter Tyrer et al., "A Study of the Clinical Effects of Phenelzine and Placebo in the Treatment of Phobic Anxiety," *Psychopharmacologia*, 32 (1973), 237–257. At 8 weeks, the difference between phenelzine and placebo was evident.
81. Thomas Ban, interview, in Ban, ed., *Oral History of Neuropsychopharmacology*, IV, 25.
82. Kurt Schneider, "Die Schichtung des emotionalen Lebens und der Aufbau der Depressionszustände" ["The Layering of Emotionl Life and the Structure of Depressive Conditions"], *Zeitschrift für die gesamte Neurologie und Psychiatrie* [Journal of Global Neurology and Psychiatry], 59 (1920), 281–286.

83. Karl Leonhard, *Aufteilung der endogenen Psychosen* [The Classification of the Endogenous Psychoses, affect-laden paraphrenia] (Berlin: Akademie-Verlag, 1957), 185–218; "die affektvolle Paraphrenie."

84. Robert Spitzer, "Explanation of Mood Disorders Classification and Criteria," March 15, 1986; APA Archives, Williams Papers, Research—DSM-III-R, binder "DSM-III revisions."

85. Gordon Parker, et al., "Issues for DSM-5: Whither Melancholia? The Case for Its Classification as a Mood Disorder," *AJP*, 167 (2010), 745–747. doi:10.1176/appi. ajp.2010.09101525

86. Ivan [Goldberg], comment, *1BOM*, June 12, 2012, 2.

87. Nardo, *1BOM*, February 15, 2012, 1.

88. William Coryell to Max Fink, April 12, 2010; Fink Papers, Stony Brook University Archive.

89. James O'Brien, comment, *1BOM*, January 28, 2015, 6.

90. Center for Behavioral Health Statistics and Quality. (2015). *Behavioral Health Trends in the United States: Results from the 2014 National Survey on Drug Use and Health* (HHS Publication No. SMA 15-4927, NSDUH Series H-50). Retrieved from http://www.samhsa.gov/ data/

91. https:// www.samhsa.gov/ data/ sites/ default/ files/ cbhsq- reports/ NSDUH DetailedTabs2017/NSDUHDetailedTabs2017.htm#tab8-1A

92. Center for Behavioral Health Statistics and Quality. (2018). *National-level Comparisons of Mental Health Estimates from the National Survey on Drug Use and Health (NSDUH) and Other Data Sources: NSDUH Methodological Report*. Rockville MD: Substance Abuse and Mental Health Services Administration. https://www. samhsa.gov/data/default/files/cbhsq-reports/NSDUHC2MentalHealthEst2018.pdf

93. H. U. Wittchen, "The Timing of Depression: An Epidemiological Perspective," *Medicographia*, 32 (2010), 115–125. https://www.medicographia.com/2010/10/ the-timing-of-depression-an-epidemiological-perspective/

94. Ronald C. Kessler et al., "Lifetime and 12-Month Prevalence of *DSM-III-R* Psychiatric Disorders in the United States," *AGP*, 31 (1994), 8–19, 12, tab. 2.

95. Bernard Carroll, *1BOM*, December 7, 2014, 5.

96. See Sarah O'Connor, "The Town the British Economy Forgot [Blackpool]." *Financial Times*, November 18–19, 2017, 18.

97. Richard I. Shader, interview, in Ban, ed., *Oral History of Neuropsychopharmacology*, VIII, 326.

98. Healy, ed., *Psychopharmacologists*, III, xix.

99. Max Fink to Ronald Pies, September 11, 2011; Fink Papers, Stony Brook University Archive.

100. Conrad Swartz to Edward Shorter, February 27, 2010.

101. Herman van Praag, "Nosologomania: A Disorder of Psychiatry," *World Journal of Biological Psychiatry*, 1 (2000), 151–158, 154.

102. Nancy C. Andreasen, "DSM and the Death of Phenomenology in America: An Example of Unintended Consequences," *Schizophrenia Bulletin*, 33 (2007), 108–112, 111.

103. Herman van Praag, interview, in Healy, ed., *Psychopharmacologists*, I, 369.

104. Gary Greenberg, "Inside the Battle to Define Mental Illness," p. 2. https://www.wired.com/2010/12/ff_dsmv/

105. Charles Medawar, "The Antidepressant Web: Marketing Depression and Making Medicines Work," *International Journal of Risk & Safety in Medicine*, 10 (1997), 75–126, 84.

106. David Healy, *Let Them Eat Prozac* (Toronto: Lorimer, 2003), 410, n. 82.

107. Michael Alan Taylor, *Hippocrates Cried: The Decline of American Psychiatry* (New York: Oxford University Press, 2013), 175.

Chapter 8

1. Edward Sutleffe, *Medical and Surgical Cases, Selected During a Practice of Thirty-Eight Years* (London: Underwood, 1824), 332–333.

2. Carl Eisdorfer, presentation, Psychopharmacologic Drugs Advisory Committee (PDAC), March 12, 1981, 50. Obtained through the Freedom of Information Act.

3. Pertofrane ad, *AJP*, 133 (1976).

4. These examples are from Jeffrey R. Lacasse et al., "Serotonin and Depression: A Disconnect between the Advertisements and the Scientific Literature," *PLOS Medicine*, 2 (12) (December 2005) 1211–1216, tab. 2, 1213. doi:10.1371/journal.pmed.0020392

5. Janet K. Acker et al., "Let's Talk About Depression: Social Workers' Use of Chemical Imbalance Explanations," *Social Work in Mental Health*, January 28, 2020. https://doi.org/10.1080/15332985.2019.1700872

6. Carlo Perris and Joseph Mendels, discussion, in Donald M. Gallant and George M. Simpson, eds., *Depression: Behavioral, Biochemical, Diagnostic and Treatment Concepts* (New York: Spectrum, 1976), 62–66. The conference was in November 1974.

7. D. L. Murphy et al., "Current Status of the Indoleamine Hypothesis of the Affective Disorders," in M. A. Lipton et al., eds., *Psychopharmacology: A Generation of Progress* (New York: Raven Press, 1978), 1235–1247.

8. Alec Coppen et al., "Inhibition of 5-Hydroxytryptamine [serotonin] Reuptake by Amitriptyline and Zimelidine and Its Relationship to Their Therapeutic Action," *Psychopharmacology*, 63 (1979), 125–129, 128.

9. Bernard J. Carroll, "Brain Mechanisms in Manic Depression," *Clinical Chemistry*, 40 (1984), 303–308, 308.

10. John Lengel to Ed West, April 15, 1991. http://www.healyprozac.com/trials/critical/docs

11. Joseph J. Schildkraut, "The Catecholamine Hypothesis of Affective Disorders: A Review of Supporting Evidence," *AJP*, 122 (1965), 509–522.

12. Ira P. Lapin and Gregory F. Oxenkrug, "Intensification of the Central Serotonergic Processes as a Possible Determinant of the Thymoleptic Effect," *Lancet*, 1 (January 18, 1969), 132–136.

13. Bernard Carroll, comment, *1BOM*, May 5, 2015, 3.

14. Jeffrey R. Lacasse and Jonathan Leo, "Serotonin and Depression: A Disconnect between the Advertisements and the Scientific Literature," *PLOS Medicine*, 2 (12) (December 2005), 1211–1216, 1213; e392. www.plosmedicine.org

15. Sandra Steingard, comment, *1BOM*, May 3, 2015, 5.

16. Robert Whitaker, quoted in *1BOM*, May 5, 2015, 1.

17. Alfred Pletscher, "The Dawn of the Neurotransmitter Era in Neuropsychopharmacology," in Thomas A. Ban et al., eds., *The Neurotransmitter Era in Neuropsychopharmacology* (Buenos Aires: Polemos/CINP, 2006), 27–37, 35.

18. On this, see Gerald Curzon, interview in Healy, ed., *Psychopharmacologists*, II, 309.

19. Barry Blackwell, *Bits and Pieces of a Psychiatrist's Life* (Philadelphia: Xlibris, 2012), 210.

20. Allen J. Frances, "Will $650 Million Solve the Mystery of Mental Illness?" *Psychology Today*, July 25, 2014.

21. John R. Smythies, discussion, in E. Beresford Davies, ed., *Depression: Proceedings of the Symposium Held at Cambridge 22 to 26 September 1959* (Cambridge UK: Cambridge University Press, 1964), 137.

22. Adam Rogers, "Star Neuroscientist Tom Insel Leaves the Google-Spawned Verily for . . . A Startup?" *Wired*, May 2017. https://www.wired.com/2017/05/star-neuroscientist-tom-insel-leaves-google-spawned-verily-startup/

23. David Korn, *Drug Development Science* (Washington DC: AAMC/FDA, 2005), 27. Korn was an official at AAMC. https://services.aamc.org/Publications/showfile.cfm?file=version

24. Michael Dazenski to Bernard Carroll, March 19, 1993; Carroll Papers, Nashville Collection, currently in Neuroscience History Archive, UCLA.

25. Venlafaxine ad, *British Journal of Psychiatry*, Jan–June 1995, 148b-c, 166.

26. FDA, PDAC, June 4, 1979, 2. National Archives, UDWW E21, 88-5-33–88-OS-0033, AC Minutes 1979.

27. Paul Hoch, discussion, in Sidney Malitz, ed., *In the Beginning—The Origin of the American College of Neuropsychopharmacology* (ACNP, 1990), B-9.

28. A. Dale Console, testimony, in *"Administered Prices—Drugs," Report of the Committee on the Judiciary, United States Senate, Made by its Subcommittee on Antitrust and Monopoly ["Kefauver Committee"], Eighty-Seventh Congress, First Session, June 27, 1961* (Washington DC: GPO, 1961), 173.

29. For excerpts of A. Dale Console's testimony, see *F-D-C Reports ("The Pink Sheet")*, June 126, 1969, 9–15, 13. June 16, 1969, 11–15, 13. The Pharmaceutical Manufacturers Association (PMA) found Console's testimony quite damaging and attempted to gaslight him, claiming that he had resigned "after a long illness" (12).

30. Jeffrey Goldstein to Andrew Goudie, undated, early November, 1997; AZ/SER 4239852; Goldstein exhibit no. 7, June 4, 2008. psychrights,org-research/Digest/NLPs/Seroquel

31. David Healy, discussion, in E. M. Tansey et al., eds., *Wellcome Witnesses to Twentieth Century Medicine* (London: Wellcome Trust, 1998), II, 195.

32. David Healy, *Pharmageddon* (Berkeley: University of California Press, 2012), 34.

33. Mark Kramer to correspondents, August 23, 2016.

34. Nardo, *1BOM*, October 11, 2016, 2.

35. Bernard Carroll elaborated this point in his comment on Phil Hickey, "DSM-5—Dimensional Diagnoses—More Conflicts of Interest," December 23, 2013, in Hickey blog, *Behaviorism and Mental Health*. Carroll comment at p. 16. http://behaviorismandmentalhealth.com/2013/12/23/dsm-5-dimensional-diagnoses-more-conflicts-of-interest/

36. Nardo, *1BOM*, August 1, 2015, 1.

37. Glen I. Spielmans and Peter I. Parry, "From Evidence-based Medicine to Marketing-based Medicine: Evidence from Internal Industry Documents," *Bioethical Inquiry*, 7 (2010), 13–29, 13. doi:10.1007/s11673-010-9208-8

38. Des Spence, "Evidence Based Medicine is Broken," *BMJ*, (2014). doi: 10.1136/bmj.g22

39. Nardo, *1BOM*, January 3, 2015, 4.

40. Mark Kramer, reply to Barry Blackwell, October 13, 2016, 9. http://inhn.org/fileadmin/user_upload/User_Uploads/INHN/FILES/Kramers-__LM_Revised_commentary_-_October_13__2016.pdf

41. Arvid Carlsson, interview by David Healy and Edward Shorter, February 27, 2007, 94.

42. Robin M. Murray, "On Collecting Meta-Analyses of Schizophrenia and Postage Stamps," *Psychol Med*, 44 (2014), 3407–3408. doi:10.1017/S0033291714000178

43. Oleh Hornykiewicz, discussion, in Gregory M. Brown et al., eds., *Neuroendocrinology and Psychiatric Disorder* (New York: Raven Press, 1984), 86–87. The conference was in 1983.

44. Oldrich Vinar summarized this work in Vinar, "The Neurotransmitter Era in Neuropsychopharmacology," in Thomas Ban et al., eds., *The Neurotransmitter Era in Neuropsychopharmacology* (Buenos Aires: Podemos/CINP, 2006), 201–210, 207.

45. Ross Baldessarini interview, in Ban, ed., *Oral History of Neuropsychopharmacology*, V, 24–25.

46. See Ian Creese, David R. Burt, and Solomon H. Snyder, "Dopamine Receptor Binding Predicts Clinical and Pharmacological Potencies of Antischizophrenic Drugs," *Science*, 192 (April 30, 1976), 481–483. For an authoritative introduction to this contentious area, see the entry "Dopamine receptor," in Frank Ayd, Jr., *Lexicon of Psychiatry, Neurology, and the Neurosciences,* 2nd ed. (Philadelphia: Lippincott Williams & Wilkins, 2000), 341–344.

47. Philip Seeman et al., "Letter: Dopamine D4 Receptors Elevated in Schizophrenia," *Nature*, 365 (September 30, 1993), 441–445.

48. Mark Kramer et al., "The Effects of a Selective D4 Dopamine Receptor Antagonist (L-745,870) in Acutely Psychotic Inpatients with Schizophrenia," *AGP*, 54 (1997), 567–572.

49. Leslie Iversen, interview, in Healy, ed., *Psychopharmacologists,* II, 344–345.

50. Melvin L. Kohn, "Reflections on the Intramural Research Program of the NIMH in the 1950s," in Ingrid G. Farreras et al., eds., *Mind, Brain, Body and Behavior: Foundations of Neuroscience and Behavioral Research at the National Institutes of Health* (Amsterdam: IOS Press, 2004), 257–266, 260.

51. Robert Cancro, "The Uncompleted Task of Psychiatry," in Thomas A. Ban et al., eds., *From Psychopharmacology to Neuropsychopharmacology in the 1980s and the Story of CINP, As Told in Autobiography* (Budapest: Animula, 2002), 237–241, 240–241.

52. Max Fink, "Remembering the Forgotten Neuroscience of Pharmaco-EEG," 10. http://inhn.org/archives/fink-collection/remembering-the-forgotten-neuroscience-of-pharmaco-eeg.html

53. Hans Berger, "Ueber das Elektroenkephalogramm des Menschen: Dritte Mitteilung" ["Electroencephalogram in Humans: Third Report"], *Archiv für Psychiatrie und Nervenkrankheiten*, 94 (1931), 16–60.

54. Martin A. Roth. "Changes in the EEG Under Barbiturate Anesthesia Produced by Electro-convulsive Treatment and Their Significance for the Theory of ECT Action." *Electroencephalography and Clinical Neurophysiology*, 3 (1951), 261–280.

55. These values are from Charles Shagass and Arthur L. Jones, "A Neurophysiological Test for Psychiatric Diagnosis: Results in 750 Patients," *AJP*, 114 (1958), 1002–1010, tab. 1, 1003.

56. Dieter Bente, Turan Itil, and E. E. Schmid, "Elektroencephalographische Studien zur Wirkungsweise des LSD 25" ["Electroencephalographic Studies on the Mechanism of LSD"], *European Neurology*, 135 (1958), 273–284.

57. Dieter Bente, "Elektroencephalographische Gesichtspunkte zur Klassifikation neuro- und thymoleptischer. Pharmaka" ["Electrocencephalographic Contributions to the Classification of Neuro- and Thymoleptic Psychopharmaceuticals"], *Pharmacology*, 5 (1961), 337–346.". For the introduction of the test, see Charles Shagass, "The Sedation Threshold: A Method for Estimating Tension in Psychiatric Patients," *Electroencephalography and Clinical Neurophysiology*, 6 (1954), 221–233.

58. Max Fink and Turan M. Itil, "Neurophysiology of Phantastica: EEG and Behavioral Relations in Man," in Daniel H. Efron, ed., *Psychopharmacology: A Review of Progress, 1957–1967* (Washington DC: NIMH/PHS, 1968), 1231–1239.

59. Max Fink, in Tom Ban et al., eds., *Reflections on Twentieth-Century Psychopharmacology* (Budapest: Animula, 2004), 663.

60. Max Fink, "A Selected Bibliography of Electroencephalography in Human Psychopharmacology, 1951–1962," *Electroencephalography and Clinical Neurophysiology*, 23 (1964), 1–68.

61. Max Fink et al., "EEG Profiles of Fenfluramine, Amobarbital and Dextroamphetamine in Normal Volunteers," *Psychopharmacologia*, 22 (1971), 369–383.

62. J Simeon et al., "Clinical and EEG Studies of Doxepin," *Psychosomatics*, 10 (1969), 14–17. See Max Fink, "Remembering the Forgotten Neuroscience of Pharmaco-EEG," 6. http://inhn.org/archives/fink-collection/remembering-the-forgotten-neuroscience-of-pharmaco-eeg.html

63. T. N. Itil et al., "Clinical and EEG Effects of GB-94, a Tetracyclic Antidepressant: EEG Model in the Discovery of a New Psychotropic Drug," *Current Ther Res Clin Exp*, 14 (1972), 395–413.

64. Max Fink, "Remembering the Forgotten Neuroscience of Pharmaco-EEG," 6. http://inhn.org/archives/fink-collection/remembering-the-forgotten-neuroscience-of-pharmaco-eeg.html

65. Turan Itil, interview, in Ban, ed., *Oral History of Neuropsychopharmacology*, IX, 175.
66. News story, *Drug and Therapeutics Bulletin*, 15 (1) (January 7, 1977), 1.
67. See Fink, in Ban et al., eds., *Reflections on Twentieth-Century Psychopharmacology*, 663–664.
68. See Fink, in Ban et al., eds., *Reflections on Twentieth-Century Psychopharmacology*, 668.
69. Adrienne Grzenda et al., "Editorial: Electroencephalographic Biomarkers for Predicting Antidepressant Response: New Methods, Old Questions," *JAMA Psychiatry*, online January 2, 2020. https://jamanetwork.com/journals/jamapsychiatry/fullarticle/2757886?guestAccessKey=c686a8ee-17e6-4c8a-a594-8314eda1e8e7&utm_source=silverchair&utm_medium=email&utm_campaign=article_alert-jamapsychiatry&utm_content=olf&utm_term=010220
70. Max Fink, "A Useful Example of Pharmaco-Electroencephalogram Science," *Journal of Clinical Psychopharmacology*, 38 (2018), 552–554, 553.
71. Bernard Carroll to Edward Shorter, personal communication, April 15, 2018.

Chapter 9

1. Karl Rickels, *A Serendipitous Life* (Evergreen CO: Notting Hill Press, 2011), 170.
2. See Roland Kuhn to Robert Domenjoz (Geigy), June 26, 1957, in Thomas A. Ban et al., eds., *From Psychopharmacology to Neuropsychopharmacology in the 1980s and the Story of CINP, As Told in Autobiography* (Budapest: Animula, 2002), 321–323.
3. A. Dale Console testimony, in *"Administered Prices," Hearings Before the Subcommittee on Antitrust and Monopoly of the Committee on the Judiciary, United States Senate, Eighty-Sixth Congress, Second Session, February 25 . . . 1960, part 18* (Washington DC: GPO, 1960), 10372.
4. Sergio Sismondo, "Key Opinion Leaders and the Corruption of Medical Knowledge: What the Sunshine Act Will and Won't Cast Light On," *Journal of Law, Medicine and Ethics*, 41 (2013), 635–643, 635–636.
5. Nardo, *1BOM*, March 12, 2011, 1.
6. Paul Lazarsfeld et al., *The People's Choice: How the Voter Makes Up His Mind in a Presidential Campaign* (New York: Duell, Sloan and Pearce, 1944).
7. "Talbot" comment, *1BOM*, November 22, 2011, 5. Her identity is known to the author.
8. Nardo, *1BOM*, October 20, 2016.
9. Sismondo, "Key Opinion Leaders" (2013), 639.
10. Johan Hoegstedt to staff, August 18, 2003; exhibit Jackson#3. psychrights.org/research/Digest/NLPs/Seroquel/
11. Thomas Ban, interview, in Healy, ed., *Psychopharmacologists*, I, 608.
12. Parexel, "Meeting Minutes," November 24, 2004; exhibit Goldstein#31. psychrights.org/research/Digest/NLPs/Seroquel/
13. Sismondo, "Key Opinion Leaders" (2013), 637–639.
14. APA Archives, Professional Affairs, box 17, folder 192.

15. "In the United States District Court for the Eastern District of Pennsylvania: United States of America v. Janssen Pharmaceutica Products, L.P.; Civil Action No. 04-cv-5184; November 4, 2013; p. 3. See Case 2:04 – cv – 01529 – TJS. Document 60, filed 11/04/13. http://psychrights.org/States/Wisconsin/WatsonvVassel/158-131125Opp2 KingInLimine.pdf

16. Benedict Carey and Gardiner Harris, "Psychiatric Group Faces Scrutiny Over Drug Industry Ties," *New York Times*, July 12, 2008. https://www.nytimes.com/2008/07/12/washington/12psych.html

17. The phrase is Mickey Nardo's. *1BOM*, September 16, 2014, 1.

18. Roy Poses, "Key Opinion Leader Services Companies: The Creation of Useful Idiots and Usefully Idiotic Organizations," *Health Care Renewal* blog, January 7, 2011.

19. Nicolas Rasmussen, "The Drug Industry and Clinical Research in Interwar America: Three Types of Physician Collaborator," *Bulletin of the History of Medicine*, 79 (2005), 50–80, 74.

20. Melody Petersen, "Madison Ave. Has Growing Role in the Business of Drug Research," *New York Times*, November 22, 2002. https://www.nytimes.com/2002/11/22/business/madison-ave-has-growing-role-in-the-business-of-drug-research.html

21. Douglas Montero, "Columbia U. Is Well Schooled On Cashing In," *New York Post*. https://nypost.com/1999/02/28/columbia-u-is-well-schooled-on-cashing-in/. The sources for the story were anonymous.

22. For reasons of discretion, I am suppressing the name of the principal investigator. I have, however, seen the correspondence in question. This letter is dated January 31, 1986.

23. Nardo, *1BOM*, September 9, 2013, 2.

24. Mark Kramer, "Commentary" on Barry Blackwell: Corporate Corruption in the Psychopharmaceutical Industry, October 13, 2016, 3. http://inhn.org/fileadmin/user_upload/User_Uploads/INHN/FILES/Kramers-__LM_Revised_commentary_-_October_13__2016.pdf

25. Daniel L. Michels, interview, June 26, 2000, 22; "History of the U. S. Food and Drug Administration," transcript in NLM, History of Medicine Division, FDA Oral History Collection.

26. Kenneth R. Feather, interview, May 7, 1997, 24–25; "History of the U. S. Food and Drug Administration," transcript in NLM, History of Medicine Division, FDA Oral History Collection.

27. Benedict Carey, "Correcting the Errors of Disclosure," *New York Times*, July 25, 2006, D5.

28. Bernard Carroll, "How It Really Works," *BMJ*, 337 (2008), 129. doi:10.1136/bmj.a788

29. Nardo, *1BOM*, November 19, 2012, 4.

30. Ray Moynihan, "Key Opinion Leaders: Independent Experts or Drug Representatives in Disguise?" *BMJ*, 336 (June 21, 2008), 1402–1403, 1402.

31. Giovanni A. Fava, "The Hidden Costs of Financial Conflicts of Interest in Medicine," *Psychotherapy and Psychosomatics*, 85 (2016), 65–70. https://doi:org/10.1159/000442694

32. Donald Klein to correspondents, November 3, 2016. See Donald F. Klein and Max Fink, "Psychiatric Reaction Patterns to Imipramine," *AJP*, 119 (1962), 432–438.

33. Roy Poses, post, *1BOM*, February 3, 2011, 4. Poses' own blog was *Health Care Renewal*.

34. Timothy S. Anderson et al., "Research Letter: Academic Medical Center Leadership on Pharmaceutical Company Boards of Directors," *JAMA*, 311 (April 2, 2014), 1353–1355.

35. Edward F. Domino, interview, in Ban, ed., *Oral History of Neuropsychopharmacology*, I, 164.

36. Nardo, *1BOM*, April 6, 2013, 2.

37. News story, *Scrip*, June 18, 2000, 22.

38. John M. Kane et al., "Efficacy and Safety of Aripiprazole and Haloperidol Versus Placebo in Patients with Schizophrenia and Schizoaffective Disorder," *Journal of Clinical Psychiatry*, 63 (2002), 763–771. https://www.ncbi.nlm.nih.gov/pubmed/12363115

39. Robert M. Berman et al., "The Efficacy and Safety of Aripiprazole as Adjunctive Therapy in Major Depressive Disorder: A Multicenter, Randomized, Double-Blind, Placebo-Controlled Study," *J Clin Psych*, 68 (2007), 843–853. https://www.ncbi.nlm.nih.gov/pubmed/17592907 See Bernard Carroll's demolition of this article in "Letter," *Journal of Clinical Psychopharmacol*, 29 (1) (2009), 90–91. doi:10.1097/JCP.0b013e318193c9b1

40. John M. Kane et al., "A Multicenter, Randomized, Double-Blind,Controlled Phase 3 Trial of Fixed-Dose Brexpiprazole for the Treatment of Adults with Acute Schizophrenia," *Schizophren Research*, 164 (May 2015), 127–135. doi:10.1016/j.schres.2015.01.038

41. C. U. Correll et al., "Efficacy and Safety of Brexpiprazole for the Treatment of Acute Schizophrenia: A 6-Week Randomized, Double-Blind, Placebo-Controlled Trial," *AJP*, 172 (2015), 870–880. doi:10.1176/appi.ajp.2015.14101275

42. On all this, see Johanna Ryan, "The Once and Future Abilify: Depot Injections for Everyone?" *Mad in America*, May 11, 2015. https://www.madinamerica.com/2015/05/the-once-and-future-abilify-depot-injections-for-everyone/

43. Name of sender confidential. Post to Edward Shorter of November 17, 2007.

44. Peter J. Whitehouse, "Why I No Longer Consult for Drug Companies," *Cult Med Psychiatry*, 32 (2008), 4–10, 9.

45. Bernard Carroll, post, *1BOM*, December 19, 2011, 5.

46. Anonymous, *1BOM*, February 20, 2013, 4.

47. Michael Göpfert, September 25, 2016, to critical-psychiatry@jiscmail.ac.uk

48. Anna Van Meter et al., "Updated Meta-Analysis of Epidemiologic Studies of Pediatric Bipolar Disorder," *J Clin Psych*, 80 (2019), e1–e11. https://www.ncbi.nlm.nih.gov/pubmed/30946542

49. Ronald Steingard, Joseph Biederman et al., "Comorbidity in the Interpretation of Dexamethasone Suppression Test Results in Children: A Review and Report," *Biological Psychiatry*, 28 (1990), 193–202.

50. David Healy, *Mania: A Short History of Bipolar Disorder* (Baltimore: Johns Hopkins University Press, 2008), 202–208. See the references on p. 282.

51. Janet Wozniak, Joseph Biederman et al., "Mania-Like Symptoms Suggestive of Childhood-Onset Bipolar Disorder in Clinically Referred Children," *Journal of the American Academy of Child and Adolescent Psychiatry*, 34 (1995), 867–876. https://doi.org/10.1097/00004583-199507000-00010

52. See the interview with Biederman collaborator Janet Frazier in Alix Spiegel, "Children Labeled 'Bipolar' May Get a New Diagnosis," NPR Newscast, February 10, 2012. https://www.npr.org/templates/story/story.php?storyId=123544191

53. Joseph Biederman, "Developmental Subtypes of Juvenile Bipolar Disorder," *Harvard Review of Psyciatry*, 3 (1995), 227–230.

54. J. A. Frazier, M. C. Meyer, J. Biederman et al., "Risperidone Treatment for Juvenile Bipolar Disorder: A Retrospective," *Journal of the American Academy of Child and Adolescent Psychiatry*, 38 (1999), 960–965. https://jaacap.org/article/S0890-8567(09)62977-4/pdf

55. Joseph Biederman et al., "Pediatric Mania: A Developmental Subtype of Bipolar Disorder?" *Biological Psychiatry*, 48 (2000), 458–466. https://www.biologicalpsychiatryjournal.com/article/S0006-3223(00)00911-2/abstract

56. David J. Rothman, "Expert Witness Report," October 15, 2010, 30–31. Available at jannel.se/Rothman.Report.pdf

57. Rothman, "Expert Witness Report," October 15, 2010, 32.

58. Alex Gorsky, deposition, May 18, 2012. https://highline.huffingtonpost.com/miracleindustry/americas-most-admired-lawbreaker/assets/documents/1/gorsky-deposition-2012.pdf?build=02281049

59. John Bruins to colleagues, November 17, 1999; in Alma Avila v. Johnson & Johnson, "Plaintiff's Response in Opposition to Non-Party Joseph Biederman, M.D.'s Motion to Quash and/or Motion for Protective Order"; Commonwealth of Massachusetts, Suffolk, SS; Superior Court Dept, Civil No., SU:CV 2008-04392-A. http://psychrights.org/research/Digest/NLPs/Risperdal/081112Opp2BiedermanQuash-Seal.pdf

60. Gahan Pandina to Biederman and MGH team, June 11, 2002, in Commonwealth of Massachusetts Suffolk.

61. Gahan Pandina to executives, March 22, 2002. in Commonwealth of Massachusetts Suffolk.

62. M. G. Aman et al., "Risperidone Disruptive Behavior Study Group," *AJP*, 159 (2002), 1337–1346.

63. Joseph Biederman et al., "Risperidone for the Treatment of Affective Symptoms in Children with Disruptive Behavior Disorder: A Post-hoc Analysis of Data from a 6-Week, Multicenter, Randomized, Double-Blind, Parallel-arm Study," *Clinical Therapeutics*, 28 (2006), 794–800. https://www.ncbi.nlm.nih.gov/pubmed/16861101

64. Gardiner Harris, "Use of Antipsychotics in Children Is Criticized," *New York Times*, November 19, 2008, A20.

65. Mark Moran, "Several Theories Try to Explain Rise in Bipolar Diagnoses," *Psychiatric News*, October 5, 2007, 18.

66. Lucette Lagnado, "Federal Health Officials Are Reviewing Antipsychotic Drug Use of Children in the Medicaid System," *Wall Street Journal*, August 11, 2013.

67. Benedict Carey and Gardiner Harris, "Psychiatric Group Faces Scrutiny Over Drug Industry Ties," *New York Times,* July 12, 2008.

68. Senator Charles Grassley to Drew Gilpin Faust and Peter L. Slavin, March 20, 2009. http://s.wsj.net/public/resource/diocuments/wsj-Major_Protocol_Violation_Letters032009.pdf

69. Xi Yu, "Three Professors Face Sanctions Following Harvard Medical School Inquiry," *Harvard Crimson,* July 2, 2011. https://www.thecrimson.com/article/2011/7/2/school-medical-harvard-investigation/

70. David A. Kessler, "Expert Report," October 2, 2012, 60–61; case ID: 100503629; Control No. 12100558; Exhibit F."

71. M. Olfson et al., "National Trends in the Office-Based Treatment of Children, Adolescents, and Adults with Antipsychotics," *AGP,* 69 (2012), 1247–1256. doi:10.1001/archgenpsychiatry.2012.647

72. Sam Gershon to correspondents, December 1, 2012.

73. Allen Frances, "Psychiatric Diagnosis Gone Wild: The 'Epidemic' of Childhood Bipolar Disorder," *Psychiatric Times,* April 8, 2010, 1–2.

74. Arnold Relman, "Improper Rewards of Research," *Boston Globe,* July 12, 2008. http://www.boston.com/bostonglobe/editorial_opinion/oped/articles/2008/07/12

75. Nardo, *1BOM,* April 4, 2012, 2.

76. Blogpost, "Say It Ain't So Joe," *FeedBlitz,* June 10, 2008.

77. Gardiner Harris and Benedict Carey, "Child Experts Fail to Reveal Full Drug Pay," *New York Times,* June 8, 2008, 1, 28.

78. Nardo, *1BOM,* August 8, 2011, 2.

79. https://www.forbes.com/sites/paulthacker/2011/09/13/how-an-ethically-challenged-researcher-found-a-home-at-the-university-of-miami/#4cf7400d5e12

80. Nardo, *1BOM,* February 14, 2011, 1.

81. Charles B. Nemeroff and Alan F. Schatzberg, *Recognition and Treatment of Psychiatric Disorders: A Psychopharmacology Handbook for Primary Care* (Washington DC: American Psychiatric Press, 1999).

82. https://www.forbes.com/sites/paulthacker/2011/09/13/how-an-ethically-challenged-researcher-found-a-home-at-the-university-of-miami/#4cf7400d5e12

83. Information in this paragraph, unless otherwise noted, is from Duff Wilson, "Drug Maker Hired Writing Company for Doctors' Book, Documents Say," *New York Times,* November 29, 2010. Corrections published December 1 and December 8, 2010.

84. Charles B. Nemeroff, ed., "Introduction: Advancing the Treatment of Mood and Anxiety Disorders: The First 10 Years' Experience with Paroxetine," *Psychopharmacology Bulletin,* Suppl. 1, 37 (2003), 6.

85. See the email exchange between Carroll and Nardo, August 24, 2015.

86. Charles B. Nemeroff, Helen S. Mayberg, Scott E. Krahl, James McNamara, Alan Frazer, Thomas R. Henry, Mark S. George, Dennis S. Charney, and Stephen K. Brannan, "VNS Therapy in Treatment-Resistant Depression: Clinical Evidence and Putative Neurobiological Mechanisms," *Neuropsychopharmacology,* 31 (2006), 1345–1355. doi:10.1038/sj.npp.1301082

87. Gardiner Harris, "Top Psychiatrist Didn't Report Drug Makers' Pay," *New York Times*, October 3, 2008. http://www.nytimes.com/2008/10/04/health/policy//04drug.html?fta=y

88. David Armstrong, "Medical Reviews Face Criticism Over Lapses," *Wall Street Journal*, July 19, 2006, B1; Benedict Carey, "Correcting the Errors of Disclosure," *New York Times,* July 25, 2006, 5.

89. Mark Hyman Rapaport [et al.], Charles B. Nemeroff, "Effects of Risperidone Augmentation in Patients with Treatment-Resistant Depression: Results of Open-Label Treatment Followed by Double-Blind Continuation," *Neuropsychopharmacology*, 31 (2006), 2505–2513. doi:10.1038/sj.npp1301113

90. Bernard Carroll, letter, on "Effects of Risperidone Augmentation in Patients with Treatment-Resistant Depression," *Nature*, November 21, 2007. https:www.nature.com/articles/1301613

91. Benedict Carey and Gardiner Harris, "Psychiatric Group Faces Scrutiny Over Drug Industry Ties," *New York Times,* July 12, 2008; David Armstrong, "Doctor Didn't Disclose Glaxo Payments, Senator Says," *Wall Street Journal*, October 4, 2008.

92. http://carlatpsychiatry.blogspot.com/2008/10/ curtains-for-nemeroff.html. Italics in original.

93. Gardiner Harris, "Top Psychiatrist Didn't Report Drug Makers' Pay," *New York Times*, October 3, 2008. http://www.nytimes.com/2008/10/04/health/policy//04drug.html?fta=y

94. Jack Gorman to Charles Nemeroff, June 12, 2000. All of the correspondence in this section is from https://www.industrydocuments.ucsf.edu/drug/results/#q=collection%3A%22paxil%20litigation%20documents%22%20AND%20case%3APaxil&col=%5B%22paxil%22%5D&h=%7B%22hideDuplicates%22%3Afalse%2C%22hideFolders%22%3Afalse%2C%22hidePrivileged%22%3Afalse%2C%22hideConfidential%22%3Afalse%2C%22hideCopyright%22%3Afalse%7D&subsite=drug&cache=true&count=43

95. See Grace Johnson at STI to Muriel Young at SmithKline, April 4, 1997. https://www/industrydocuments.ucsf.edu/drug/docs

96. See Muriel Young to Grace Johnson, May 19, 1997. https://www/industry-documents.ucsf.edu/drug/docs

97. Baum Hedlund to Donald Wright, June 25, 2012, 4. This letter is available at http://blogs.nature.com/news/files/2012/06/Jay-Amsterdam-today-filed-a-24-page-complaint-with-the-Office-of-Research-Integrity-at-the-US-National-Institutes-of-Health.pdf

98. "U.S. to Probe Emory, Nemeroff," emorywheel.com, March 7, 2009. http://www.emorywheel,com/detail.php?n=26733

99. U.S. to Probe Emory, 11.

100. Meredith Wadman, "Paxil Study Under Fire," *Nature*, 475 (July 14, 2011), 153. http://www.nature.com/news/2011/110712/full/475153a,html

101. Jack Gorman to Charles Nemeroff, June 12, 2000. https://www/industrydocuments.ucsf.edu/drug/docs.

102. See Baum Hedlund to Donald Wright, June 25, 2012, 18. http://blogs.nature.com/news/files/2012/06/Jay-Amsterdam-today-filed-a-24-page-complaint-with-the-Office-of-Research-Integrity-at-the-US-National-Institutes-of-Health.pdf. Gorman appeared as a coauthor in at least one article ghosted by Sally Laden, which is to say that her name appears in the author line! D. S. Charney, C. B. Nemeroff, L. Lewis, S. K. Laden, J. M. Gorman, E. M. Laska, M. Borenstein, C. L. Bowden, A. Caplan, GJ, D. L. Evans, B. Geller, L. RE. Grabowski, J. Herson, N. H. Kalin, P. E. Keck, Jr., I. Kirsch, K. R. Krishnan, D. J. Kupfer, R. W. Makuch, F. G. Miller, H. Pardes, R. Post, M. M. Reynolds, L. Roberts, J. F. Rosenbaum, D. L. Rosenstein, D. R. Rubinow, A. J. Rush, N. D. Ryan, G. S. Sachs, A. F. Schatzberg, S. Solomon, Consensus Development Panel, "National Depressive and Manic-Depressive Association Consensus Statement on the Use of Placebo in Clinical Trials of Mood Disorders," *AGP*, 59 (2002), 262–270. On Gorman's role as a "paid consultant to GlaxoSmithKline," see Brendan I. Koerner, "Disorders Made to Order," *Mother Jones*, July/August 2002. https://www.motherjones.com/politics/2002/07/disorders-made-order/

103. Melody Petersen, "Madison Ave. Has a Growing Role in the Business of Drug Research," *New York Times*, November 22, 2002. https://www.nytimes.com/2002/11/22/business/madison-ave-has-growing-role-in-the-business-of-drug-research.html

104. Brendan Koerner, "Disorders Made to Order: Pharmaceutical Companies Have Come Up with a New Strategy to Market Their Drugs: First Go Out and Find a New Mental Illness, Then Push the Pills to Cure It," *Mother Jones*, July/August, 2002, 58–63, 81.

105. The *Wall Street Journal* reported a session sponsored by SmithKline in March 2000 in Naples, Florida, where Nemeroff was listed as one of two speakers, "to train doctors 'on the efficacy of Paxil and the PsychNet presentation.' Doctors were paid $2,500 per talk." David Armstrong, "U.S. Probes Emory Doctor's Glaxo Ties," *Wall Street Journal*, February 26, 2009.

106. Laden to Nemeroff, March 5, 1999. https://www/industrydocuments.ucsf.edu/drug/docs

107. Baum Hedlund, "Dr Amsterdam's Timeline re Publication of Paxil Bipolar Study 352 Without His Knowledge," July 8, 2011.

108. John Romankiewicz to staff, June 13, 2000. https://www/industrydocuments.ucsf.edu/drug/docs.

109. Charles B. Nemeroff, Dwight L. Evans, Laazlo Gyulai, Gary S. Sachs, Charles L. Bowden, Ivan P. Gergel, Rosemary Oakes, Cornelius D. Pitts, "Double-Blind, Placebo-Controlled Comparison of Imipramine and Paroxetine in the Treatment of Bipolar Depression," *AJP*, 158 (6) (June 2001), 906–912. The latter three authors were SmithKline staff.

110. Baum Hedlund to Donald Wright, Office of Research Integrity, DHHS, June 25, 2012, 2.

111. Nardo, *IBOM*, November 29, 2012, 2.

112. Sally Laden to Cornelius Pitts at SmithKline, June 27, 2001. https://www/industrydocuments.ucsf.edu/drug/docs

113. Baum Hedlund to Donald Wright, June 25, 2012, 7.

114. Dwight L. Evans and Dennis S. Charney, "Mood Disorders and Medical Illness: A Major Public Health Problem," *Biological Psychiatry*, 54 (2003), 177–180. https://www.biologicalpsychiatryjournal.com/article/S00006-3223(03)00639-5/abstract These events, plus a long trail of consequences, were documented in the Project on Government Oversight (POGO) at http://www.pogo.org/pogofiles/letters/publichealth-ph-iis-20101129.html See also Baum Hedlund letter to Donald Wright, Office of Research Integrity, July 8, 2011. http://psychrights.org/Research/Digest/Science4Sale/110708EthicsComplaintAgainstEvansGyualaiNemeroffSachsBowdenetal.pdf

115. Paul Basken, "U. of Pennsylvania Absolves Psychiatry Chairman of Ghostwriting Complaint," *Chronicle of HIgher Education*, February 29, 2012. https://www.chronicle.com/article/U-of-Pennsylvania-Absolves/130977

116. Robert Rubin comment in Nardo, *1BOM*, April 7, 2014, 3.

117. http://s.wsj.net/public/resources/documents/SenateLetter081003.pdf

118. B. Carroll, "Walk the Walk," *Health Care Renewal* blog, April 6, 2013. http://hcrenewal.blogspot.com/2013/04/walk-walk-for-some-time-jeremiad-theme.html

119. Kenneth R. Feather, interview, May 7, 1997, 26; "History of the U.S. Food and Drug Administration," transcript in the NLM, History of Medicine Division, FDA Oral History Collection.

Chapter 10

1. Louis Lasagna, "Clinical Trials of Drugs from the Viewpoint of the Academic Investigator (a Satire)," *Clinical Pharmacology and Therapeutics*, 18 (1975), 629–633, 632.

2. Paul Leber interview manuscript, June 9, 2008, 28. I am grateful to Dr. Healy for showing me in advance a copy of this interview. *Psychopharmacologists*, II.

3. Harry M. Marks, *The Progress of Experiment: Science and Therapeutic Reform in the United States, 1900–1990* (New York: Cambridge University Press, 1997), 130.

4. J. T. Hart, discussion, "The Medical Use of Psychotropic Drugs: A Report of a Symposium, Sponsored by the Department of Health and Social Security and held at University College, Swansea on 1–2 July 1972," *Journal of the Royal College of General Practitioners*, Suppl. no. 2, 23 (1973), 73.

5. Jonathan O. Cole, interview, in Ban, ed., *Oral History of Neuropsychopharmacology*, X, 47.

6. William G. Goodrich, interview, October 15, 1986, 2 of 12; FDA Oral History Program, NLM. https://www.fda.gov/media/87084/download; http://www.fda.gov/oc/history/oralhistories/goodrich/part2.html

7. See John P. Swann, "Sure Cure: Public Policy on Drug Efficacy Before 1962," in Gregory J. Higby et al., eds., *The Inside Story of Medicines: A Symposium* (Madison WI: American Institute of the History of Pharmacy, 1997), 223–261.

8. Paul Leber, interview, in Ban, ed., *Oral History of Neuropsychopharmacology*, VIII, 239–240.

9. W. Leigh Thompson, ""Dix, Cent, Mille: Proof of Principle with $10 Million, 100 Patients, and 1000 Days," in Allen Cato et al., eds., *Clinical Drug Trials and Tribulations*, 2nd ed. (New York: Dekker, 2002), 93–111.

10. Louis Lasagna, "Congress, the FDA, and New Drug Development Before and After 1962," *Perspectives in Biology and Medicine*, 12 (1989), 322–343, 337.

11. A. L. Cochrane, *Effectiveness and Efficiency* (London: Nuffield Provincial Hospitals Trust, 1971), 11.

12. Jerome Y. Lettvin and Walter Pitts, "A Mathematical Theory of the Affective Psychoses," *Bulletin of Mathematical Biophysics*, 5 (1943), 139–148.

13. Jerome Lettvin, in Larry R. Squires, ed., *The History of Neuroscience in Autobiography* (New York: Academic Press, 1998), II, 224–243, 228.

14. Alexandre Moreau de Jonnès, presentation, *Annales médico-psychologiques*, 2 (1843), 302.

15. Jean-Pierre Falret, *Des Maladies Mentales* [On Mental Illness] (Paris: Baillière, 1864), xlii–xliii.

16. Friedrich Jolly, discussion, in "XIX. Versammlung der südwestdeutschen Irrenärzte am 27. und 28. Oktober 1888 zu Karlsruhe" ["Meting of the Southwest German Psychiatrists on 27-28 October in Karlsruhe"], *Allgemeine Zeitschrift für Psychiatrie* [General Journal of Psychiatry], 46 (1889), 48.

17. See Yifeng Lieu et al., "Recruitment and Retention Strategies in Mental Health Trials," *PLOS One*, Aug 29, 2018. https://doi.org/10.1371/journal.pone.0203127

18. Etienne Esquirol, "De l'épilepsie" (1815), reprinted in Esquirol, ed., *Des Maladies Mentales* (Paris: Baillière, 1838), I, 318–319.

19. John T. G. Nichols, "The Misuse of Drugs in Modern Practice," *Boston Medical and Surgical Journal*, 129 (September 14, 1893), 261–264, 263.

20. J. Burns Amberson et al., "A Clinical Trial of Sanocrysin in Pulmonary Tuberculosis," *American Review of Tuberculosis*, 24 (1931), 401–435.

21. Francis H. K. Green, "The Clinical Evaluation of Remedies," *Lancet*, 267 (November 27, 1954), 1085–1090, 1088.

22. Linford Rees, interview, in Healy, ed., *Psychopharmacologists*, II, 175.

23. Linford Rees and G. M. King, "Desoxycortone Acetate and Ascorbic Acid in the Treatment of Schizophrenia," *Journal of Mental Science [British Journal of Psychiatry]*, 97 (1951), 376–380.

24. Ralph W. Gerard, "European Tour, Survey of Science in Relation to Neuropsychiatry (1934–35)," Ralph W. Gerard Collection at Department of Special Collections, University of California at Irvine Libraries, Box II-D, p. 176.

25. Mindel C. Sheps, "The Clinical Value of Drugs: Sources of Evidence," *J Public Health*, 51 (1961), 647–654, 651. The paper was delivered at a conference in 1960.

26. Daniel Shaw, discussion, in Joseph D. Cooper, ed., *The Philosophy of Evidence* (Washington DC: Interdisciplinary Communication Associates, 1972), 280. Vol. 3 in the series *Philosophy and Technology of Drug Assessment*, sponsored by the Smithsonian Institution. The conference was held in 1971.

27. Medical Research Council, "Streptomycin in the Treatment of Tuberculous Meningitis," *Lancet,* 1 (1948), 582–596.

28. The concept of "randomization" comes to us from agricultural studies in 1920s. First double-blind trial was Amberson, 1931 (see Abraham M. Lilienfeld, "Ceteris Paribus: The Evolution of the Clinical Trial," *Bulletin of the History of Medicine,* 56 (1982), 1–18, 14, 17. On the history of blind assessment and placebo controls, see Ted J. Kaptchuk, "Intentional Ignorance," *Bulletin of the History of Medicine,* 72 (1998), 389–433. These are not part of the narrative of trials in psychopharmacology.

29. See Mark Parascandola, "Clinical Trials: New Developments and Old Problems," in Gregory J. Higby et al., eds., *The Inside Story of Medicines: A Symposium* (Madison WI: American Institute of the History of Pharmacy, 1997), 201–214, 204–207.

30. Allan Broadhurst, interview, in Healy, ed., *Psychopharmacologists,* I, 113–115.

31. Hutchinson, discussion, in Nathan S. Kline, ed., "Research in Psychiatry with Special Reference to Drug Therapy," *Psychiatric Research Reports of the American Psychiatric Association,* 9 (March 1958), 72–73.

32. Joel Elkes and Charmian Elkes, "Effect of Chlorpromazine on the Behaviour of Chronically Overactive Psychotic Patients," *BMJ,* 2 (September 4, 1954), 560–576. Around this time, at the All Saints Hospital in Birmingham Charmian Elkes conducted her own randomized controlled trial of the rauwolfia alkaloids, including reserpine, on 50 inpatients with a mixture of serious diagnoses. She used the patients as their own controls. Staff were also blinded. The rauwolfia alkaloids did quite well compared to chlorpromazine, although the rauwolfia trial itself may have been conducted prior to the chlorpromazine trial and the comparison inserted afterward by Mayer-Gross. Somewhat oddly, Charmian Elkes' trial was first reported by Willi Mayer-Gross in October 1955 at Jean Delay's big conference in Paris on chlorprom-azine. He gave her full credit. See W. Mayer-Gross, "Intervention," in Jean Delay, *Colloque International sur la Chlorpromazine et les Médicaments Neuroleptiques en Thérapeutique Psychiatrique, Paris, 20, 21, 22 Octobre 1955* (Paris: Doin, 1956), 776–778. Elkes then reported her own trial in "Rauwolfia Alkaloids and Reserpine in the Treatment of the Chronic Psychotic Patient," in *J Mental Sci,* 103 (1957).

33. Charmian Elkes, Rauwolfia Alkaloids and Reserpine in the Treatment of the Chronic Psychotic Patient," *J Mental Sci,* 103 (1957), 464–474.

34. Linford Rees and Carl Lambert, "A Controlled Study of the Value of Chlorpromazine in the Treatment of Anxiety-Tension States," in Jean Delay, ed., *Colloque International sur la Chlorpromazine et les Médicaments Neuroleptiques en Thérapeutique Psychiatrique* (Paris: Doin, 1956), 247–249. Rees's other two papers at this meeting were also cross-over studies. The main publication of the anxiety paper was Linford Rees, "The Value and Limitations of Chlorpromazine in the Treatment of Anxiety States," *J Ment Sci,* 101 (1955), 834–840.

35. David Lewis Davies and Michael Shepherd, "Reserpine in the Treatment of Anxious and Depressed Patients," *Lancet*, 2 (July 16, 1955), 117–120.

36. Michael Shepherd interview, in Healy, ed., *Psychopharmacologists*, II, 245.

37. [George Pickering, Clinical Psychiatry Committee of the Medical Research Council, "Clinical Trial of the Treatment of Depressive Illness," *BMJ*, I (April 3, 1965), 881–886.

38. Nicholas Kopeloff and Clarence O. Cheney, "Studies in Focal Infection: Its Presence and Elimination in the Functional Psychoses," *AJP*, 79 (1922), 139–155.

39. Leonard A. Dub and Louis A. Lurie, "Use of Benzedrine in the Depressed Phase of the Psychotic State," *Ohio State Med J*, 35 (1939), 39–45.

40. Leo E. Hollister, interview, in Ban, ed., *Oral History of Neuropsychopharmacology*, IX, 144–145.

41. See L. E. Hollister et al., "Chlorpromazine Alone and With Reserpine. Use in the Treatment of Mental Diseases," *Calif Med*, 83 (1955), 218–221.

42. Leo E. Hollister, interview, in Ban, ed., *Oral History of Neuropsychopharmacology*, IX, 138–139.

43. Louis Lasagna, "A Combination of Hypnotic Agents," *J Pharmacol and Expmtl Ther*, 111 (1954), 9–20.

44. Louis Lasagna, "A Study of Hypnotic Drugs in Patients with Chronic Diseases," *Journal of Chronic Diseases*, 3 (1956), 122–133.

45. John L. Hampson, David Rosenthal, and Jerome D. Frank, "A Comparative Study of the Effect of Mephenesin and Placebo on the Symptomatology of a Mixed Group of Psychiatric Outpatients," *Johns Hopkins Hospital Bulletin*, 95 (1954), 170–177.

46. See, for example, the short paper by Robert Hall at Agnew State Hospital in Agnew, California. It is unknown if Dr. Hall received support from the company. Smith, Kline & French Laboratories, ed., *Chlorpromazine and Mental Health: Proceedings of the Symposium Held Under the Auspices of Smith, Kline & French Laboratories, June 6, 1955, Warwick Hotel, Philadelphia, Pennsylvania* (Philadelphia: Lea & Febiger, 1955), 64–68.

47. [Jonathan Cole, The National Institute of Mental Health Psychopharmacology Service Center Collaborative Study Group, "Phenothiazine Treatment in Acute Schizophrenia," *AGP*, 10 (1964), 246–261.

48. Milton Greenblatt et al., "Differential Response of Hospitalized Depressed Patients to Somatic Therapy," *AJP*, 120 (1964), 935–943.

49. John Clancy, Abram Hoffer, John Lucy, Humphrey Osmond, John Smythies, and Ben Stefaniuk, "Design and Planning in Psychiatric Research as Illustrated by the Weyburn Chronic Nucleotide Project," *Menninger Clinic Bulletin*, 18 (1954), 147–153. The study was not widely cited and Erika Dyck, who wrote the standard monograph on the later LSD experiments at Weyburn, did not mention Clancy Dyck, *Psychedelic Psychiatry: LSD from Clinic to Campus* (Baltimore: Johns Hopkins University Press, 2008).

50. Donald Klein, comment, *1BOM*, July 5, 2012, 5. For an example of this great raft of scholarship, see Donald F. Klein and Max Fink, "Psychiatric Reaction Patterns to Imipramine," *AJP*, 119 (1962), 432–438.

51. Rachel Klein, interview, in Ban, ed., *Oral History of Neuropsychopharmacology*, VII, 306.

52. Mogens Schou, "Phases in the Development of Lithium Treatment in Psychiatry," in Fred Samson et al., eds., *The Neurosciences: Paths of Discovery* (Boston: Birkhäuser, 1991), II, 149–166, 153.

53. M. Schou et al., "The Treatment of Manic Psychoses by the Administration of Lithium Salts," *Journal of Neurology, Neurosurgery and Psychiatry*, 17 (1954), 250–260.

54. J. R. B. Ball and L. G. Kiloh, "A Controlled Trial of Imipramine in Treatment of Depressive States," *BMJ*, 2 (November 21, 1959), 1052–1055.

55. David Healy, interview of Paul Leber, ms. p. 22.

56. Louis Lasagna, interview, in Healy, ed., *Psychopharmacologists*, II, 136–137.

Chapter 11

1. Charles Mackay, *Memoirs of Extraordinary Popular Delusions and the Madness of Crowds* (London: Routledge, 1869), I, 262.

2. Barbara J. Mason, James H. Kocsis, Allen J. Frances, and J. John Mann, "Amoxapine versus Amitriptyline for Continuation Therapy of Depression," *Journal of Clinical Psychopharmacology*, 10 (1990), 338–343.

3. Leo E. Hollister, "Drugs for Emotional Disorders," *JAMA*, 234 (December 1, 1975), 942–947, 944.

4. Nardo, *1BOM*, December 19, 2011, 3.

5. Gordon Parker, "Clinical Trials of Antidepressant Medications Are Producing Meaningless Results," *British Journal of Psychiatry*, 183 (2003), 102–104, 103.

6. Mark Kramer, comment, on Barry Blackwell, "Corporate Corruption in the Psychopharmaceutical Industry" (version of September 1, 2016), 72. http://inhn.org/controversies/barry-blackwell-corporate-corruption-in-the-psychopharmaceutical-industry.html

7. Mark Kramer, reply to Barry Blackwell, October 13, 2016, 26. http://inhn.org/fileadmin/user_upload/User_Uploads/INHN/FILES/Kramers-__LM_Revised_commentary_-_October_13__2016.pdf

8. Bernard Carroll to correspondents, May 17, 2008.

9. "The Imipramine Dossier," in Thomas A. Ban et al., eds., *From Psychopharmacology to Neuropsychopharmacology in the 1980s and the Story of CINP, As Told in Autobiography* (Budapest: Animula, 2002), 326. Vol. 3 of the series *The History of Psychopharmacology and the CINP*. Kuhn's memory has recently been tarnished in Switzerland by activists who reproach him for not having sought "consent" from his patients, even though in Switzerland in the 1950s this kind of explicit consent was unheard of. It is worth pointing out that Kuhn's patients did give implicit consent, based, as Carroll put it, "on the therapeutic relationship [which] matters far more than a legalistic 6-page informed consent document." Bernard Carroll to Edward Shorter, May 22, 2017.

10. Fritz Freyhan, "Selection of Patients," in Jonathan O. Cole and Ralph W. Gerard, eds., *Psychopharmacology: Problems in Evaluation* (Washington DC: National Academy of Science—National Research Council, 1959), 383. The conference was in 1956.

11. Malcolm Lader, discussion, in Michael R. Trimble, ed., *Benzodiazepines Divided: A Multidisciplinary Review* (Chichester: Wiley, 1983), 42.

12. Jules Angst, interview, in David Healy, ed., *Psychopharmacologists,* I, 287–307, 291.

13. Leo Hollister, interview, in Ban, ed., *Oral History of Neuropsychopharmacology,* I, 50.

14. PricewaterhouseCoopers, *Pharma 2005: An Industrial Revolution in R&D* (1998), 14. www.pwcglobal.com/gx/eng/ins-sol/spec-int/eeo/pwc_pharmar6d2005.pdf

15. David Healy, "Some Continuities and Discontinuities in the Pharmacotherapy of Nervous Conditions Before and After Chlorpromazine and Imipramine," *History of Psychiatry,* 11 (2000), 393–412, 407.

16. Paul Hoch and Theodore Rothman, discussion, in Sidney Malitz, ed., *In the Beginning—The Origin of the American College of Neuropsychopharmacology* (American College of Neuropsychopharmacology, 1990), B-26.

17. Paul Leber, ms. of interview, June 9, 2008, 31. This portion of the interview was not included in the published version in Healy, ed., *Psychopharmacologists,* II, 607–622.

18. Paul Janssen, interview, in Healy, eds., *Psychopharmacologists,* II, 49–50.

19. Bernard Carroll, post, *1BOM,* April 1, 2013, 4.

20. A. L. Cochrane, *Effectiveness and Efficiency* (London: Nuffield Provincial Hospitals Trust, 1971), 23.

21. Alvan Feinstein, discussion, in Joseph D. Cooper, ed., *The Philosophy of Evidence* (Washington DC: Interdisciplinary Communication Associates, 1972). This was vol. 3 in the series *Philosophy and Technology of Drug Assessment,* sponsored by the Smithsonian Institution. The conference was held in 1971.

22. Alvan Feinstein, discussion, in Joseph D. Cooper, ed., *The Efficacy of Self-Medication* (Washington DC: Interdisciplinary Communication Associates, 1973), 146. This was vol. 4 in the series *Philosophy and Technology of Drug Assessment,* sponsored by the Smithsonian Institution.

23. Alvan Feinstein in Cooper, ed., *The Efficacy of Self-Medication,* 146.

24. William M. Wardell and Louis Lasagna, *Regulation and Drug Development* (Washington DC: American Enterprise Institute for Public Policy Research, 1975), 39.

25. Amos Tversky and Daniel Kahneman, "Belief in the Law of Small Numbers," *Psychological Bulletin,* 76 (1971), 105–110, 110. For an update, see Shitij Kapur and Marcus Munafò, "Small Sample Sizes and a False Economy for Psychiatric Clinical Trials," *JAMA Psychiatry,* March 27, 2019. doi:10.1001/jamapsychiatry.2019.0095

26. Robert Temple, "How FDA Currently Makes Decisions on Clinical Studies," *Clinical Trials,* 2 (2005), 276–281, 277.

27. Michael Alan Taylor, *Hippocrates Cried: The Decline of American Psychiatry* (New York: Oxford University Press, 2013), 68–69. See Chmura Kraemer, "Is It Time to Ban the *P* Value?" *JAMA Psychiatry,* online August 2, 2019. doi:10.1001/jamapsychiatry.2019.19.1965

28. Gordon Parker, "Evaluating Treatments for the Mood Disorders: Time for the Evidence to Get Real?" *Australian and New Zealand Journal of Psychiatry*, 38 (2004), 408–414, 412–413.

29. See James J. McGough et al., "Estimating the Size of Treatment Effects: Moving Beyond *P* Values," *Psychiatry*, 6 (2009), 21–29.

30. News story, *Scrip*, June 26, 2002, 20.

31. David Healy to Edward Shorter, September 1, 2008.

32. Donald F. Klein, "The Loss of Serendipity in Psychopharmacology," *JAMA*, 299 (March 5, 2008), 1063–1065, 1064.

33. Paul Leber, discussion, PDAC, March 12, 1981, I, 205. Obtained through the Freedom of Information Act.

34. "Draft. Hoechst-Roussel Pharmaceuticals Inc. Protocol for Study of Nomifensine Maleate," 2; attached to Michael A. Pierro (Hoecht-Roussel) to Bernard Carroll, May 21, 1976; in Carroll Papers, Nashville Division, at UCLA Neuroscience History Archive.

35. For a critique that really discredits the entire STAR*D enterprise, see H. Edmund Pigott et al., "Efficacy and Effectiveness of Antidepressants: Current Status of Research," *Psychother and Psychosom*, 79 (2010), 267–279. doi:10.1159/000318293 H. Edmund Piggott, "STAR*D: A Tale and Trail of Bias," *Ethical Human Psychology and Psychiatry*, 13 (2011), 6–28. doi:10.1891/1559-4343.13.1.6 H. Edmund Pigott, "The STAR*D Trial: It is Time to Reexamine the Clinical Beliefs That Guide the Treatment of Major Depression," *Canadian Journal of Psychiatry*, 60 (2015), 9–13. doi:10.1177/070674371506000104

36. John T. Aquino, "Whistleblower Claims Forest Bribed Study's Investigator to Favor Celexa," *Bloomberg*, February 1, 2012. This article, later taken down from the web, was quoted at *1BOM*, February 2, 2012, 1.

37. For this re-analysis, see Irving A. Kirsch et al., "Do Outcomes of Clinical Trials Resemble Those 'Real World' Patients? A Reanalysis of the STAR*D Data Set," *APA PsycNET*, 2018. https://psycnet.apa.org/record/2018-45831-001

38. Leo E. Hollister, interview, in Ban, ed., *Oral History of Neuropsychopharmacology*, IX, 152.

39. Harry Gold et al., "The Xanthines (Theobromine and Aminophylline) in the Treatment of Cardiac Pain," *JAMA*, 108 (June 26, 1937), 2173–2179.

40. Jürgen Margraf et al., "How 'Blind' Are Double-Blind Studies?" *Journal of Consulting and Clinical Psychology*, 59 (1991), 184–187, 186.

41. Seymour Fisher and Roger P. Greenberg, "How Sound is the Double-Blind Design for Evaluating Psychotropic Drugs?" *Journal of Nervous and Mental Diseases*, 181 (1993), 345–350, 348.

42. Benjamin Brody et al., "Antidepressant Clinical Trials and Subject Recruitment: Just Who Are Symptomatic Volunteers?" *AJP*, 168 (2011), 1245–1247, 1245.

43. See Burton J. Goldstein, interview, in Ban, ed., *Oral History of Neuropsychopharmacology*, IV, 136–137.

44. News story, *Scrip sic,* July/August 2002, 32.

45. Samuel Gershon, discussion, PDAC, March 13, 1981, II–115. Obtained through the Freedom of Information Act.

46. Mark Kramer, comment, on Barry Blackwell, "Corporate Corruption in the Psychopharmaceutical Industry" (2016 version), 83, September 1, 2016, INHN. org.   http://inhn.org/controversies/barry-blackwell-corporate-corruption-in-the-psychopharmaceutical-industry.html

47. Bernard Carroll, discussion, PDAC, November 6, 1980, 117–118. Obtained through the Freedom of Information Act.

48. "Major depression" ad, *Toronto Star*, September 19, 2007, A12. On professional patients, see Benjamin Brody et al., "Antidepressant Clinical Trials and Subject Recruitment: Just Who Are Symptomatic Volunteers?" *AJP*, December 1, 2011. https://doi.org/10.1176/appi.ajp.2011.11060864

49. See Manfred Ackenheil, interview, in Ban, ed., *Oral History of Neuro-psychopharmacology*, VIII, 8.

50. Robert Temple, discussion, PDAC, April 8, 2009, 230–231.

51. Herbert Meltzer, discussion, PDAC, July 25, 1995, 52. Obtained through the Freedom of Information Act.

52. Robert Temple, discussion, PDAC, July 19, 1993, 189. Obtained through the Freedom of Information Act.

53. Nardo, *1BOM*, December 23, 2011, 2. http://1boringoldman.com/index.php/2011/12/03/16794   http://1boringoldman.com/index.php/2011/12/03/the-grand-prize/ Cf. Brody et al., "Antidepressant Clinical Trials and Subject Recruitment," *AJP* (2011).

54. Robert J. Temple, "Special Study Designs: Early Escape, Enrichment, Studies in Non-responders," *Communications in Statistics—Theory and Methods*, 23(2) (1994), 499–531. https://www.tandfonline.com/doi/abs/10.1080/03610929408831269

55. Aaron Levin, "'Serendipity' Endangered in Psychiatric Research," [an interview with Donald Klein], *Psychiatric News*, April 18, 2008. Journalistic paraphrase of Klein's comments. For a critical assessment of this technique, see, however, Jonah Campbell and Nicholas B. King, "'Unsettling Circularity': Clinical Trial Enrichment and the Evidentiary Politics of Chronic Pain," *BioSocieties*, 12 (2016), 191–216. https://link.springer.com/article/10.1057/biosoc.2016.7

Chapter 12

1. Mark Kramer, comment, on Barry Blackwell, "Corporate Corruption in the Psychopharmaceutical Industry" (version of September 1, 2016), 80. http://inhn.org/controversies/barry-blackwell-corporate-corruption-in-the-psychopharmaceutical-industry.html

2. Abraham Heller et al., "Effectiveness of Antidepressant Drugs: A Triple-Blind Study Comparing Imipramine, Desipramine, and Placebo," *AJP*, 127 (1971), 1092–1095. For the assertion that this is the first, see Laura J. Hirschbein, "Science, Gender, and the Emergence of Depression in American Psychiatry, 1952–1980," *Journal of the History of Medicine*, 61 (2006), 200. https://doi.org/10.1093/jhmas/jrj037

3. Exchange in PDAC, July 15, 1996, 291–293. Obtained through the Freedom of Information Act.

4. Duncan W. Vere, "Ethics of Clinical Trials," in C. S. Good, ed., *The Principles and Practice of Clinical Trials* (Edinburgh: Churchill, 1976), 3–12, 10.

5. Max Fink, interviewed by Edward Shorter and David Healy, October 25, 2002, 17.

6. C. M. Beasley, Jr., et al., "Fluoxetine and Suicide: A Meta-analysis of Controlled Trials for Treatment of Depression," *BMJ*, 303 (1991). https://doi.org/10.1136/bmj.303.6804.685

7. Mark Olfson and Steven C. Marcus, "Decline in Placebo-Controlled Trial Results Suggests New Directions for Comparative Research," *Health Affairs*, 32 (2013). https://www/healthaffairs.org/doi/full/10.1377/hlthaff.2012.1353

8. J. M. Kane [Zucker-Hillside], et al., "A Multicenter, Randomized, Double-blind, Controlled Phase 3 Trial of Fixed-Dose Brexpiprazole for the Treatment of Adults with Acute Schizophrenia," *Schizophrenia Research*, 164 (2015), 127–135. doi:10.1016/j.schres.2015.01.038

9. C. U. Correll [Zucker-Hillside] et al., "Efficacy and Safety of Brexpiprazole for the Treatment of Acute Schizophrenia: A 6-Week Randomized, Double-Blind, Placebo-Controlled Trial," *AJP*, 172 (2015). doi:10.1176/appi.ajp.2015.14101275

10. Nardo, *1BOM*, May 7, 2015, 1.

11. Andy Forbes et al., "A Long-Term, Open-Label Study to Evaluate the Safety and Tolerability of Brexpiprazole as Maintenance Treatment in Adults with Schizophrenia," *International Journal of Neuropsychopharmacol*, 21 (2018), 433–441. doi:10.1093/ijnp/pyy002

12. Nardo, *1BOM*, February 7, 2014, 1.

13. News story, *Scrip*, January 16 (1996), 17.

14. Bernard Carroll to Lowell I. Goodman (Wyeth Ayerst Laboratories), November 2, 1992; Carroll Papers, Nashville Division, UCLA Neuroscience History Archive.

15. News stories, *F-D-A Reports ("The "Pink Sheet"),* April 6, 1998, 16; June 15, 1998, 15.

16. Frank Davidoff et al., "Sponsorship, Authorship and Accountability," *Canadian Medical Association Journal*, 165 (September 18, 2001), 786–788, 786.

17. Mark Kramer to correspondents, May 15, 2017.

18. Bernard Carroll, comment, *1BOM*, March 12, 2013, 3.

19. George M. Simpson, interview, in Ban, ed., *Oral History of Neuropsychopharmacology*, IX, 298.

20. Rosa Ahn et al., "Financial Ties of Principal Investigators and Randomized Controlled Trial Outcomes: Cross Sectional Study," *BMJ*, 356 (2017), 1–9. doi:10.1136/bmj.i6770

21. Richard Lawrence to distribution, February 12, 1997, exhibit 13; document AZSER10628743 at psychrights.org-/research/Digest/NLPs/Seroquel

22. Jay Amsterdam to correspondents, May 6, 2017.

23. David O. Antonuccio et al., "Antidepressants: A Triumph of Marketing Over Science?" *Prevention & Treatment*, article 25, posted July 15, 2002, 2. http://journals.apa.org/prevention/volume5/pre0050025c.html

24. David Healy, *Let Them Eat Prozac* (Toronto: Lorimer, 2003), 81, 132, 229, and passim.

25. J. R. Wittenborn, ed., "Guidelines for Clinical Trials of Psychotropic Drugs, June 1, 1977," *Pharmakopsychiatrie*, 10 (1979), 205–231, 221.

26. Wayne Katon, discussion, in "Cost of Depression in the 1990s and the Benefits of Appropriate Treatment," *Journal of Clinical Psychiatry*, 51, Suppl. (June 1990), see 12–81, 37.

Chapter 13

1. Michael Alan Taylor, *Hippocrates Cried: The Decline of American Psychiatry* (New York: Oxford University Press, 2013), 66.
2. Haskell J Weinstein testimony, in *"Administered Prices," Hearings Before the Subcommittee on Antitrust and Monopoly of the Committee on the Judiciary, United States Senate, Eighty-Sixth Congress, Second Session, February 25 . . . 1960, part 18* (Washington DC: GPO, 1960), 10259–10260.
3. Claude C. Hopkins, My Life in Advertising (New York: Harper, 1927), 38–39, 73–74.
4. Bernard Carroll, post, *1BOM*, September 20, 2012, 2.
5. Steve Lucas, comment, *1BOM*, August 23, 2013, 2.
6. David M. Moreau, preface, in Barrie G. James, *The Future of the Multinational Pharmaceutical Industry to 1990* (London: Associated Business Programmes, 1977), xii.
7. Alan Schwarz, "The Selling of Attention Deficit Disorder," *New York Times*, December 14, 2013. https://www.nytimes.com/2013/12/15/health/the-selling-of-attention-deficit-disorder.html
8. Jay Amsterdam to Donald Klein and correspondents, April 4, 2019.
9. Bernard Carroll comment, *1BOM,* September 25, 2015, 3.
10. Tone Jones, testimony, State of Texas v. Janssen, LP, January 18, 2012, 12. http://1boringoldman.com/texas-transcripts/2012-01-18%20State%20v.%20Janssen%20Vol%207-1.pdf#page=5
11. United States' Complaint, United States District Court for the District of Massachusetts, US *ex rel.* Greg Thorpe et al v. GlaxoSmithKline PLC, C.A. No. 11-10398-RWZ17-19. https://www.justice.gov/sites/default/files/opa/legacy/2012/07/02/us-complaint.pdf
12. Harold A. Pincus et al., "Psychiatric Patients and Treatments in 1997," *AGP*, 56 (1999), 441–449, 448.
13. Nardo, *1BOM*, February 15, 2014, 1.
14. Don Kartzinel, discussion, FDA, Neurologic Drugs Advisory Committee, October 12, 1977, 247; US National Archives, HD –WW, E18, box 13.
15. John M. Davis, discussion, PDAC, March 21, 1977, 37–39. Obtained through the Freedom of Information Act.
16. *Physicians' Desk Reference*, 1985, p. 1977.
17. On DESI, see Edward Shorter, *Before Prozac: The Troubled History of Mood Disorders in Psychiatry* (New York: Oxford University Press, 2009), 126–149.
18. Steven Brill, "America's Most Admired Lawbreaker," 48. http://highline.huffingtonpost.com/miracleindustry/americas-most-admired-lawbreaker
19. News story, *Scrip*, March 4, 1997, 9.
20. "Seroquel PR Plan 2001," February 2001; SQ1ED00244315. Online: psychrights.org-/research/Digest/NLPs/Seroquel/ Documents cited in this section are from this source.
21. Memo from Simon Hagger, global brand manager, Seroquel, to Seroquel Global Brand Team, August 7, 2003. AZSER 10068202, Goldstein, exhibit no. 44.

22. S. Nassir Ghaemi, "Toward a Hippocratic Psychopharmacology," *Canadian Journal of Psychiatry*, 53 (2008), 189–196, 189. By "non-Hippocratic" Ghaemi meant the philosophy that, "only some, not all, diseases should be treated and, even then, treatments should enhance the natural healing process, not serve as artificial cures." doi:10.1177/070674370805300309

23. *1BOM*, March 25, 2011, 3.

24. Frank Ayd, discussion ["a speaker from the panel"], *In the Beginning: The Origin of the American College of Neuropsychopharmacology* (ACNP, 1990—privately printed), B33–B34.

25. Nardo, *1BOM*, May 1, 2014, 4.

26. Bernard Carroll, comment, *1BOM*, February 19, 2011, 5.

27. E. Beresford Davies, discussion, in John Marks and C. M. B. Pare, eds., *The Scientific Basis of Drug Therapy in Psychiatry: A Symposium at St. Bartholomew's Hospital in London, 7th and 8th September, 1964* (Oxford: Pergamon, 1965), 182.

28. Fritz Freyhan, "Clinical Effectiveness of Tofranil in the Treatment of Depressive Psychoses," *Journal of the Canadian Psychiatric Association*, 4 (suppl) (1959), S86–S99.

29. Jules Angst, interview, in Healy, ed., *Psychopharmcologists*, I, 287–307, 297.

30. News story, *Scrip*, May 27–29, 1998, 15.

31. Leila Abboud, "Should Family Doctors Treat Serious Mental Illness?" *Wall Street Journal*, March 24, 2004, D1.

32. Mike Bandick, memo on "ZYPREXA—Primary Care. Strategy and Implementation Overview," August 2000. http://industrydocuments.library.ucsf.edu/drug/docs/nlvn0217

33. Tone Jones, testimony, State of Texas v. Janssen, January 18, 2012, 14.

34. In the United States District Court for the Eastern District of Pennsylvania. United States of America v. Janssen Pharmaceutica, November 4, 2013, 27–28. http://highline.huffingtonpost.com/miracleindustry/americas-most-admired-lawbreaker/assets/documents/5/highlighted-us-complaint-pa.pdf?build=01121512

35. See Jan Robinson (Audio Visual Medical Marketing Inc.) to Carolyn Robinowitz (APA), August 22, 1980; APA Archives, Education, box 36, folder 453. Robinson: "The DSM-III Symposia were planned to be conferences which taught the use of DSM-III. They were never planned as fundraising ventures for the APA."

36. Ben Wallace-Wells, "Bitter Pill: How the Pharmaceutical Industry Turned a Flawed and Dangerous Drug into a $16 Billion Bonanza, *Rolling Stone*, February 5, 2009, 13–15.

37. Nardo, *1BOM*, January 3, 2014

38. Thomas R. Insel and Remi Quirion, "Psychiatry as a Clinical Neuroscience Discipline," *JAMA*, 294 (November 2, 2005), 2221–224.

39. Donald Klein to correspondents, May 5, 2013.

40. Peter Skrabanek, "Nonsensus Consensus," *Lancet*, June 16, 1990. doi:https://doi.org/10.1016/0140-6736(90)91460-R

41. Haskell J. Weinstein, testimony, in *"Administered Prices," Hearings Before the Subcommittee on Antitrust and Monopoly of the Committee on the Judiciary, United*

States Senate, Eighty-Sixth Congress, Second Session, February 25 . . . 1960, part 18 (Washington DC: GPO, 1960), 10245.

42. Frank Ayd, Jr., discussion, in Sidney Malitz, ed., *In the Beginning: The Origin of the American College of Neuropsychopharmacology* (Nashville: ACNP, 1990), B-8.

43. Michael Alan Taylor, *Hippocrates Cried: The Decline of American Psychiatry* (New York: Oxford University Press, 2013), 67.

44. Jan Robinson (AV/MDF) to Henry H. Work (APA), July 2, 1980; APA Archives, Professional Affairs, box 17, folder 192.

45. Jan Robinson (Audio Visual Medical Marketing) to Carolyn Robinowitz (APA deputy medical director), August 22, 1980; APA Archives, Education, box 36, folder 453.

46. Dr. Henry H. Work to Jack White, June 10, 1980; APA, Professional Affairs, box 17, folder 192, Pharmaceutical Companies. On this correspondence, see also APA Archives, Education, box 36, folder 453.

47. American Psychiatric Association, "Minutes of Meeting with Representatives of Pharmaceutical Companies," June 9, 1980; APA Archives, Professional Affairs, box 17, folder 192, "Pharmaceutical Companies."

48. David Healy, *Let Them Eat Prozac: The Unhealthy Relationship between the Pharmaceutical Industry and Depression* (New York: New York University Press, 2004), 122.

49. Henry H. Work to Richard Dudley (Roche), October 3, 1980; APA Archives, Professional Affairs, box 17, folder 192.

50. See the Minutes of the June 9 meeting, attached to Henry Work to Jack White, June 10, 1980; APA Archives, Professional Affairs, box 17, folder 192.

51. I was given in confidence a copy of the "Sponsorship & Exhibit Prospectus," of the CINP Congress, Montreal, June 23–27, 2002.

52. Ed Roseman, "Where the Changing Promotional Mix Is Headed," *Medical Marketing and Media*, 24 (6) (June 1989), 10–20, 18–19.

53. Melody Petersen, "Madison Ave. Has Growing Role in the Business of Drug Research," *New York Times*, November 22, 2002. https://www.nytimes.com/2002/11/22/business/madison-ave-has-growing-role-in-the-business-of-drug-research.html

54. Benedict Carey and Gardiner Harris, "Psychiatric Group Faces Scrutiny Over Drug Industry Ties," *New York Times*, July 12, 2008.

55. Francis T. Roberts letter to Senator Humphrey, October 28, 1963, 2524; in *"Interagency Coordination in Drug Research and Regulation," Hearings Before the Subcommittee on Reorganization and International Organizations of the Committee on Government Operations, United States Senate, Eighty-Eighth Congress, First Session, June 19, 1963, part 5* (Washington DC: GPO, 1964).

56. Roberts letter to Senator Humphrey, October 28, 1963, 2524.

57. Mike Luby et al., "The Best-Sellers List: The 2007 Sales and Marketing Quality Ranking," *Pharmaceutical Executive*, 27 (3) (March 2007), 82–90.

58. News story, *F-D-A Reports ("The Pink Sheet")*, October 26, 1970, TG-10.

59. Adriane Fugh-Berman et al., "Following the Script: How Drug Reps Make Friends and Influence Doctors," *PLOS Medicine*, 4 (4) (April 2007), e150. www.plosmedicine.org

60. Jeffrey A. Mattes, "Letter: Evidence-Based Promotion," *AJP*, online December 22, 2014. https://doi.org/10.1176/ajp.161.10.1928

61. Frank Berger, "My Biography" (2014), 63–64. http://inhn.org/ebooks/frank-m-berger-my-biography.html

62. Rufus L. McQuillan, *Is the Doctor In? The Story of a Drug Detail Man's Fifty Years of Public Relations with Doctors and Druggists* (New York: Exposition Press, 1963), 138.

63. Walter Modell, testimony, in *"Administered Prices," Hearings Before the Subcommittee on Antitrust and Monopoly of the Committee on the Judiciary, United States Senate, Eighty-Sixth Congress, Second Session, February 25 . . . 1960, part 18* (Washington DC: GPO, 1960), 11607.

64. Melvin R. Gibson, "Editorial," *Am J Pharma Ed*, 23 (1959), 461–466, 465.

65. Nardo, *1BOM*, January 21, 2012, 1.

66. Stephanie Saul, "Gimme an Rx! Cheerleaders Pep Up Drug Sales," *New York Times*, November 28, 2005, A1.

67. Gardiner Harris et al., "Its Rivals in Funk, Novartis Finds a Way to Thrive," *Wall Street Journal*, August 23, 2002, 1.

68. Valerie Robinson, testimony, State of Texas v. Janssen, LP, January 18, 2012, 138, 140–141, 148–149. http://1boringoldman.com/texas-transcripts/2012-01-18%20 State%20v.%20Janssen%20Vol%207-1.pdf#page=5

69. Alan Breier to Lilly executives, November 9, 1999. http://industrydocuments.library. ucsf.edu/drug/docs/gnvn0217

70. Beasley to Lilly executives, October 10, 2000. http://industrydocuments.library.ucsf. edu/drug/docs/hpvn0217

71. Beasley to Lilly executives, October 10, 2000. http://industrydocuments.library.ucsf. edu/drug/docs/hpvn0217

72. C. E. Koro et al., "Assessment of Independent Effect of Olanzapine and Risperidone on Risk of Diabetes Among Patients with Schizophrenia: Population Based Nested Case-Control Study," *BMJ*, 325 (2002), 243.

73. Robert Baker to Beasley, October 10, 2000. http://industrydocuments.library.ucsf. edu/drug/docs/jpvn0217

74. Thomas M. Brodie to Baker, October 9, 2000. http://industrydocuments.library.ucsf. edu/drug/docs/zyvn0217

75. Elvis A. Rivera [on Zyprexa Brand Team] to Katherine A. Armington et al., November 20, 2001. http://industrydocuments.library.ucsf.edu/drug/docs/nlun0217

76. Correspondence between Rivera and Armington and Illram Wildgust and Nell Archer, October 14, 2001. http://industrydocumentslibrary.ucsf.edu/drug/docs/ ghbn0217

77. Arvid Carlsson, interview with David Healy and Edward Shorter, February 27, 2007, 84.

78. http://www.badfaithinsurance.org/reference/PH/0006c.htm

79. https://www.integrativepsychiatry.net/psychiatric_drugs_on_the_couch.html

80. https://www.propublica.org/article/dollars-for-docs-the-top-earners

81. David Healy to Edward Shorter, May 16, 2008.

82. Barry Blackwell, "Corporate Corruption in the Pharmaceutical Industry," 1. http://inhn.org/controversies/barry-blackwell-corporate-corruption-in-the-psychopharmaceutical-industry-revised.html

83. "Talbot," comment, *1BOM*, March 12, 2011, 5. The identity of Talbot is known to the author.

84. Kirstine Adam and Ian Oswald, "Can a Rapidly-Eliminated Hypnotic Cause Daytime Anxiety." *Pharmacopsychiatry,* 22 (1989), 115–119. doi:10.1055/s-2007-1014592. PMID 2748714. See Ian Oswald interview in Healy, ed., *Psychopharmacologists,* III, 467-468. See also Gina Kolata, "Maker of Sleeping Pill Hid Data On Side Effects, Researchers Say," *New York Times,* January 20, 1992. News story, *Scrip,* January 29, 1992, 6.

85. *"Administered Prices, Drugs," Senate Subcommittee on Antitrust and Monopoly,* June 27, 1961, 199.

86. Leemon McHenry, "On the Origin of Great Ideas: Science in the Age of Big Pharma," *Hastings Center Report,* November–December 2005, 17–19, 17.

87. Roy M. Poses, "A Cautionary Tale: The Dysfunction of American Health Care," *European Journal of Internal Medicine,* 14 (2003), 123–130.

88. Roy Poses, *Health Care Renewal,* February 2, 2013, 2.

89. John J. A. Tumas to colleagues, December 6, 1999; document AZSER12916365 at psychrights.org-/research/Digest/NLPs/Seroquel

90. See Alex Berenson, "Drug Files Show Maker Promoted Unapproved Use," *New York Times,* December 18, 2006. https://www.nytimes.com/2006/12/18/business/18drug.html

91. Healy letter, *BMJ,* May 14, 2015, 1.

92. Evidence in this paragraph comes from David A. Kessler, "Expert Report" filed October 2, 2012, Exhibit F in Texas v Janssen, LP The letter from the Excerpta Medica staffer to Findling is dated August 2000; Exhibit F. http://freepdfhosting.com/a6e96eb7f0.pdf

93. Herman C. B. Denber, "Notes from Another Time and Place," in Thomas A. Ban et al., eds., *The Rise of Psychopharmacology and the Story of CINP* (Budapest: Animula, 1998), 368–371, 371.

94. Nathan S. Kline, "Editorial: Relation of Psychiatry to the Pharmaceutical Industry," *AMA Archives of Neurology and Psychiatry,* 77 (1957), 613–615, 614.

95. Haskell J. Weinstein, testimony, in *"Administered Prices," Hearings Before the Subcommittee on Antitrust and Monopoly of the Committee on the Judiciary, United States Senate, Eighty-Sixth Congress, Second Session, February 25 . . . 1960, part 18* (Washington DC: GPO, 1960), 10244.

96. "Paxil and Adolescent Depression (Study 329): Scientific Presentations/Meetings Strategy" (Philadelphia, November 4, 1997). http://industrydocuments.library.ucsf.edu/drug/docs/ylfw0217

97. Cover sheet attached to Gahan Pandina to staff, February 20, 2002. https://highline.huffingtonpost.com/miracleindustry/americas-most-admired-lawbreaker/assets/documents/7/Plaintiff-Exhibit-55.pdf When the creation appeared in 2003, the list of authors had grown considerably.

98. Robert L. Findling, Vivek Kusumakar, Denis Daneman, Thomas Moshang, Goedele De Smedt, and Carin Binder, "Prolactin Levels During Long-Term Risperidone Treatment in Children and Adolescents," *Journal of Clinical Psychiatry*, 64 (2003), 1362–1369. It is unclear if much of this paper was ghosted.

99. "Seroquel PR Plan 2001," February 2001; see the appended "Seroquel International Media Schedule—2001, 3. https://jimedwardsnrx.files.wordpress.com/2009/05/birkett09.pdf

100. Nardo, *1BOM*, November 29, 2012, 1.

101. Sergio Sismondo, "Key Opinion Leaders and the Corruption of Medical Knowledge: What the Sunshine Act Will and Won't Cast Light On," *Journal of Law, Medicine & Ethics*, 41 (Fall 2013), 635–643, 639.

102. Leemon McHenry, "Of Sophists and Spin-Doctors: Industry-Sponsored Ghostwriting and the Crisis of Academic Medicine," *Mens Sana Monographs*, 8 (1) (2010), 129–145, 131. The "182" statistic is from 2001.

103. See the deposition of former FDA Commissioner David A. Kessler, filed October 2, 2012, 48–51, Exhibit F. Texas v Janssen, LP; case ID: 100503629; control no.: 12100558.

104. Kessler deposition, 48–51.

105. Kessler deposition, 51–52. See also Dinesh Mittal . . . Henry A Nasrallah, "Risperidone in the Treatment of Delirium: Results from a Prospective Open-Label Trial," *Journal of Clinical Psychiatry*, 65 (2004), 662–667. https://www.psychiatrist.com/JCP/article/Pages/2004/v65n05/v65n0510.aspx

106. Rothman, Expert Witness Report, 45–46.

107. "Seroquel PR Plan, 2001," 12–13. https://jimedwardsnrx.files.wordpress.com/2009/05/birkett09.pdf

108. Bernard Carroll, comment, *1BOM*, April 28, 2011, 4.

109. Charles B. Nemeroff et al., "VNS Therapy in Treatment-Resistant Depression: Clinical Evidence and Putative Neurobiological Mechanisms," *Neuropsychopharmacology*, 31 (2006), 1345–1355. The acknowledgement of Laden's "editorial support" is on p. 38.

110. Nardo, *1BOM*, April 29, 2011, 1-2. On Sally Laden as the evident ghostwriter, see Daniel Carlat, "Vagus Nerve Stimulation and Depression: Conflict of Interest's 'Perfect Storm'?" *Psychiatric Times*, 23 (December 1, 2006). https://www.psychiatrictimes.com/articles/vagus-nerve-stimulation-and-depression-conflict-interests-perfect-storm/page/0/2
    Van Os's paper following the meeting—his second paper on the subject—acknowledged "an unrestricted grant from AstraZeneca." Jim van Os, "Evaluation of the Two-Way Communication Checklist as a Clinical Intervention," *BJP*, 184 (2004), 79–83, 83.

111. Bernard Carroll, comment on Ed Silverman blog, *Pharmalot*, "UPenn Looks the Other Way at Ghostwriting," *Pharmalot*, March 1, 2012.

112. David Healy, Letter: "Transparency and Trust," *BMJ*, 329 (December 4, 2004), 1345. doi:https://doi.org/10.1136/bmj.329.7478.1345

113. David Healy, "The Dilemmas Posed by New and Fashionable Treatments," *Advances in Psychiatric Treatment*, 7 (2001), 322–327, 324.

114. David Healy, "Shaping the Intimate: Influences on the Experience of Everyday Nerves," *Social Studies of Science*, 34 (2004), 219–245, 230. doi:10.1177/0306312704042620

115. David Healy, blog post "Brand Fascism," April 30, 2013, 4. davidhealy.org

116. Surendra Kelwala, letter, *Psychiatric News*, June 21, 2002, 33.

117. Lewis Morris, et al., "The Agenda for Continuing Medical Education – Limiting Industry's Influence," *NEJM*, 361 (December 17, 2009), 2478–2482, 2478.

118. Bernard Carroll, "Variations on a Theme of Sleaze," *Health Care Renewal*, January 22, 2008, 5. http://hcrenewal.blogspot.ca/2008/01/variations-on-theme-of-sleaze.html

119. Melvin Sabshin, *Changing American Psychiatry: A Personal Perspective* (Washington DC: American Psychiatric Publishing, 2008), 194.

120. Videotape deposition of Alex Gorsky, May 18, 2012. In the Court of Common Pleas, First Judicial District of Pennsylvania, Civil Trial Division, In re: Risperdal Litigation: March Term, 2010217-218. Link at 9/16/2015, 4:01:02 PM, in Steven Brill, "America's Most Admired Lawbreaker," *Huffington Post* (2015, 39). http://highline.huffingtonpost.com/miracleindustry/americas-most-admired-lawbreaker/

121. Henry Nasrallah, "Sponsored CME: Do Drug Companies Influence the Content?" *Current Psychiatry*, August 2007, 17–18. Readers' letters, *Current Psychiatry*, October 2007, 14–19.

122. The exchange is in *"False and Misleading Advertising (Prescription Tranquilizing Drugs),"* Hearings Before a Subcommittee of the Committee ion Government Operations, House of Representatives, Eighty-Fifth Congress, Second Session, February 1958 (Washington DC: US GPO, 1958), 122.

123. News story, *F-D-C Reports ("The Pink Sheet")*, October 14, 1974, 12.

124. News story, *Scrip*, July 29, 1992, 16.

125. Arnold S. Relman, "Separating Continuing Medical Education from Pharmaceutical Marketing," *JAMA*, 285 (April 18, 2001), 2009–2012.

126. News story, *Scrip*, August 24, 1993, 13.

127. "Tortured Soul," *BMJ*, October 22, 1994, 309. doi:https://doi.org/10.1136/bmj.309.6961.1093

128. Paul Glader, "From the Maker of Effexor: Campus Forums on Depression," *Wall Street Journal*, October 10, 2002, B1.

129. Charles D. May, "Selling Drugs by 'Educating' Physicians," *Journal of Medical Education*, 36 (1961), 1–23, 15, 21.

130. Max Fink, interview, in Ban, ed., *Oral History of Neuropsychopharmacology*, IX, 104.

131. Mark S. Kramer, "Commentary" on Barry Blackwell: Corporate Corruption in the Psychopharmaceutical Industry, October 13, 2016, 4. http://inhn.org/fileadmin/user_upload/User_Uploads/INHN/FILES/Kramers

132. Nardo, *1BOM*, November 1, 2012, 2.

Chapter 14

1. Nardo, *1BOM*, September 27, 2012, 3.
2. Richard Smith, "Medical Journals Are an Extension of the Marketing Arm of Pharmaceutical Companies," *PLOS Medicine*, 2(5) (May 2005), e138. www.plosmedicine.org
3. David Healy et al., "Interface Between Authorship, Industry and Science in the Domain of Therapeutics," *British Journal of Psychiatry*, 183 (2003), 22–27.
4. Nardo, *1BOM*, November 1, 2012, 1–2.
5. Bernard Carroll, "Sertraline and the Cheshire Cat in Geriatric Depression," *AJP* (April 1, 2004). https://doi.org/10.1176/appi.ajp.161.4.759
6. The "marketing plan" definition of it is Nardo's, *1BOM*, October 21, 2012, 2.
7. Max Fink, interview by Edward Shorter and David Healy, October 2002, 24; Haskell J. Weinstein, testimony, in *"Administered Prices," Hearings Before the Subcommittee on Antitrust and Monopoly of the Committee on the Judiciary, United States Senate, Eighty-Sixth Congress, Second Session, February 25 . . . 1960, part 18* (Washington DC: GPO, 1960), 10245.
8. "Talbot" comment, *1BOM*, September 16, 2011, 5. Talbot was the pseudonym of an experienced medical writer whose identity is known to the author.
9. Charles B. Nemeroff, "Use of Atypical Antipsychotics in Refractory Depression and Anxiety," *Journal of Clinical Psychiatry*, 66(Suppl. 8) (2005), 13–21. The issue also contained supportive articles by C. B. Keller and A. M. H. Pollack.
10. Leemon McHenry, "Villains and Heroes: Academic Thuggery." https://davidhealy.org/villains-and-heroes-academic-thuggery/
11. Kenneth R. Feather, interview, May 7, 1997, 32; "History of the U. S. Food and Drug Administration," transcript in NLM, History of Medicine Division, FDA Oral History Collection.
12. Goldine C. Gleser, "Psychometric Contributions to the Assessment of Patients," in Daniel H. Efron, ed., *Psychopharmacology: A Review of Progress, 1957–1967* (Washington DC: GPO, 1968), 1029–1037, 1031. PHS Pub. No. 1836.
13. Haskell J. Weinstein, testimony, in *"Administered Prices," Report of the Committee on the Judiciary, United States Sensate, Made by Its Subcommittee on Antitrust and Monopoly, June 27, 1961* (Washington DC: GPO, 1961), 182.
14. Erick H. Turner et al., "Selective Publication of Antidepressant Trials and Its Influence on Apparent Efficacy," *New England Journal of Medicine*, 358 (2008), 252–260. doi:10.1056/NEJMsa065779
15. Jay Amsterdam to correspondents, July 20, 2019.
16. Benedict Carey, "Researchers Find Bias in Drug Trial Reporting," *New York Times*, January 17, 2008, A18.
17. Frank Ayd, Jr., interview, in Healy, ed. *Psychopharmacologists*, I, 106.
18. Lisa Cosgrove, "Under the Influence: The Interplay among Industry, Publishing, and Drug Regulation," *Accountability in Research*, 23 (2016), 257–279; 264. http://dx.doi.org/10.1080/08989621.2016.1153971
19. On this, see Nardo, *1BOM*, May 20, 2016, 1–2.

20. Brett J. Deacon and Glen I. Spielmans, "Is the Efficacy of 'Antidepressant' Medications Overrated?" in Scott O. Lilienfeld and Irwin D. Waldman, eds., *Psychological Science Under Scrutiny* (New York: Wiley, 2017), 250–270, 257.

21. Jay D. Amsterdam and Leemon B. McHenry, "The Paroxetine 352 Bipolar Study Revisited: Deconstruction of Corporate and Academic Misconduct," *Journal of Scientific Practice and Integrity*, 1 (2019), 1–12, 10. doi:10.35122/jospi.2019.958452

22. Marcia Angell, "Is Academic Medicine for Sale?" *New England Journal of Medicine*, 342 (May 18, 2000), 1516–1518.

23. Jack Gorman, associate editor of the *American Journal of Psychiatry*, to Nemeroff, June 12, 2000. https://www.industrydocuments.ucsf/#id=ft Marcia Angell, "Is Academic Medicine for Sale?" *New England Journal of Medicine*, 342 (May 18, 2000), 1516–1518.

24. Sally Laden to Charles Nemeroff, October 31, 2000. https://www.industrydocuments. ucsf.edu/drug/docs/#id=nshk0228

25. Karen Dineen Wagner, Adelaide S. Robb, Robert L. Findling, Jianquing Jin, Marcelo M. Gutierrez, and William E. Heydorn, "A Randomized, Placebo-Controlled Trial of Citalopram for the Treatment of Major Depression in Children and Adolescents," *AJP*, 161 (2004), 1079–1083. https://psycnet.apa.org/record/2004-16538-018

26. Jon N. Jureidini, Jay D. Amsterdam and Leemon B. McHenry, "The Citalopram CIT-MD-18 Pediatric Depression Trial: Deconstruction of Medical Ghostwriting, Data Mischaracterisation and Academic Malfeasance," *International Journal of Risk & Safety in Medicine*, 28 (2016), 33–43. doi:10.3233/JRS-160671

27. Jay D. Amsterdam, Leemon B. McHenry, and Jon N. Jureidini, "Industry-corrupted Psychiatric Trials," *Psychiatria Polska*, 51 (2017), 993–1008. doi:https://doi.org/ 10.12740/PP/80136

28. Jay Amsterdam to correspondents, January 23, 2018.

29. Kristin Riding et al., "Reporting Bias in Drug Trials Submitted to the Food and Drug Administration: Review of Publication and Presentation," *PLOS Medicine*, 5 (November 2008), 1567. www,plosmedicibne.org

30. Paul Lovinger at Wayne State University School of Medicine, testimony, in "Competitive Problems in the Drug Industry," *Hearings Before the Subcommittee on Monopoly of the Select Committee on Small Business, United States Senate, Ninetieth Congress—Second Session, Part 10 (December 11, 1968–January 23, 1969* (Washington DC: GPO, 1969), 3998.

31. Bernard Carroll, letter, "Aripiprazole in Refractory Depression?" *Journal of Clinical Psychopharmacology*, 29 (2009), 90–91. The original report was Ronald N. Marcus et al., "The Efficacy and Safety of Aripiprazole as Adjunctive Therapy in Major Depressive Disorder," *J Clin Psychopharm*, 28 (2008), 156–165.

32. Jureidini, Amsterdam, McHenry, "Background Notes." http://1boringoldman.com/ index.php/background-notes/#

33. http://inhn.org/controversies/barry-blackwell-corporate-corruption-in-the-psychopharmaceutical-industry/jay-d-amsterdam-leemon-b-mchenry-and-jon-n-jureidinis-commentary-industry-corrupted-psychiatric-trials.html For the Richard Smith article in 2005, see "Medical Journals Are an Extension of the Marketing Arm of Pharmaceutical Companies," *PLOS Medicine*, 2(5): e138.

34. Mark Kramer, "Commentary" on Barry Blackwell: Corporate Corruption in the Psychopharmaceutical Industry, October 13, 2016, 25–26. http://inhn.org/fileadmin/ user_upload/User_Uploads/INHN/FILES/Kramers-__LM_Revised_commentary_ -_October_13__2016.pdf

35. David Healy, "The Dilemmas Posed by New and Fashionable Treatments," *Advances in Psychiatric Treatment*, 7 (2001), 322–327, 325. https://www.cambridge.org/core/ journals/advances-in-psychiatric-treatment/article/dilemmas-posed-by-new-and- fashionable-treatments/3B662F08015B7160B43329AB544F164E

36. Floyd Garrett, post of April 2, 2007, to psycho-pharm@psycom.net. In the post, Garrett quoted Goldberg.

Chapter 15

1. Paul Leber, interview, in Ban, ed., *Oral History of Neuropsychopharmacology*, VIII, 227.

2. Louis Lasagna, discussion, in Craig D. Burrell, ed., *Drug Assessment in Ferment: Multinational Comparisons* (Washington DC: Smithsonian Institution, 1976), 149. The conference was in 1973.

3. Louis Lasagna and William M. Wardell, "The FDA, Politics, and the Public," *JAMA*, 232 (April 14, 1975), 141–142, 142.

4. Melody Petersen, "Who's Minding the Drugstore?" *New York Times*, June 29, 2003, 1–3. Gardiner Harris, "At FDA Strong Drug Ties and Less Monitoring," *New York Times*, December 6, 2004, A1, A20. See also Alison Bass, *Side Effects* (Chapel Hill: Algonquin Books, 2008), 141–142.

5. Jonathan J. Darrow et al., "FDA Approval and Regulation of Pharmaceuticals, 1983– 2018," *JAMA*, 323 (2020), 164–176. doi:10.1001/jama.2019.20288

6. William M. Wardell and Louis Lasagna, *Regulation and Drug Development* (Washington DC: American Enterprise Institute for Public Policy Research, 1975).

7. Louis Lasagna, "Research Regulation, and Development of New Pharmaceuticals: Past, Present, and Future, Part I," *American Journal of Medical Science*, 263 (1972), 9–19, 16.

8. Paul Leber, discussion, PDAC, July 25, 1995, 108–109. Obtained through the Freedom of Information Act.

9. See John P. Swann, "Sure Cure: Public Policy on Drug Efficacy Before 1962," in Gregory J. Higby et al., eds., *The Inside Story of Medicines: A Symposium* (Madison WI: American Institute of the History of Pharmacy, 1997), 223–261.

10. For a careful history of these regulatory changes, see Suzanne White Junod, *FDA and Clinical Drug Trials: A Short History*. US Food and Drug Administration. 2008 www. fda.gov

11. Joseph F. Sadusk, Jr., to Commissioner, October 15, 1964; Federal Archives, UD-WW635, 88 – 7Q, 4049, Gen Subject Files, 1964 (box 280), 505.5.

12. The best guide to the history of the agency in these years is Wallace F. Janssen, inter-view, January 30–31, 1984; in "History of the U. S. Food and Drug Administration,"

transcript in NLM, History of Medicine Division, FDA Oral History Collection. See also https://www.fda.gov/about-fda/virtual-exhibits-fda-history/brief-history-center-drug-evaluation-and-research—which does not even mention Goddard.

13. Lowrie M. Beacham, interview, August 28, 1985, 5; "History of the U. S. Food and Drug Administration," transcript in NLM, History of Medicine Division, FDA Oral History Collection.

14. Donald C. Healton, interview, June 19, 1995, 58; "History of the U. S. Food and Drug Administration," transcript in NLM, History of Medicine Division, FDA Oral History Collection.

15. http://www.foxnews.com/video-search/m/21485444/medication_nation. htm?q=dougl Laughren said in a deposition that Forest approached him about 5 months after he left FDA (Deposition, January 27, 2017, 81).

16. See Robert Temple, discussion, PDAC, November 1, 2018, 234.

17. Ronald Kartzinel, discussion, PDAC, November 14, 1978, 291–292. Obtained through the Freedom of Information Act.

18. Paul Leber, interview, in Healy, ed., *Psychopharmacologists*, II, 612.

19. David Healy, "Psychopharmacology in the New Medical State," in Healy et al., eds., *Psychotropic Drug Development* (London: Chapman & Hall, 1996), 13–40, 34.

20. Hillary Lee, discussion, PDAC, December 3, 1981, I-163. Yet FDA had already embraced in general the DSM-III criteria. See Paul Leber, PDAC, February 6, 1980, 191–192. He endorsed DSM-III criteria for antidepressant trials at the meeting of November 6, 1980, 192. But then he later said "We are not tied to DSM-III, you know. You don't have to go on the market with a DSM-III diagnosis." PDAC, December 4, 1981, II-170. The issue of "depression" was clearly in flux at FDA in these years.

21. John Overall, discussion, PDAC, December 4, 1981, II-177. All the PDAC transcripts were obtained through the Freedom of Information Act.

22. News story, *F-D-C Reports ("The Pink Sheet"),* February 7, 2000, 27.

23. Paul Leber, ms. interview with David Healy, June 9, 2008, 25. I am grateful to Dr. Healy for sharing a copy of the ms. with me.

24. Robert Temple, discussion, PDAC, November 1, 2018, 378.

25. Paul Leber, discussion, PDAC (Workshop), January 31, 1985, 52. Obtained through the Freedom of Information Act.

26. Paul Leber, interview, in Ban, ed., *Oral History of Neuropharmacology*, VIII, 228.

27. Paul Leber, discussion, PDAC, September 27, 1994, 197–198.

28. Robert Temple, discussion, PDAC, September 14, 2004 (Day 2), 45.

29. Samuel Maldonado, discussion, PDAC, February 2, 2004, 332. http://www.fda.gov/ohrrms/dockets/ac/04/transcripts/4006T1.pdf

30. See Paul Leber to Roy Baranello, Jr. (Wyeth), August 23, 1996; NDA 18-140/S-003; FDA CDER, Approval Package for Ativan (lorazepam), September 5, 1997. http://www.fda.gov/cder/foi/nda/97/018140ap_5003.pdf

31. Paul Leber, discussion, PDAC, November 6, 1980, 108–109.

32. Leo Hollister, interview, in Ban, ed., *Oral History of Neuropsychopharmacology*, I, 50.

33. Paul Leber, interview by David Healy, June 9, 2008, 30. I am grateful to Dr Healy for making a copy of this interview available to me.

34. Donald Klein to correspondents, April 15, 2017.

35. John Nardo, *1BOM*, June 11, 2013, 1–2.

36. "An Interview with Morris Fishbein, M.D.," March 12, 1968, 63. Transcript in NLM, History of Medicine Division, FDA Oral History Collection.

37. Malcolm R. Stephens interview, December 4, 1984, 92. FDA Collection, National Library of Medicine.

38. Thomas Laughren, presentation, PDAC, February 2, 2004, 235–236, 243. http://www.fda.gov/ohrms/dockets/ac/04/transcripts/4006T1.pdf

39. Robert Temple to Stephanie Barba, RW Johnson Pharmaceutical Research Institute, December 29, 1995. www.fda.gov/cder/foi/nda/96/020505_s000_Topamax.htm

40. Michael Alan Taylor, *Hippocrates Cried: The Decline of American Psychiatry* (New York: Oxford University Press, 2013), 73.

41. FDA, "Establishment Inspection Endorsement," March 10, 1976; National Archives, RG88, UD-WW, E15, 88 82-64, box 32.

42. News story, *Scrip*, May 13, 1994, 21.

43. A. Dale Console, Senate testimony, summarized in *F-D-C Reports ("The Pink Sheet")*, June 16, 1969, 15.

44. https://caselaw.findlaw.com/ca-court-of-appeal/1820626.html

45. Theodore C. Maraviglia, interview, September 11, 1981, 22–23; "History of the U. S. Food and Drug Administration," transcript in NLM, History of Medicine Division, FDA Oral History Collection.

46. *"Preclinical and Clinical Testing by the Pharmaceutical Industry." Part 5: Hearings on Examinations of the Process of Drug Testing and the FDA's Role in the Regulation and Conditions Under Which Such Testing is Carried out, Subcommittee on Health and Scientific Research of the Committee on Human Resources, 95th Congress (1978).* For a review of the several such hearings, see Marc A. Rodwin, "Independent Drug Testing to Ensure Drug Safety and Efficacy," *Journal of Health Care Law and Policy*, 18 (2015), 45–84. http://digitalcommons.law.umaryland.edu/jhclp/vol18/iss1/3

47. L. F. Fabre et al., "Sertraline Safety and Efficacy in Major Depression: A Double-Blind Fixed-Dose Comparison with Placebo," *Biological Psychiatry*, 38 (1995), 592–602.

48. Nardo, *1BOM*, February 17, 2013, 5.

49. News story, *F-D-C Reports ("The Pink Sheet")*, December 8, 1997, T-G, 4.

50. *Physicians' Desk Reference*, 1980, 1485–1487.

51. Leo Hollister, discussion, in Hollister, ed., "Valium: A Discussion of Current Issues," *Psychosomatics*, 18 (1977), 44–58, 57. He was referring to the physicians' "package in-sert," as published in *Physicians' Desk Reference (PDR)*. For the label on imipramine, see *PDR*, 1980, 907–911.

Chapter 16

1. Bernard Carroll, comment, *1BOM*, February 22, 2015, 4.

2. Daniel W. Cathell, *The Physician Himself and What He Should Add to the Strictly Scientific* (Baltimore: Bailey, 1882), 146.

3. See Petra Brhlikova et al., "Global Burden of Disease Estimates of Depression—How Reliable is the Epidemiological Evidence?" *Journal of the Royal Society of Medicine*, 104 (2011), 25–35. doi:10.1258/jrsm.2010.100080

4. Carroll, comment, *1BOM*, February 15, 2013, 5.

5. Roger P. Greenberg, "Reflections on the Emperor's New Drugs," *Prevention & Treatment*, article 27, vol. 5, posted July 15, 2002. http://journals.apa.org/prevention/volume5/pre0050027c.html

6. Paul Leber, discussion, PDAC, June 10, 1982, 141.

7. Charles Barber, *Comfortably Numb: How Psychiatry Is Medicating a Nation* (New York: Vintage Books, 2008), 24.

8. Paul Leber, PDAC, February 24, 1983, I-157 to I-158. Obtained through the Freedom of Information Act.

9. Leigh Thompson to Allen Weinstein, February 7, 1990. http://healyprozac.com/Trials/CriticalDocs/thompson070290.htm

10. News story, *Scrip*, March 2, 1993, 7.

11. Alec Coppen, "Potentiation of the Antidepressant Effect of a Monoamine-Oxidase Inhibitor by Tryptophan," *Lancet*, 1 (January 12, 1963). doi: https://doi.org/10.1016/S0140-6736(63)91084-5

12. See David Healy, *Let Them Eat Prozac: The Unhealthy Relationship Between the Pharmaceutical Industry and Depression* (New York: New York University Press, 2004).

13. News story, *Scrip*, April 28, 1995, 11. CNS drugs were 35 percent of Lilly's pharma sales, and Prozac was 91 percent of Lilly's CNS sales.

14. News story, *Scrip*, February 6, 1996, 8.

15. News story, *Scrip*, April 28, 1995, 23.

16. David O. Antonuccio et al., "Antidepressants: A Triumph of Marketing Over Science?" *Prevention & Treatment*, 5 (2002), 1–13, 7.

17. [Name redacted], Professor of Psychiatry to IH Slater (Lilly Research Laboratories), December 24, 1979. http://www.healyprozac.com/trials/criticaldocs

18. News story on reboxetine, *Scrip*, April 28, 1999, 25.

19. See N. Freemantle et al., "Predictive Value of Pharmacological Activity for the Relative Efficacy of Antidepressant Drugs," *BJP*, 177 (2000), 292–302,

20. Seroxat ad, *BJP*, 158 (January–June 1991), 374b-c.

21. David Healy, *Pharmageddon* (Berkeley: University of California Press, 2012), 35.

22. Gary D. Tollefson and Jerrold F. Rosenbaum, "Selective Serotonin Reuptake Inhibitors," in Alan F. Schatzberg and Charles B. Nemeroff, eds., *Textbook of Psychopharmacology*, 2nd ed. (Washington DC: American Psychiatric Press, 2005), 219–237, 228.

23. NCHS, *Advance Data from Vital and Health Statistics*, 322 (July 2001), 27, tab. 18.

24. Mark Olfson et al., "National Trends in the Outpatient Treatment of Depression," *JAMA*, 287 (January 9, 2002), 203–209.

25. George Simpson, interview, Healy, ed., *Psychopharmacologists*, II, 302.

26. Giovanni A. Fava, "The Hidden Costs of Financial Conflicts of Interest in Medicine," *Psychotherapy and Psychosomatics*, 85 (2016), 65–70. https://www.karger.com/Article/FullText/442694

27. S. M. Schappert, "Office Visits to Psychiatrists: United States, 1989–90." *Advance Data from Vital and Health Statistics*, 237 (December 28, 1993) (Hyattsville MD: NCHS, 1993), tab. 14, 13.

28. David Healy to Edward Shorter, May 16, 2008.

29. Robert Temple, discussion, PDAC, February 2, 2004, 388. http://www.fda.gov/ohrms/dockets/ac/04/transcriprts/4006T1.pdf

30. Max Hamilton, discussion, in Jules Angst, ed., *Classification and Prediction of Outcome of Depression* (Stuttgart: Schattauer, 1974), 284. The symposium was in 1973.

31. Robert Temple, discussion, PDAC meeting, April 8, 2009, 307.

32. See David Healy et al., "Enduring Sexual Dysfunction After Treatment with Antidepressants, 5a-reductase Inhibitors and Isotretinoin: 300 Cases" (2018). https://content.iospress.com/articles/international-journal-of-risk-and-safety-in-medicine/jrs744l Christopher Lane, "Post-SSRI Sexual Dysfunction Recognized as Medical Condition" (January 14, 2019). https://www.psychologytoday.com/ca/blog/side-effects/201906/post-ssri-sexual-dysfunction-recognized-medical-condition

33. Jeffrey R. Vittengl, "Poorer Long-Term Outcomes among Persons with Major Depressive Disorder Treated with Medication" [letter], *Psychotherapy and Psychosomatics*, 86 (2017), 302–304, 303.

34. Jay Amsterdam to correspondents, October 31, 2017.

35. Jules Angst, "Severity of Depression and Benzodiazepine Co-medication in Relationship to Efficacy of Antidepressants in Acute Trials. A Meta-analysis of Moclobemide Trials," *Human Psychopharmacology*, 8 (1993), 401–407.

36. News story, *F-D-C Reports ("The Pink Sheet"),* June 4, 1990, 11–12.

37. Harriett Speight (Wyeth's medical systems manager) to Bernard Carroll, February 2, 1996; in Nashville Division of Carroll Papers, at the UCLA Neuroscience History Archives.

38. Mark Kramer, February 17, 2017; attached to Jay Amsterdam to correspondents, February 17, 2017.

39. Nardo, *1BOM*, June 28, 2012, 2.

40. On this, see Edward Shorter, *What Psychiatry Left Out of the DSM-5: Historical Mental Disorders Today* (New York: Routledge, 2015).

41. Thomas A. Ban, "RDoC in Historical Perspective," February 19, 2015. http://inhn.org/perspectives/thomas-a-ban-the-rdoc-in-historical-perspective.html

42. Mark S. Kramer, "Commentary" on Barry Blackwell: Corporate Corruption in the Psychopharmaceutical Industry, October 13, 2016, 17. http://inhn.org/fileadmin/user_upload/User_Uploads/INHN/FILES/Kramers-__LM_Revised_commentary_-_October_13__2016.pdf

43. Glen D. Mellinger and Mitchell B. Balter, "Prevalence and Patterns of Use of Psychotherapeutic Drugs: Results from a 1979 National Survey of American Adults," in G. Tognoni et al., eds., *Epidemiological Impact of Psychotropic Drugs* (Amsterdam: Elsevier, 1981), 117–135, 126, tab. 2.

44. News story, *Scrip*, February 15, 1991, 23, 19.

45. Paxil ad, *AJP*, March 1993, A17.

46. Nardo, *1BOM*, March 24, 2012, 2.

47. News story, *Scrip*, April 13, 1995, 17.

48. National Center for Health Statistics, "Utilization of Ambulatory Medical Care by Women: United States, 1997–98," Data from the National Health Care Survey; 38, tab. 14; Vital and Health Statistics, ser 13, no. 149 (Hyattsville MD: NCHS, July 2001). DHHS Pub No. (PHS) 2001-1720.

49. T. J. Moore et al., "Adult Utilization of Psychiatric Drugs and Differences by Sex, Age, and Race," *JAMA Internal Medicine*, 177 (2017), 274–275.

50. Jerome D. Frank, "Psychotherapy: The Restoration of Morale," *AJP*, 131 (1974), 271–274. doi:https://ajp.psychiatryonline.org/doi/abs/10.1176/ajp.131.3.271

51. Carroll, post, *1BOM*, January 7, 2015, 5–6.

52. Leo Alexander, "The Psychiatric Armamentarium," *Diseases of the Nervous System*, 20 (1959), 75–78, 75.

53. David Healy, "Winging It: Antidepressants and Plane Crashes." https://davidhealy.org/winging-it-antidepressants-and-plane-crashes/

54. J. Read et al., "Adverse Emotional and Interpersonal Effects Reported by New Zealanders While Taking Antidepressants," *Psychiatry Research*, 216 (2014), 67–73. doi:10.1016/j.psychres.2014.01.042

55. See Berend Olivier and Jan Mos, "Behavioural Pharmacology of the Serenic Eltoprazine," *Drug Metabolism and Drug Interactions* 8 (1990), 31–83. https://www.ncbi.nlm.nih.gov/pubmed/2091890

56. Donald Klein to correspondents, April 18, 2018.

57. Joseph Guislain, *Traité sur les Phrénopathies* [Treatise on the Phrenopathies] (Brussels: Établissement Quai au Pont, 1833), x–xi, 20.

58. Michael Sullivan, discussion, PDAC, November 1, 2018, 208–209.

59. Bernard J. Carroll, "Brain Mechanisms in Manic Depression," *Clinical Chemistry*, 40/2 (1994), 303–308.

60. See Elias Patetsos, "Treating Chronic Pain with SSRIs: What Do We Know?" *Pain Research and Management* (2016). doi:10.1155/2016/2020915

61. For critiques of antidepressant trials, see David O. Antonuccio et al., "Raising Questions About Antidepressants," *Psychotherapy and Psychosomatics*, 68 (1999), 3–14; and Irving Kirsch et al., "The Emperor's New Drugs: An Analysis of Antidepressant Medication Data Submitted to the U.S. Food and Drug Administration," *Prevention & Treatment*, art. 23, posted July 15, 2002. https://scholar.google.com/scholar_lookup?journal=Prevention+and+Treatment&title=Theemperor's+new+drugs:+An+analysis+of+antidepressant+medication+datasubmitted+to+the+U.S.+Food+and+Drug+Administration&volume=5&publication_year=2002&pages=23&

62. Michael A. Sugarman et al., "The Efficacy of Paroxetine and Placebo in Treating Anxiety and Depression: A Meta-Analysis of Change on the Hamilton Rating Scales," *PLOS One*, August 27, 2014. doi:10.137/journal.pone.0106337 See also Nardo, *1BOM*, September 3, 2014, 1–2.

63. Leslie Iversen, interview, Healy, ed., *Psychopharmacologists*, II, 344.

64. Phoebe Danziger, "The Language of Suicide," *JAMA*, 320, no. 24 (2018), 2537–2538. doi:10.1001/jama.2018.19199

65. Jay Amsterdam to colleagues, July 7, 2019. Jay D. Amsterdam and Thomas T. Kim, "Prior Antidepressant Treatment Trials May Predict a Greater Risk of Depressive Relapse During Antidepressant Maintenance Therapy," *Journal of Clinical Psychopharmacology*, 39 (2019), 344–350.

66. J. Alexander Bodkin, discussion, PDAC, November 1, 2018, 296.

67. Soren H. Sindrup et al., "Antidepressants in the Treatment of Neuropathic Pain," *Basic & Clinical Pharmacology & Toxicology*, 96 (2005), 399–409.

68. Adrienne J. Lindblad et al., "Antidepressants in the Elderly," *Canadian Family Physician*, 65 (2019). https://www.cfp.ca/content/65/5/340

69. Mark S. Kramer, "Commentary" on Barry Blackwell: Corporate Corruption in the Psychopharmaceutical Industry, October 13, 2016, 33. http://inhn.org/fileadmin/user_upload/User_Uploads/INHN/FILES/Kramers-__LM_Revised_commentary_-_October_13__2016.pdf

70. S. P. Roose et al., "Comparative Efficacy of Selective Serotonin Reuptake Inhibitors and Tricyclics in the Treatment of Melancholia," *AJP*, 151 (1994), 1735–1739.

71. Jan Fawcett et al., "Efficacy Issues With Antidepressants," *Journal of Clinical Psychiatry*, 58, Suppl 6. (1997), 32–39, 35, tab. 2, citing data from a previous study.

72. Gordon Parker et al., "Are the Newer Antidepressant Drugs as Effective as Established Physical Treatments? Results from an Australasian Clinical Panel," *Australian and New Zealand Journal of Psychiatry*, 33 (1999), 874–881.

73. Gordon Parker to correspondents, April 28, 2013. See Gordon Parker, "Differential Effectiveness of Newer and Older Antidepressants Appears Mediated by an Age Effect on the Phenotypic Expression of Depression," *Acta Psychiatrica Scandinavica*, 106 (2002), 168–170.

74. Michael Alan Taylor, *Hippocrates Cried: The Decline of American Psychiatry* (New York: Oxford University Press, 2013), 80–81.

75. Nardo, *1BOM*, October 4, 2011, 4–5.

76. Steve Balt, "Assessing and Enhancing the Effectiveness of Antidepressants," *Psychiatric Times*, June 13, 2014. https://www.psychiatrictimes.com/psychopharmacology/assessing-and-enhancing-effectiveness-antidepressants

77. David Healy, "Prozac and SSRIs: Twenty-Fifth Anniversary," Healy blog, February 6, 2013. https://davidhealy.org/prozac-and-ssris-twenty-fifth-anniversary/2

78. Sam Gershon to correspondents, May 8, 2017.

79. Mario Maj, "Preface," in Maj et al., eds., *Psychiatric Diagnosis and Classification* (Chichester: Wiley, 2002), ix.

80. https://davidhealy.org/something-happened-to-science-and-to-us/

81. David Healy, "The Marketing of 5-Hydroxytryptamine [serotonin]: Depression or Anxiety?" *BJP*, 158 (1991), 737–742, 740.

82. Prozac ad, *BJP*, 1656 (July–December 1994), back cover of October issue; Prozac ad, *AJP*, 153 (1996).

83. News story, *F-D-C Reports ("The Pink Sheet")*, 52 (20) (May 14, 1990), T&G1. The NDA was later withdrawn.

84. https://www.thepharmaletter.com/article/prozac-approved-for-ocd-in-usa

85. News story, *Scrip*, May 8, 1994, 28.

86. News story, *Scrip*, November 18, 1998, 23.

87. News story, *Scrip*, July 12, 2000, 18.

88. News story, *Scrip*, May 24, 2002, 24.

89. News story, *Scrip*, July 30, 1996, 6. "59 percent" for the second quarter of 1996.

90. See Brendan I. Koerner, "Disorders Made to Order," *Mother Jones*, July/ August 2002. https://www.motherjones.com/politics/2002/07/disorders-made-order/ Tempting though it is to dismiss "general anxiety disorder" as yet another disease created by the pharmaceutical industry—in this case GlaxoSmithKline for the benefit of Paxil sales—the fact remains that, historically, anxiety disorders have been very common, especially in "mixed anxiety-depression," and are in no sense a figment created by Pharma.

91. Thomas Newman, discussion, PDAC, September 14, 2004, 338–339. Obtained through the Freedom of Information Act.

92. Max Fink to correspondents, April 15, 2018.

93. Carroll to correspondents, April 15, 2018.

94. News story, *Scrip*, April 9, 1996, 21.

95. Max Fink, interview, in Ban, ed., *Oral History of Psychopharmacology*, IX, 92.

96. See, for example, Steve Balt, "Assessing and Enhancing the Effectiveness of Antidepressants," *Psychiatric Times*, June 13, 2014, which takes the various clinical studies absolutely at face value as though they were all bricks in a solid scientific wall. https://www.psychiatrictimes.com/psychopharmacology/assessing-and-enhancing-effectiveness-antidepressants

97. Brief, Baum-Hedlund for Laura A. Plumlee v. Pfizer, Inc, United States District Court for the Northern District of California, San Jose Division, filed January 30, 2013, pp. 19–20. http://www.baumhedlundlaw.com/pdf/zoloft-class-action-efficacy-lawsuit.pdf

98. Nadia Iovieno et al., "Residual Symptoms After Remission of Major Depressive Disorder with Fluoxetine and Risk of Relapse," *Depression and Anxiety*, 28 (2011), 137–144.

99. Irving Kirsch et al., "Listening to Prozac but Hearing Placebo: A Meta-Analysis of Antidepressant Medication," *Prevention & Treatment*, 1, article 0002a. http://journals.apa.org/prevention/volume1/pre0010002a.html See also Irving Kirsch, "The Emperor's New Drugs: An Analysis of Antidepressant Medication Data, Submitted to the US Food and Drug Administration," *Prevention & Treatment*, 5 (2002), 1–11, and Irving Kirsch, *The Emperor's New Drugs: Exploding the Antidepressant Myth* (New York: Basic Books, 2010).

100. Brett J. Deacon and Glen I. Spielmans, "Is the Efficacy of 'Antidepressant' Medications Overrated?" in Scott O. Lilienfeld and Irwin D. Waldman, eds., *Psychological Science Under Scrutiny* (New York: Wiley, 2017), 250–270, 261.

101. Donald Klein, "Listening to Meta-Analysis but Hearing Bias," *Prevention & Treatment*, 1, article 0006c, posted June 26, 1998. http://journals.apa.org/prevention/volume1/pre0010006c.html

102. Gordon Parker, "Evaluating Treatments for the Mood Disorders: Time for the Evidence to Get Real," *Australian and New ZealandJournal of Psychiatry*, 38 (2004), 408–414.

103. Robert Whitaker, "Do Antidepressants Work? A People's Review of the Evidence." https://www.madinamerica.com/2018/03/do-antidepressants-work-a-peoples-review-of-the-evidence/

104. Baron Shopsin, interview, in Ban, ed., *Oral History of Neuropsychopharmacology*, V, 340.

105. See data on "mood disorders" in Søren Dalsgaard et al., "Incidence Rates and Cumulative Incidences of the Full Spectrum of Diagnosed Mental Disorders in Childhood and Adolescence," *JAMA Psychiatry*, 77 (2020), 155–164, 158, fig. 1(c), where the curve takes off steeply in girls around age 12, and in boys at age 13. doi:10.1001/jamapsychiatry.2019.3523

106. Jay Amsterdam to correspondents, March 8, 2018.

107. Bach X. Tran et al., "Indices of Change, Expectations, and Popularity of Biological Treatments for Major Depressive Disorders between 1988 and 2017: A Scientometric Analysis," *International Journal of Environment Research and Public Health*, 16 (2019), 2255. doi:10.3390/ijerp16132255

108. Evelyn Pringle, "SSRI Pushers Under Fire," *Scoop*. January 2, 2009. http://www.scoop.co.nz/stories/HL0901/500008.htm

109. Peter Gøtzsche, "Why I Think Antidepressants Cause More Harm Than Good," *Lancet Psychiatry*, July 2014. doi:https://www.thelancet.com/journals/lanpsy/article/PIIS2215-0366(14)70280-9/fulltext

110. Jay Amsterdam to correspondents, February 17, 2017.

111. Thomas C. Baghai et al., "General and Comparative Efficacy and Effectiveness of Antidepressants in the Acute Treatment of Depressive Disorders: A Report by the WPA Section of Pharmacopsychiatry," *European Archives of Psychiatry and Clinical Neuroscience*, 261, Suppl. 3 (2011), S207–245, S230–231.

112. Robert Temple, discussion, PDAC, April 8, 2009, 223. Laughren soon left the FDA to begin consulting for Forest some months later.

113. See MDL Docket Nr. 907, USDC, SD. of Indiana, PZ 65 451 ff. The document is attached to Dorothy Dobbs to FDA, December 17, 1984, exhibit Stark 6. The cover sheet is "Request: To provide additional summary information about concomitant medications used in the controlled studies." There follow 22 tables showing, for each patient and each trialist, the concomitant drugs. This document may be accessed at www.healyprozac.com/Trials/CriticalDocs/default.htm, under the tab "Dobbs." On the coadministration question, see Charles Medawar, "The Antidepressant Web: Marketing Depression and Making Medicines Work," *International Journal of Risk & Safety in Medicine*, 10 (1997), 75–126, 86.

114. Escobar–Tollefson exchange, PDAC, September 20, 1991, 251–252. http://www.fda.gov/ohrms/dockets/ac/prozac/2443T1.pdf

115. David Drachman, discussion comment, PDAC, March 13, 1981, II-76. Obtained through the Freedom of Information Act.

116. David Healy, "The Empire of Humbug: Not So Bad Pharma," April 23, 2013, 3. https://davidhealy.org/the-empire-of-humbug-not-so-bad-pharma/

117. Benjamin Crocker, email to psycho-pharm@psycom.net, May, 2, 2008.

118. Bernard Carroll, post, *1BOM*, May 20, 2014, 2–3.

119. Jamie Reidy, *Hard Sell: The Evolution of a Viagra Salesman* (Kansas City: Andrews McMeel, 2005), 49–50.

120. Sara Rimer, "With Millions Taking Prozac, A Legal Drug Culture Arises," *New York Times*, December 13, 1993, C1, 11.

121. "Tom," a psychiatrist, post, *1BOM*, March 13, 2014, 8.

122. Ted Mauger, note, August 16, 2008. psych_pharm@hotmail.com

123. Heather Mallick, "A Tip for Growing Old with Grace," *Globe and Mail*, January 5, 2002, F7.

124. David Healy, *Let Them Eat Prozac: The Unhealthy Relationship between the Pharmaceutical Industry and Depression* (New York: New York University Press, 2004), 264.

125. Ramin Mojtabai and Mark Olfson, "Proportion of Antidepressants Prescribed Without a Psychiatric Diagnosis is Growing," *Health Affairs*, 30 (2011). https://doi.org/10.1377/hlthaff.2010.1024

126. *Newsweek*, February 7, 1994, cover, 41.

127. Michael W. Miller, "Listening to Eli Lilly: Prozac Hysteria Has Gone Too Far," *Wall Street Journal*, March 31, 1994, B1.

Chapter 17

1. Nardo, *1BOM*, April 29, 2011, 2.

2. Eyes wide with greed, the drug makers may have been overestimating the size of the genuine depression market in children and adolescents. A careful Danish study found the incidence of mood disorders among girls to be 2.5 percent, boys 1.1 percent. The fears of parents and clinicians to the contrary notwithstanding, these are not enormous figures. (Far more girls were "anxious," and ADHD was the commonest diagnosis in boys.) Soren Dalsgaard et al., "Incidence Rates and Cumulative Incidences of the Full Spectrum of Diagnosed Mental Disorders in Childhood and Adolescence, *JAMA Psychiatry* 2019. doi:10.1001/jamapsychiatry.2019.3523

3. For an overview, see Nardo, *1BOM*, October 16, 2014, 3–4. The literature seems to have been almost entirely ghosted, and "author" Karen Dineen Wagner came in for some of Nardo's criticism.

4. See "Protocol/CRF Approval," December 5, 1992. http://industrydocuments.library.ucsf.edu/drug/docs/qjfw0217 "Minutes of the Adolescent Unipolar Depression Conference Call," December 21, 1992. http://industrydocuments.library.ucsf.edu/drug/docs/pjfw0217

5. Dolores Kong and Alison Bass, "Case at Brown Leads to Review," *Boston Globe*, October 8, 1999. See also Bass's gripping book, *Side Effects: A Prosecutor, a Whistleblower, and a Bestselling Antidepressant on Trial* (Algonquin Books: Chapel Hill, 2008).

6. Matt R. Battin to Sally Laden, April 25, 2001. https://www.justice.gov/archives/opa/documents-and-resources-july-2-2012-glaxosmithkline-gsk-press-conference

7. Marcia Angell, "Is Academic Medicine for Sale?" *New England Journal of Medicine*, 342 (May 18, 2000), 1516–1518, 1516. https://www.nejm.org/doi/full/10.1056/NEJM200005183422009

8. See Martin Keller to Catherine Sohn (SKB), March 19, 1993. http://industrydocuments.library.ucsf.edu/drug/docs/zjfw0217

9. See "Paxil Advisory Board Meeting: A Proposal for One Psychiatric Advisory Board Meeting," October 1, 1993. http://industrydocuments.library.ucsf.edu/drug/docs/lhfw0217

10. Martin B. Keller et al., "Efficacy of Paroxetine in the Treatment of Adolescent Major Depression: A Randomized, Controlled Trial," *Journal of the American Academy of Child and Adolescent Psychiatry* 40 (2001), 762–772. The Wikipedia account is also informative: https://en.wikipedia.org/wiki/Study_329 This is the most widely discussed trial in history. For an overview, see David Healy, *Children of the Cure: Missing Data, Lost Lives and Antidepressants* (Samizdat Health Writers' Co-operative Inc., May 2020).

11. Gerald Klerman, discussion, in Joseph D. Cooper, ed., *The Philosophy of Evidence* (Washington DC: Interdisciplinary Communication Associates, 1972), 274. The conference was in 1971. This was part of a series in "The Interdisciplinary Communications Program," of The Smithsonian Institution.

12. This was the first point made by one of the reviewers to whom JAMA sent the paper. http://industrydocuments.library.ucsf.edu/drug/docs/mlfw0217

13. Sally Laden, deposition, In the United States District Court for the Eastern District of Pennsylvania, Case no. C-06-03186 MJJ, March 15, 2007, 127. pogoarchives.org/m/ph/sally-laden-sti-deposition-20070315.pdf

14. See [Sally Laden] "Response to Queries from Mina Dulcan, Editor JAACAP," January 5, 2001; "modified by Dr Rachel Klein. We regret that the revised version has never been published." http://industrydocuments.library.ucsf.edu/drug/docs/rfgw0217

15. Memo on "Paroxetine 329 Final Reporting and Analysis Plan," from R. Oakes (SKB) to staff, September 1, 1995, 5–6. .http://industrydocuments.library.ucsf.edu/drug/docs/kjfw0217

16. See Norbert Kerr, "HARKing: Hypothesizing After the Results are Known," *Personality and Social Psychology Review*, 2 (1998), 196–217, *IBQM*, January 4 2016 1–2

17. United States District Court, District of Massachusetts, United States of America v. GlaxoSmithKline LLC, July 2, 2012, 13. https://www.justice.gov/archives/opa/documents-and-resources-july-2-2012-glaxosmithkline-gsk-press-conference See also https://www.justice.gov/sites/default/files/opa/legacy/2012/07/02/us-complaint.pdf

18. See Kristina Fiore, "New Analysis of Paxil Data: Were Adverse Events Downplayed?" *Medpage Today*, September 16, 2015. http://www.medpagetoday.com/Psychiatry/GeneralPsychiatry/53583

19. See the list of over 100 projects that STI conducted for SKB, 1998 being the first date on the list. https://www.industrydocuments.ucsf.edu/drug/docs/#id=znxl0228

20. "Paroxetine Study 329: Top Line Results," January 21, 1998; attached to Kate Beebe (SKB) to Neal Ryan, February 4, 1998. http://industrydocuments.library.ucsf.edu/drug/docs/skfw0217

21. Rachel Kline to Martin Keller et al., April 9, 1999. http://industrydocuments.library.ucsf.edu/drug/docs/rlfw0217

22. "Adolescent Depression, Study 329: Proposal for a Journal Article," sent to Ivan Gergel at SKB, from Sally K. Laden and John A. Romankiewicz at Scientific Therapeutics Information, Inc, April 3, 1998. http://industrydocuments.library.ucsf.edu/drug/docs/npfw0217

23. See Laden, deposition, Sally Laden, deposition, In the United States District Court for the Eastern District of Pennsylvania, March 15, 2007, 18; in Cheryl J Cunningham and William F Williams, vs SmkithKline Beecham Corporation, C A No. 06-3022-TJS.

24. Keller et al., "Paroxetine and Imipramine Treatment of Adolescent Depression: A Randomized, Controlled Trial," Draft I, December 18, 1998. http://industrydocuments.library.ucsf.edu/drug/docs/ksfw0217

25. Neal Ryan to James P. McCafferty, May 14, 1998. http://industrydocuments.library.ucsf.edu/drug/docs/yfgw0217

26. James P. McCafferty to Neal Ryan, October 13, 1998. http://industrydocuments.library.ucsf.edu/drug/docs/mzfw0217

27. Jackie Westaway to staff, October 14, 1998. It was actually Julie Wilson who wrote the "Position Piece on the phase III clinical studies" attached. http://industrydocuments.library.ucsf.edu/drug/docs/syfw0217

28. Oliver Dennis (The Medicine Group) to Scott Sproull (the Paxil project manager), January 21, 1999. http://industrydocuments.library.ucsf.edu/drug/docs/jgfw0217

29. "Attachment 3: Chronology of Publications/Presentations/Posters on Pediatric Efficacy and Safety Data." http://industrydocuments.library.ucsf.edu/drug/docs/fhgw0217

30. Martin Keller to Sally Laden, February 11, 1999. http://industrydocuments.library.ucsf.edu/drug/docs/rhfw0217

31. Martin B. Keller to co-authors, February 22, 1999. http://industrydocuments.library.ucsf.edu/drug/docs/phfw0217

32. Karen Dineen Wagner to Martin B. Keller et al., April 2, 1999. http://industrydocuments.library.ucsf.edu/drug/docs/fmfw0217 On Wagner's role in these events, see Nardo, 1BOM, October 16, 2014, 3.

33. James P. McCafferty to Sally Laden, March 9, 1999. http://industrydocuments.library.ucsf.edu/drug/docs/sfgw0217

34. Holly White (Cohn and Wolfe) to Sheila Hood (SKB), March 5, 2001. http://industrydocuments.library.ucsf.edu/drug/docs/pggw0217

35. Martin B. Keller et al., "Efficacy of Paroxetine in the Treatment of Adolescent Major Depression: A Randomized Controlled Trial," *Journal of the American Academy of Child and Adolescent Psychiatry*, 40 (2001), 762–772. https://study329.org/wp-content/uploads/2015/04/Study-329-original-published.pdf

36. Raza Silveira et al., letter, *Journal of the American Academy of Child and Adolescent Psychiatry*, 41 (November 2002), 1270. https://www.jaacap.org/arrticle/S0890-8567(09)60627-4/fulltext

37. Ed Zaleski (Department of Psychiatry, Brown University) to Sally Laden, Jim McCafferty, February 14, 2002. http://industrydocuments.library.ucsf.edu/drug/docs/rpfw0217

38. Martin Keller to Jim McCafferty, Sally Laden, February 18, 2002. http://industry-documents.library.ucsf.edu/drug/docs/qpfw0217

39. For an explicit statement of Laden's authorship of this and another letter, see James McCafferty to Karen Wagner et al., September 14, 2001. In another note, Ed Zaleski, the secretary at Brown University Department of Psychiatry, said "Attached is a copy of a fax sent to Dr. Keller requesting a response for a letter to the editor. Dr. Keller has asked that I give this to you to respond to." Zaleski to Laden, December 17, 2001. http://industrydocuments.library.ucsf.edu/drug/docs/qzfw0217 ppfw0217

40. Martin B. Keller and Neal D. Ryan, letter, *Journal of the American Academy of Child and Adolescent Psychiatry,* 41 (November 2002), 1271. https://www.jaacap.org/arrticle/S0890-8567(09)60628-6/fulltext

41. The cover sheet of Draft IV is at http://industrydocuments.library.ucsf.edu/drug/docs/zqfw0217

42. Robert N. Golden, Charles B. Nemeroff, Paul McSorley, Cornelius D. Pitts, and Eric M Dubé, "Efficacy and Tolerability of Controlled-Release and Immediate-Release Paroxetine in the Treatment of Depression," *Journal of Clinical Psychiatry*, 63, (2002), 577–584. https://www.psychiatrist.com/JCP/article/Pages/2002/v63n07/v63n0707.aspx

43. Robert N. Golden, Charles B. Nemeroff, Paul McSorley, Cornelius D. Pitts, and Eric M Dube, "Efficacy and Tolerability of Controlled-Release and Immediate-Release Paroxetine in the Treatment of Depression," *Journal of Clinical Psychiatry*, 63 (2002), 577–584. https://www.psychiatrist.com/JCP/article/Pages/2002/v63n07/v63n0707.aspx

44. http://industrydocuments.library.ucsf.edu/drug/docs/zqfw0217

45. Nardo, *1BOM*, November 29, 2012, 2.

46. Kimberly Yonkers, "Paroxetine Treatment of Mood Disorders in Women: Premenstrual Dysphoric Disorder and Hot Flashes," *Psychopharmacology Bulletin* 37 (2003), 135–147.

47. "Paroxetine Treatment of Mood Disorders in Women: Premenstrual Dysphoric Disorder and Hot Flashes, authored by Kimberly A. Yonkers . . . Prepared by: C. Gloria Mao, Sally K. Laden, Scientific Therapeutics Information." Draft I, March 24, 2003. http://industrydocuments.library.ucsf.edu/drug/docs/tggw0217

48. James C. Ballenger, Jonathan R. T. Davidson, Yves Lecrubier, David J. Nutt, Randall D. Marshall, Charles B. Nemeroff, Arieh Y. Shalev, and Rachel Yehuda, "Consensus Statement Update on Posttraumatic Stress Disorder from the International Consensus Group on Depression and Anxiety," *Journal of Clinical Psychiatry*, 65 Suppl. 1 (2004), 55–62.

49. James C. Ballenger et al., "Consensus Statement Update on Posttraumatic Stress Disorder From the International Consensus Group on Depression and Anxiety,"

prepared by Sally K. Laden, Scientific Therapeutic Information, Inc., Draft I, April 30, 2003, "for publication in a supplement to: *Journal of Clinical Psychiatry*." http://industrydocuments.library.ucsf.edu/drug/docs/rsfw0217

50. "Authored by D. Jeffrey Newport, Zachary N. Stowe," "for submission to: *Psychopharmacology Bulletin*. Edited by: Sally K. Laden, STI." "Draft I, January 14, 2003." http://industrydocuments.library.ucsf.edu/drug/docs/nggw0217

51. D. Jeffrey Newport and Zachary N. Stowe, "Clinical Management of Perinatal Depression: Focus on Paroxetine," *Psychopharmacology Bull*, 37 (Spring 2003), Suppl. 1148–1166,

52. Dwight L. Evans and Dennis S. Charney, "Editorial: Mood Disorders and Medical Illness: A Major Public Health Problem," *Biological Psychiatry*, 54 (2003), 177–180.
    "We acknowledge Sally K. Laden for editorial support." Attached to July 28, 2003 document. referenc #53. See below.

53. Sally Laden to Eric Dubé at GSK, July 28, 2003. http://industrydocuments.library.ucsf.edu/drug/docs/txgw0217 PAR070321651

54. Nardo, *1BOM*, December 20, 2013, 6.

55. Sally K. Laden to Eric Dubé (GSK), July 28, 2003. She had now founded her own firm, "MSE Communications." http://industrydocuments.library.ucsf.edu/drug/docs/txgw0217

56. Sally Laden to Eric Dubé (GSK), July 28, 2003. http://industrydocuments.library.ucsf.edu/drug/docs/sxgw0217

57. Sally Laden to Charles B. Nemeroff, February 4, 1997. http://industrydocuments.library.ucsf.edu/drug/docs/zgfw0217

58. Charles B. Nemeroff and Alan F. Schatzberg, *Recognition and Treatment of Psychiatric Disorders: A Psychopharmacology Handbook for Primary Care* (Washington DC: American Psychiatric Press, 1999), vii.

59. This fraud did evoke some resonance. See Paul Thacker, "American Psychiatric Association Spooked about Ghostwriting," *The Project on Government Oversight (POGO) Blog*, April 5, 2011. https://pogoblog.typead.com/pogo/2011/04/american-psychiatric-association-spooked-about-ghostwriting.html; Bernard Carroll, post, "Who You Gonna Believe?" *Health Care Renewal*, April 5, 2011. http://hcrenewal.blogspot.com/2011/04/who-you-gonna-believe-html

60. http://blogs.nature.com/news/files/2012/06/Jay-Amsterdam-today-filed-a-24-page-complaint-with-the-Office-of-Research-Integrity-at-the-US-National-Institutes-of-Health.pdf p 7.

61. See Jay D. Amsterdam and Leemon B. McHenry, "The Paroxetine 352 Bipolar Trial: A Study in Medical Ghostwriting," *International Journal of Risk & Safety in Medicine*, 24 (2012), 221–231. doi:10.3233/JRS-2012-0571 See also J. D. Amsterdam and L. B. McHenry, "The Paroxetine 352 Bipolar Study Revisited: Deconstruction of Corporate and Academic Misconduct," *Journal of Scientific Practice and Integrity*, 1 (2019) 1–12. doi:10.35122/jospi.2019.958452 See also the excellent summary of these developments: Peter Simons, "The Whistleblower and Penn: A Final Accounting of Study 352." https://www.madinamerica.com/2019/12/the-whistleblower-and-penn-a-final-accounting-of-study-352/

62. Bob Roehr, "Professor Files Complaint of Scientific Misconduct Over Allegation of Ghostwriting," *BMJ*, 343 (2011), 343. doi:10.1136/bmj.d4458 See also http://blogs.nature.com/news/files/2012/06/Jay-Amsterdam-today-filed-a-24-page-complaint-with-the-Office-of-Research-Integrity-at-the-US-National-Institutes-of-Health.pdf

63. Nardo, *1BOM*, November 29, 2012.

64. Ed Silverman, "Ghosts in the Pharma Attic," *Pharmalot*, June 12, 2012.

65. Keller, *Journal of the American Academy of Child and Adolescent Psychiatry* (2001), 763.

66. Dwight L. Evans and Dennis S. Charney, "Mood Disorders and Medical Illness: A Major Public Health Problem," *Biological Psychiatry*, 54 (2003), 177–180. https://www.biologicalpsychiatryjournal.com/article/S0006-3223(03)00639-5/abstract

67. Charles B. Nemeroff et al., "VNS Therapy in Treatment-Resistant Depression: Clinical Evidence and Putative Neurobiological Mechanisms," *Neuropsychopharmacology*, 31 (2006), 1345–1355. doi:10.1038/sj.npp.1301082

68. *Journal of the American Academy of Child and Adolescent Psychiatry*, compilation of reviewers' comments, August 16, 2000, reviewer #1. https://www.justice.gov/archives/opa/documents-and-resources-july-2-2012-glaxosmithkline-gsk-press-conference

69. Ed Silverman, "Ghosts in the Pharma Attic," *Pharmalot*, June 12, 2012.

70. Sally Laden to John Romankiewicz et al., December 14, 2000. https://www.industrydocuments.ucsf.edu/drug/docs/#id=snxl0228

71. Deirdre Zuccarello to D. Sheehan (copy to Sally Laden), September 13, 2000. http://industrydocuments.library.ucsf.edu/drug/docs/qnfw0217

72. Zachary Hawkins to "All Sales Representatives Selling *Paxil*," August 16, 2001. http://industrydocuments.library.ucsf.edu/drug/docs/zmfw0217

73. Sally K. Laden, deposition, In the United States District Court for the Eastern District of Pennsylvania, the Estate of Scott Randall v. SmithKline Beecham Corporation, C A No 06-3022-TJS, March 15, 2007, 108–115. pogoarchives.org/m/ph/sally-laden-sti-deposition-20070315.pdf

74. David Duff to investigators, May 10, 1999. http://industrydocuments.library.ucsf.edu/drug/docs/nlfw0217

75. James P. McCafferty to Sally Laden, July 19, 1999. http://industrydocuments.library.ucsf.edu/drug/docs/kzfw0217

76. Bernard Carroll, comment, *1BOM*, September 10, 2015, 3.

Chapter 18

1. Walter Brown, interview, Ban, ed., *Oral History of Neuropsychopharmacology*, V, 55.

2. Leo E. Hollister, "Strategies for Research in Clinical Psychopharmacology," in Herbert Y. Meltzer, ed., *Psychopharmacology: The Third Generation of Progress* (New York: Raven Press, 1987), 31–38, 32.

3. See the first ad for Mellaril, *New York State Journal of Medicine*, 59 (1959), 2517–2522.

4. News story, *Scrip*, August 25, 2000, 20.

5. For a deconstruction of the whole "atypical" notion, see Tim Kendall, "The Rise and Fall of the Atypical Antipsychotics," *BJP*, 199 (2011), 266–268. https://pdfs. semanticscholar.org/30bd/5d63d40b09d211039eb3f081abb14259b78e.pdf

6. Robert Temple to Mr. Prettyman, National Center for Drugs and Biologics, FDA, December 19, 1983; Federal Archives, UD–O4W, E3, accession 88-89-16, box 28.

7. Leo Hollister, "Strategies for Research in Clinical Psychopharmacology," in Herbert Y. Meltzer, ed., *Psychopharmacology: The Third Generation of Progress* (New York: Raven Press, 1987), 31–38, 31.

8. Heinrich Gross and E. Langner, "Das Wirkungsprofil eines chemisch neuartigen Breitband-Neuroleptikums der Dibenzodiazepingruppe" ["The impact profile of a chemically novel broad-band neuroleptic of the dibenzodiazepine group"], *The Wiener Medizinische Wochenschrift*, 116 (1966), 815–816. This is the Heinrich Gross who was accused of practicing euthanasia on children as a psychiatrist during the Nazi period. Incredibly, he was honored in Austria after the war, even though insiders knew that many of the sections of children's brain tissue he was continually analyzing came from a hospital where the children were killed.

9. But see Li Chun-Rong et al., "Clozapine-induced Tardive Dyskinesia in Schizophrenic Patients Taking Clozapine as a First-line Antipsychotic Drug," *World Journal of Biological Psychiatry*, 10 (2009), 919–924. https://pubmed.ncbi.nlm.nih. gov/19995222

10. Jules Angst, "Fifty Years in Psychiatry," in Thomas Ban, et al., eds., *Reflections on Twentieth-Century Psychopharmacology* (Budapest: Animula, 2004), 195–201, 197–198.

11. Jules Angst et al., "Ergebnisse eines Doppelblindversuches von HF 1854" [Results of a Double-blind trial of HF 1854], *Pharmakopsych*, 4 (1971), 192–200. HF 1854 is clozapine. See also Angst, "Das klinische Wirkungsbild von Clozapin" ["The clinical-effectiveness picture of Clozapine'], *Pharmakopsych*, 4 (1971), 201–211.

12. Hanns Hippius, interview, in Healy, ed., *Psychopharmacologists*, I, 202–203.

13. Günther Stille and Hanns Hippius, "Kritische Stellungnahme zum Begriff der Neuroleptika (anhand von pharmakologischen und klinischen Befunden mit Clozapin)" ["Critical review of the concept of neurolepetics given the example of pharmacological and clinical findings with Clozapine"], *Pharmakopsych*, 4 (1971), 182–191.

14. According to Robert Temple, PDAC, March 23, 2006, 174.

15. Hanns Hippius, interview, in Healy, ed., *Psychopharmacologists*, I, 202–203.

16. News story, *Scrip*, August 15, 1990, 25.

17. John Kane, discussion, PDAC, April 26, 1989, 168–169. Obtained through the Freedom of Information Act.

18. George Simpson, interview, in Healy, ed., *Psychopharmacologists*, II, 299.

19. See Meltzer, autobiography, in Ban, ed., *Oral History of Psychopharmacology*, IX, 260. He said that his various observations in the mid-1980s "led Sandoz to develop the drug."

20. John Kane et al., "Clozapine for the Treatment-Resistant Schizophrenic: A Double-blind Comparison with Chlorpromazine," *AGP*, 45 (1988), 789–796.

21. See Kristian Wahlbeck et al., "Letter: Sponsored Drug Trials Show More-Favourable Outcomes," *BMJ*, 318 (February 13, 1999), 465.

22. On the history of clozapine, see John Crilly, "The History of Clozapine and Its Emergence in the US Market: A Review and Analysis," *History of Psychiatry*, 18 (2007), 39–60.

23. Thomas Laughren, comment, PDAC, April 26, 1989, 79–80.

24. Alfred Goodman Gilman et al., eds., *Goodman and Gilman's The Pharmacological Basis of Therapeutics*, 8th ed. (New York: McGraw-Hill, 1990), 391.

25. Alan A. Baumeister and Jennifer L. Francis, "Historical Development of the Dopamine Hypothesis of Schizophrenia," *Journal of the History of the Neurosciences*, 11 (2002), 265–277, 274.

26. Paul Leber, discussion, PDAC, July 24, 1995, 69. Obtained through the Freedom of Information Act.

27. Frank J. Ayd, Jr., interview, in Ban, ed., *Oral History of Psychopharmacology*, X, 41.

28. Pierre Simon, interview, in Healy, ed., *Psychopharmacologists,* III, 527.

29. Alan J. Gelenberg, "Antipsychotics, Typical and Atypical," *Biological Therapies in Psychiatry Newsletter*, 17 (11) (November 1994), 42–43.

30. John Kane, discussion, PDAC, June 16, 2003, 124.

31. Paul Leber, discussion, PDAC, July 25, 1995, 60.

32. David Healy, personal communication, January 10, 2009.

33. Thomas J. Moore et al., "Serious Adverse Drug Events Reported to the Food and Drug Administration, 1998–2005," *Archives of Internal Medicine*, 167 (2007), 1752–1759.

34. Paul Janssen, interview with David Healy, manuscript transcript, 17–18. I am grateful to Dr. Healy for sharing this transcript with me.

35. David Healy, interview of Paul Leber, June 9, 2008, 21. I am grateful to Dr. Healy for letting me see a copy of this manuscript.

36. Carol Tamminga and John Kane, discussion, PDAC, July 24, 1995, 60–61. Obtained through the Freedom of Information Act.

37. Paul Leber, discussion, PDAC, July 25, 1995, 31. Obtained through the Freedom of Information Act.

38. See David Cunningham Owens, "What CATIE Did: Some Thoughts on Implications Deep and Wide," *Psychiatric Services*, 59 (5) (May 2008), 530–533.

39. Risperdal ad, *BJP*, 163 (July–December 1993), 19b-c.

40. Risperdal ad, *AJP*, 158 (October 2001), A22. The ad mentioned only the Janssen name but not Risperdal. The point was to gullet the competition.

41. Risperdal ad, *AJP*, 161 (January 2004), A9–15.

42. Zyprexa ad, *AJP*, 158 (February 9, 2001), ad pages.

43. Miranda Chakos et al., "Effectiveness of Second-Generation Antipsychotics in Patients with Treatment-Resistant Schizophrenia: A Review and Meta-Analysis of Randomized Trials," *AJP*, April 1, 2001. https://ajp.psychiatryonline.org/doi/10.1176/appi.ajp.158.4.518

44. For a complete list, see https://www.ncbi.nlm.nih.gov/books/NBK169721/table/T1

45. Carl Salzman, discussion, PDAC, July 25, 1995, 122. Obtained through the Freedom of Information Act.

46. For the development of Seroquel (quetiapine), see Edward Warawa, interview, in Healy, ed., *Psychopharmacologists*, III, 508–518.

47. See Nardo, *1BOM*, February 14, 2011, 2.

48. Documents cited in this section may be found at http://psychrights.org/research/Digest/NLPs/Seroquel/ See "parent directory."

49. Richard Lawrence to distribution, February 12, 1997, exhibit #13. http://psychrights.org/research/Digest/NLPs/Seroquel/

50. Nardo, *1BOM*, February 14, 2011, 3.

51. Lisa Arvanitis to distribution, August 13, 1997, exhibit #10. http://psychrights.org/research/Digest/NLPs/Seroquel

52. Christopher T. Maurer to Team, October 2, 2002; Campbell, exhibit #13l. http://psychrights.org/research/Digest/NLPs/Seroquel/

53. William Hess to team, June 23, 2003; Piano, exhibit #27l. http://psychrights.org/research/Digest/NLPs/Seroquel/

54. Johan Hoegstedt to executives, August 18, 2003; Jackson exhibit #3. http://psychrights.org/research/Digest/NLPs/Seroquel/

55. See correspondence attached to Edward Repp to team, February 19, 2004; Repp exhibit #42. http://psychrights.org/research/Digest/NLPs/Seroquel/

56. Nardo, *1BOM*, October 4, 2011, 3.

57. Lauren Duby to Parexel team, December 2, 2005; Macfadden exhibit, #69. http://psychrights.org/research/Digest/NLPs/Seroquel/

58. "Oral Deposition of Wayne Macfadden." In the United States District Court, Middle District of Florida, Orlando Division, in re: Seroquel Products Liability Litigation,306–307, 716–733; Case no. 6:06-md-01769-ACC-DAB, exhibit A. http://psychrights.org/Research/Digest/NLPs/Seroquel/090303Docs/Ghostwriting%20Lim%20Resp.%20Ex%20A.pdf

59. United States District Court, Middle District of Florida, Orlando Division, in re: Seroquel Products Liability Litigation. All Unnamed Plaintiffs v. AstraZeneca Pharmaceuticals [2009], 11. Sales figures on 7. http://psychrights.org/research/Digest/NLPs/Seroquel/InReSeroquelMasterComplaint.pdf

60. Stephen R. Marder and Richard C. Meibach, "Risperidone in the Treatment of Schizophrenia," *AJP*, 151 (1994), 825–835, 834.

61. Videotape deposition of Alex Gorsky, May 18, 2012. In the Court of Common Pleas, First Judicial District of Pennsylvania, Civil Trial Division, In re: Risperdal Litigation: March Term, 2010217-218. Link at: Steven Brill, "America's Most Admired Lawbreaker," Huffington Post (2015, 231). http://highline.huffingtonpost.com/miracleindustry/americas-most-admired-lawbreaker/

62. Ben Wallace-Wells, "Bitter Pill: How the Pharmaceutical Industry Turned a Flawed and Dangerous Drug into a $16 Billion Bonanza," *Rolling Stone*, February 5, 2009, 13.

63. Bernard Carroll, comment, *1BOM*, September 1, 2011, 4.

64. Lilly company document, quoted in *1BOM*, October 15, 2011, 2.

65. Matt Keats, January 24, 2009, to psycho-pharm@psycom.net

66. Jay Amsterdam to colleagues, August 4, 2019.

67. John Geddes et al., "Atypical Antipsychotics in the Treatment of Schizophrenia: Systematic Overview and Meta-Regression Analysis," *BMJ*, 321 (December 2, 2000), 1371–1376, 1371.

68. Marvin S. Swartz et al., "What CATIE Found: Results from the Schizophrenia Trial," *Psychiatric Services*, 59 (5) (May 2008), 500–506. https://www.ncbi.nlm.nih.gov/pmc/articles/PMC5033643/

69. Marie N. Stagnitti, "Trends in the Use and Expenditures for the Therapeutic Class Prescribed Psychotherapeutic Agents and All Subclasses, 1997 and 2004," *Medical Expenditure Panel Survey, Statistical Brief #163 of the Agency for Healthcare Research and Quality*, February 2007, Fig. 1.

70. James Van Norman testimony; State of Texas, ex rel. Allen Jones, Plaintiffs, v. Janssen . . . Defendants. Travis County Texas, January 11, 2012, 176–178. The proceedings are at: http://1boringoldman.com/index.php/2012/01/26/the-trial/

71. Nardo, *1BOM*, July 2, 2013, 3. Nardo said, "While the trend line is not significant . . . it's hard to look at that graph and not see the price of a little efficacy being a lot of weight gain (maybe metabolic syndrome)."

72. T. E. Goldberg et al., "Cognitive Improvement After Treatment with Second-Generation Antipsychotics Medications in First-Episode Schizophrenia: Is It a Practice Effect?" *AGP*, 64 (2007), 1115–1122.

73. Mark Moran, "Study Questions 'Real World' Benefits of Newer Antipsychotics," *Psychiatric News*, November 16, 2007, 1, 24.

74. Peter B. Jones et al., "Randomized Controlled Trial of the Effect on Quality of Life of Second- vs First-Generation Antipsychotic Drugs in Schizophrenia: Cost Utility of the Latest Antipsychotic Drugs in Schizophrenia Study (CUTLASS 1)," *AGP*, 63 (2006), 1079–1087.

75. Mark Moran, "Experts Square Off Across Antipsychotic Generation Gap," *Psychiatric News*, July 1, 2005, 1, 48.

76. George Simpson, interview, in Ban, ed., *Oral History of Neuropsychopharmacology*, IX, 299.

77. Scott W. Woods et al., "Incidence of Tardive Dyskinesia with Atypical Versus Conventional Antipsychotic Medications: A Prospective Cohort Study," *Journal of Clinical Psychiatry*, 71 (2010), 463–474, 469.

78. Silvio Garattini, interview, in Ban, ed., *Oral History of Psychopharmacology*, III, 214.

79. Leo Hollister, interview, in Ban, ed., *Oral History of Neuropsychopharmacology*, IX, 161–162.

80. Peter Tyrer and Tim Kendall, "The Spurious Advance of Antipsychotic Drug Therapy," *Lancet*, 373 (9657) (January 3, 2009), 4–5. doi:10.1016/S0140-6736(08)61765-1

81. Stefan Leucht et al., "Second-Generation Versus First-Generation Antipsychotic Drugs for Schizophrenia: A Meta-Analysis," *Lancet*, 373 (9657) (January 3, 2009), 31–41. doi:10.1016/S0140-6736(08)61764-X

82. Robert Farley, "Drug Research: To Test or To Tout?" April 12, 2008. www.psychrights.org/Articles/080413RFarleyTestOrToutStPetTimes.htm

83. William T. Carpenter, Jr., interview, in Ban, ed., *Oral History of Neuropsychopharmacology*, V, 81.

84. On the huge literature on the psychopathology of schizophrenia, very helpful is Michael Alan Taylor and Nutan Atre Vaidya, *Descriptive Psychopathology: The Signs and Symptoms of Behavioral Disorders* (New York: Cambridge UP, 2009) and Michael Alan Taylor, *The Fundamentals of Clinical Neuropsychiatry* (New York: Oxford UP, 1999).

85. Jay Amsterdam to correspondents, June 1, 2017.

86. Nardo, *1BOM*, September 30, 2015, 2.

87. "Preliminary Data from InfoScriber's Clinical Pharmacology Network (CPN)," *CPN press release*, February 20, 2001. http://headlines.mentalhealthnet.ord/inf/

88. Daniel M. Hartung et al., "Patterns of Atypical Antipsychotic Subtherapeutic Dosing Among Oregon Medicaid Patients," *Journal of Clinical Psychiatry*, August 26, 2008, e1–e8, https://pubmed.ncbi.nlm.nih.gov/19192436/

89. Jay Amsterdam to correspondents, January 7, 2018.

90. Ivan Goldberg to psycho-pharm@psycom.net, December 24, 2007.

91. Steven Brill, "America's Most Admired Lawbreaker," *Huffington Post* (2015), 39. http://highline.huffingtonpost.com/miracleindustry/americas-most-admired-lawbreaker/

92. https://www.drugs.com/news/releases-q4-sales-top-100-u-s-abilify-overtakes-nexium-top-sales-43016.html

93. Helen C. Kales et al., "Mortality Risk in Patients with Dementia Treated with Antipsychotics Versus Other Psychiatric Medications," *AJP*, 164 (2007), 1568–1576. https://www.researchgate.net/profile/Francesca_Cunningham/publication/5947085_Mortality_Risk_in_Patients_With_Dementia_Treated_With_Antipsychotics_Versus_Other_Psychiatric_Medications/links/00b7d52ca9a5435eaf000000.pdf

94. See, In the United States District Court for the Eastern District of Pennsylvania. United States of America v. Janssen Pharmaceutica. November 4, 2013, 11–22. http://highline.huffingtonpost.com/miracleindustry/americas-most-admired-lawbreaker/assets/documents/5/highlighted-us-complaint-pa.pdf?build=01121512 On the sales increase, see "Geriatrics Market Share" slide, in slide deck "LTC Group Update to MCC," 12/15/1999; document no, JNJ 289711. https://www.justice.gov/archives/opa/documents-and-resources-november-4-2013-johnson-johnson-jj-press-conference Document Massachusetts #4.

95. News story, *Scrip*, April 20, 2005, 23.

96. In the United States District Court for the Eastern District of Pennsylvania, University States of America v. Janssen Pharmaceutica Products, November 13, 2013, 11. http://highline.huffingtonpost.com/miracleindustry/americas-most-admired-lawbreaker/assets/documents/5/highlighted-us-complaint-pa.pdf?build=01121512 This was a civil, not a criminal, action.

97. "LTC/Geriatrics: 2001 Business Plan," #12. https://www.justice.gov/archives/opa/documents-and-resources-november-4-2013-johnson-johnson-ii--press-conference

98. United States District Court, District of Massachusetts, United States of America v. Johnson & Johnson, Civil Action no. 07-10288-RGS, document 81, January 15, 2010, page 1. https://www.justice.gov/archives/opa/documents-and-resources-november-4-2013-johnson-johnson-ii--press-conference

99. In the United States District Court for the Eastern District of Pennsylvania, United States of America v. Janssen Pharmaceutica, "Information," November 4, 2013, 27–28. http://highline.huffingtonpost.com/miracle-industry/americas-most-admired-lawbreaker/assets/documents/5/highlighted-us-complaint-pa.pdf?build=01121512

100. Samuel Gershon, "Events and Memories," INHN Educational Series 3, Collated 12, 24–25. http://inhn.org/biographies/samuel-gershon-events-and-memories/samuel-gershon-events-and-memories-8-neuropathology.html

101. Alex Gorsky deposition, May 18, 2012, 156, 162, 186. https://highline.huffingtonpost.com/miracleindustry/americas-most-admired-lawbreaker/assets/documents/1/gorsky-deposition-2012.pdf?build=02281049

102. See "Janssen: Record of FDA Contact," March 3, 2000; #14; RISP-REM-1702684. https://www.justice.gov/archives/opa/documents-and-resources-november-4-2013-johnson-johnson-ii-press-conference

103. Linmarie Sikich et al., "Double-Blind Comparison of First- and Second-Generation Antipsychotics in Early-Onset Schizophrenia and Schizo-affective Disorder: Findings From the Treatment of Early-Onset Schizophrenia and Schizophrenia Spectrum Disorders (TEOSS) Study," *AJP* 2008. https://doi.org/10.1176/appi.ajp.2008.08050756

104. Nardo, *1BOM*, March 24, 2011, 4.

105. Benedict Carey, "Study of Newer Antipsychotics Finds Risks for Youths," *New York Times*, September 15, 2008, A17. This is also the source of information on the increase in prescribing of SGAs, 1994–2004.

106. Mark Kramer, "Commentary" on Barry Blackwell, "Corporate Corruption in the Psychopharmaceutical Industry" (2016), October 13, 2016, 95–96, in INHN; http://inhn.org/fileadmin/user_upload/User_Uploads/INHN/FILES/Kramers

107. Lucette Lagnado, "U.S. Probes Use of Antipsychotic Drugs on Children; Federal Health Officials Are Reviewing Antipsychotic Drug Use on Children in the Medicaid System," *Wall Street Journal*, August 1, 2013.

108. Martin Schumacher, personal communication to Edward Shorter, June 11, 2020.

109. Bernard Carroll to correspondents, June 13, 2018.

110. Bernard Carroll, comment, *1BOM*, March 15, 2013, 5.

111. Robert B. Ostroff and J. Craig Nelson, "Risperidone Augmentation of Selective Serotonin Reuptake Inhibitors in Major Depression," *Journal of Clinical Psychiatry*, 60 (1999), 256–259.

112. C. B. Nemeroff, G. M. Gharabawi, C. M. Canuso, T. Mahmoud, A. Loescher, I. Turkoz et al., "Augmentation with Risperidone in Chronic Resistant Depression: A Double-blind Placebo-controlled Maintenance Trial" [abstract], *Neuropsychopharmacology*, 29, Suppl. 1 (2004), S159.

113. Charles Nemeroff, "Use of Atypical Antipsychotics in Refractory Depression and Anxiety," *Journal of Clinical Psychiatry*, 66, Suppl. 8 (2005), 13–21.

114. Mark Hyman Rapaport…Charles B. Nemeroff, "Effects of Risperidone Augmentation in Patients with Treatment-Resistant Depression: Results of Open-Label Treatment Followed by Double-Blind Continuation" *Neuropsychopharmacology*, 31 (2006), 2505–13 https://www.nature.com/articles/1301113

115. Bernard Carroll, letter, "Effects of Risperidone Augmentation in Patients with Treatment-Resistant Depression:," *Neuropsychopharmacology*, 33 (2008), 2546–2547. https://www.nature.com/articles/1301613

116. Gabor I. Keitner, Steven J. Garlow, Christine E. Ryan, Philip T. Ninan, David A. Solomon, Charles B. Nemeroff, and Martin B. Keller, "A Randomized, Placebo-Controlled Trial of Risperidone Augmentation for Patients with Difficult-to-Treat Unipolar, Non-psychotic Major Depression," *Journal of Psychiatric Research*, 43 (2009), 205–214. doi:10.1016/j.psychires.2008.05.003 All authors were listed as "supported by an InvestigatorInitiated Grant from Janssen Pharmaceutica."

117. Mark H. Pollack, "Comorbid Anxiety and Depression," *Journal of Clinical Psychiatry*, 66, Suppl. 8 (2005), 22–29.

118. Bernard Carroll, comment, *1BOM*, October 4, 2011, 4.

119. Nardo, *1BOM*, February 14, 2011, 2.

120. Bernard Carroll, letter, "Antipsychotic Drugs for Depression?" *AJP*, 167 (2010), 216–217. For a shattering account of the thinness of the evidence base on behalf of using aripiprazole in bipolar disorder, see Alexander C. Tsai, Nicholas Z. Rosenlicht, Jon N. Jureidini, Peter I. Parry, Glen I. Spielmans, and David Healy, "Aripiprazole in the Maintenance Treatment of Bipolar Disorder: A Critical Review of the Evidence and Its Dissemination into the Scientific Literature," *PLOS Medicine*, May 3, 2011. https://doi.org/10.137/journal.prmed.1000434

121. Bernard Carroll, comment, *1BOM,* March 15, 2013.

122. Nardo, *1BOM*, December 31, 2015, 2.

Chapter 19

1. The TMAP proceedings cited in this section are at: http://1boringoldman.com/index.php/2012/01/26/the-trial/

2. Allen Jones, untitled document, revised January 20, 2004. http://psychrights.org/Drugs/AllenJonesTMAPJanuary20.pdf

3. But he did attend the meeting in 1996 where the guidelines were presented. Texas v Janssen, January 12, 2012, 17.

4. Texas v. Janssen, January 10, 2012, 104.

5. Texas v. Janssen, January 10, 107–108.

6. [Rothman Report], David J. Rothman, "Expert Witness Report," October 15, 2010, 14–16. Texas v. Janssen, January 10, 2012, 103. jannel.se/Rothman.Report.pdf

7. Texas v. Janssen, January 10, 2012, 188.

8. [Rothman Report], "Expert Witness Report," October 15, 2010, 14.

9. Texas v. Janssen, January 10, 2012, 26.

10. There is in fact a whole literature on such guidelines. See David A. Kahn, John P. Docherty, Daniel Carpenter, and Allen Frances, "Consensus Methods in Practice and Guidelines Development: A Review and Description of a New Method," *Psychopharmacology Bulletin*, 33 (1997), 631–639. John Rush and Allen Frances,

"Expert Consensus Guideline Series: Treatment of Psychiatric and Behavioral Problems in Mental Retardation," *American Journal of Mental Retardation*, 105 (2000), 159–228.

11. Joseph P. McEvoy, Patricia L. Scheifler, and Allen Frances, "The Expert Consensus Guideline Series: Treatment of Schizophrenia, 1999," *Journal of Clinical Psychiatry*, 60, Suppl. 11 (1999), 1–80, 75.

12. Texas v. Janssen, January 12, 2012, 16.

13. See Nardo, *1BOM*, June 1, 2011, 1. On "wholesale," see Rothman Report, 19

14. Rothman Report, 30.

15. Craig Malisow, "Down the Hatch," *Houston Press*, December 14, 2011.

16. Malisow, "Down the Hatch."

17. Rothman Report, 24.

18. John A. Chiles, Alexander L. Miller, M. Lynn Crismon, John Rush, Amy S. Krasnoff, Steven S. Shon, "The Texas Medication Algorithm Project: Development and Implementation of the Schizophrenia Algorithm," at: http://dx.doi..org/10.1176/ps.50.1.69 According to the *Houston Press,* Lynn Crismon had received from Janssen "at least $61,000"; Alexander Miller, $82,000; and John Chiles, $151,254.

19. Rothman Report, 25.

20. State of Texas v. Janssen, January 12, 2012, 109–111.

21. Melody Petersen, "Making Drugs, Shaping the Rules," *New York Times*, February 1, 2004.

22. Steven Brill, "America's Most Admired Lawbreaker," *Huffington Post*, September 16, 2015, 21; http://highline.huffingtonpost.com/miracleindustry/americas-most-admired-lawbreaker/

23. State of Texas v. Janssen, January 9, 2012, 79.

24. State of Texas v. Janssen, January 10, 2012, 9.

25. Melody Petersen, "Making Drugs, Shaping the Rules," *New York Times*, February 1, 2004. Jones testimony in Texas v. Janssen, January 12, 2012, 79–81.

26. Texas v. Janssen, January 11, 2012, 181–183.

27. Nardo, *1BOM*, March 17, 2012, 1.

28. Tone Jones, testimony, State of Texas v. Janssen, January 18, 2012, 12.

29. Nardo, *1BOM,* January 21, 2012, 1.

Chapter 20

1. John Gregory, *Lectures on the Duties and Qualifications of a Physician* (London: Strahan, 1770), 41.

2. Nardo, *1BOM,* January 10, 2012, 4.

3. Thomas Detre, interview, in Ban, ed., *Oral History of Neuropsychopharmacology*, X, 55. The beginnings were in the 1970s.

4. Philip Solomon, "Introduction," in P. Solomon, ed., *Psychiatric Drugs: Proceedings of a Research Conference Held in Boston* (New York: Grune & Stratton, 1966), 1–2, 1.

5. Peter Tyrer, "The End of the Psychopharmacological Revolution," *British Journal of Psychiatry*, 201 (2018). https://doi.org/10.1192/bjp.201.2.168

6. James O'Brien, comment, *1BOM*, February 7, 2016, 8.

7. Editorial, *Journal of the Royal College of Physicians*, 11 (1977), 217–218, 218.

8. Nardo, *1BOM*, September 8, 2015, 1.

9. Nardo, *1BOM*, March 17, 2012, 1.

10. Susanna Every-Palmer, "How Evidence-Based Medicine Is Failing Due to Biased Trials and Selective Publication," *Journal of Evaluation in Clinical Practice*, 20 (2014). https://onlinelibrary.wiley.com/doi/full/10.1111/jep.12147

11. Mark Kramer, "Commentary" on Barry Blackwell: Corporate Corruption in the Psychopharmaceutical Industry, October 13, 2016, 9–10. http://inhn.org/fileadmin/user_upload/User_Uploads/INHN/FILES/Kramers-__LM_Revised_commentary_-_October_13__2016.pdfcommentaries,inhn.com

12. Arvid Carlsson, "Monoamines of the Central Nervous System: A Historical Perspective," in Herbert Y. Meltzer, ed., *Psychopharmacology: The Third Generation of Progress* (New York: Raven Press, 1987), 39–48, 46.

13. [name redacted], post of January 30, 2007, to psycho-pharm@psycom.net

14. Rick Mullin, "Cost to Develop New Pharmaceutical Drug Now Exceeds $2.5B," *Scientific American*, November 24, 2014. https://www.scientificamerican.com/article/cost-to-develop-new-pharmaceutical-drug-now-exceeds-2-5b/

15. H. Christian Fibiger, "Editorial: Psychiatry, The Pharmaceutical Industry, and the Road to Better Therapeutics," *Schizophrenia Bulletin*, 38 (2012), 649–650.

16. Martin Schumacher, personal communication, June 6, 2020.

17. https://www.ddw-online.com/therapeutics/p216813-the-great-neuro-pipeline-brain-drain-why-big-pharma-hasn-t-given-up-on-cns-disorders.html

18. Jun Yan, "APF Convenes Unique Pipeline Summit," *Psychiatric News*, April 6, 2012, 1, 34.

19. https://www.drugtopics.com/drug-topics/content/top-200-drugs-retail-sales-2000

20. https://www.fiercepharma.com/special-report/top-20-drugs-by-2018-u-s-sales

21. Erika Reis-Arndt, "25 Jahre Arzneimittelforschung: Neue pharmazeutische Wirkstoffe 1961–1985" ["25 Years of Medication Research: New Pharmaceutica Agents"], *Pharma Dialog*, April 1987, 3–26, 22 tab. 6. "Neue Wirkstoffe: Neurotonika" [New Agents: Neurotonics].

22. Jule P. Miller, III (Biloxi MS), "30 Years of Psychiatry with No Fundamental Progress," *Current Psychiatry*, 14 (2015), 46.

23. Barry Blackwell, *Bits and Pieces of a Psychiatrist's Life* (Philadelphia: Xlibris, 2012), 210.

24. Bernard Carroll to correspondents, January 5, 2017.

25. James O'Brien, post, *1BOM*, October 28, 2014, 12.

26. David Healy, "Serotonin and Depression: The Marketing of a Myth," *BMJ*, April 21, 2015. doi:10.1136/bmj.h1771

27. Len Cook, interview, in Ban, ed., *Oral History of Psychopharmacology*, I, 138–139.

28. Bernard Carroll, post, *1BOM*, October 28, 2014, 8.

29. Mark Kramer to correspondents, June 5, 2016.

30. Nardo, *1BOM*, April 12, 2012, 3–4.

31. Joseph J. Schildkraut, "The Catecholamine Hypothesis of Affective Disorders: A Review of Supporting Evidence," *AJP*, 122 (1965), 509–522.

32. Arvid Carlsson, interview by David Healy and Edward Shorter, February 28, 2007, 19. See Arvid Carlsson et al., "Effect of Chlorpromazine or Haloperidol on Formation of 3-Methoxytyramine and Normetanephrine in Mouse Brain," *Acta Pharmacol et Toxicol* [Acta Pharmacologica et Toxicologica], 20 (1963), 140–144.

33. Alfred Burger, "Medicinal Chemistry· A Personal View," in Corwin Hansch, ed., *Comprehensive Medicinal Chemistry* (Oxford: Pergamon Press, 1990), I, 1–5, 4.

34. Frank M. Berger, interview, in Ban, ed., *Oral History of Neuropsychopharmacology*, IX, 55.

35. Solomon Snyder, interview, Healy, ed., *Psychopharmacologists*, III, 234–235.

36. Donald Klein to correspondents, January 7, 2017

37. Jay Amsterdam to correspondents, January 8, 2017.

38. Joshua Gordon, "New Hope for Treatment-Resistant Depression: Guessing Right on Ketamine." https://www.nimh.nih.gov/about/director/messages/2019/new-hope-for-treatment-resistant-depression-guessing-right-on-ketamine.shtml

39. Lisa Stockbridge to Todd McIntyre (Janssen regulatory affairs), January 5, 1999. https://www.justice/gov/archives/opa/documents-and-resources-november-4-2013-johnson-johnson-ii-press-conference

40. *Physicians' Desk Reference*, 2001, 1580.

41. Erik Turner to correspondents, January 8, 2017.

42. George Beaumont, discussion, in E. M. Tansey et al., eds., *Wellcome Witnesses to Twentieth Century Medicine* (London: Wellcome Trust, September 1998), II, 196.

43. Leo Hollister interviewing George A. Aghajanian, in Ban, ed., *Oral History of Neuropsychopharmacology*, II, 186.

44. A. O. Oluyomi, K. P. Datla, and G. Curzon, "Effects of the (+) and (-) Enantiomers of the Antidepressant Drug Tianeptine on 5-HTP-Induced Behavior," *Neuropharmacology*, 36 (1997), 383–387.

45. Martin Schumacher, personal communication, June 6, 2020.

46. Thomas A. Ban, interview, Healy, ed., *Psychopharmacologists*, I, 619.

47. Sam Gershon to correspondents, January 8, 2017. Representative of this work is S. Gershon, L. J. Hekimian, A. Floyd, and L. E. Hollister, "Methylparatyrosine (AMP) in Schizophrenia," *Psychopharmacology*, 11 (1967), 189–194.

48. Marta Peciña et al., "Endogenous Opioid System Dysregulation in Depression: Implications for New Therapeutic Approaches," *Molecular Psychiatry*, 24 (2019), 576–587.

49. "Neuroskeptic," in *1BOM*, May 4, 2016, 1.

50. This particular finding is from Charles Shagass and Arthur L. Jones, "A Neurophysiological Test for Psychiatric Diagnosis: Results in 750 Patients," *AJP*, 114 (1958), 1002–1010, tab. 1, 1003.

51. Jay Amsterdam to correspondents, March 28, 2017.

52. Nathan S. Kline, "Manipulation of Life Patterns with Drugs," in Wayne O. Evans and Nathan S. Kline eds., *Psychotropic Drugs in the Year 2000* (Springfield: Charles C Thomas, 1971), 69–85, 69.

53. Amsterdam to correspondents, May 13, 2017.

54. Blackwell, *Bits and Pieces*, 210.

55. Roy Poses, *Health Care Renewal*, April 6, 2013. http://hcrenewal.blogspot,ca/2013/04/walk-walk-for-some-time-jeremiad-theme.html

56. On dismantling "schizophrenia" into "subgroups" of psychosis, see Dominic B. Dwyer et al., "An Investigation of Psychosis Subgroups with Prognostic Validation and Exploration of Genetic Underpinnings: The PsyCourse Study," *JAMA Psychiatry*, February 12, 2020. https://jamanetwork.com/journals/jamapsychiatry/fullarticle/2760515?guestAccessKey=d3b6d1fd-363d-4b00-8cde-05c03a3dc2bd&utm_source=silverchair&utm_medium=email&utm_campaign=article_alert-jamapsychiatry&utm_content=olf&utm_term=021220

57. Manfred Bleuler, "Comparison of Drug-Induced and Endogenous Psychoses in Man," in P. B. Bradley et al., eds., *Neuropsychopharmacology: Proceedings of the First International Congress of Neuro-pharmacology (Rome, September 1958)* (Amsterdam: Elsevier, 1959), 161–165, 164–165.

58. Gerald L. Klerman, "Future Prospects for Clinical Psychopharmacology," in Herbert Y. Meltzer, ed., *Psychopharmacology: The Third Generation of Progress* (New York: Raven Press, 1987), 1699–1705, 1702–1703.

59. Nancy C. Andreasen, "Positive and Negative Symptoms: Historical and Conceptual Aspects," in N. C. Andreasen, ed., *Schizophrenia: Positive and Negative Symptoms and Syndromes; Modern Problems in Pharmacopsychiatry* (Basel: Karger, 1990), vol. 24, 1–42, 1.

60. Conan Kornetsky, interview, in Ban, ed., *Oral History of Neuropsychopharmacology*, VI, 162–163.

61. Conan Kornetsky, "Hyporesponsivity of Chronic Schizophrenic Patients to Dextroamphetamine," *AGP*, 33 (1976), 1425–1428.

62. George M. Simpson, interview, in Ban, ed., *Oral History of Neuropsychopharmacology*, IX, 312.

63. Jan Fawcett, quoted in Nardo to correspondents, March 14, 2014.

64. Caroline White, "Brain Circuitry Model for Mental Illness Will Transform Management, NIH mental health director," *BMJ*, September 1, 2011, 343. https://doi.org/10.1136/bmj.d5581

65. Thomas Ban, http://inhn.org/no_cache/home/central-office-cordoba-unit/education/thomas-a-ban-neuropsychopharmacology-in-historical-perspective-education-in-the-field-in-the-post-neuropsychopharmacology-era/bulletin-75-the-confounding-of-education-with-marketing.html?sword_list%5B0%5D=the&sword_list%5B1%5D=postneuropsychopharmacology&sword_list%5B2%5D=era

66. Nardo, *1BOM*, August 12, 2011, 1–2.

67. Jay Amsterdam to correspondents, April 9, 2019.

68. PDAC, July 25, 1995, 73–76. Obtained through the Freedom of Information Act.

69. Mayer Brezis, "Big Pharma and Health Care: Unsolvable Conflict of Interests between Private Enterprise and Public Health," *The Israeli Journal of Psychiatry and Related Sciences*, 45 (2008), 83–94, 84, 86.

70. Mark Kramer, "Commentary" on Barry Blackwell: Corporate Corruption in the Psychopharmaceutical Industry, October 13, 2016, 5. http://inhn.org/fileadmin/user_upload/User_Uploads/INHN/FILES/Kramers-__LM_Revised_commentary_-_October_13__2016.pdf

Chapter 21

1. *Scrip Magazine,* note, February 2000, 57.
2. Ivan Goldberg, post of March 2, 2008. psycho-pharm@psycom.net
3. Max Fink to correspondents, June 19, 2019.
4. Ross Baldessarini interview with Edward Shorter and Max Fink, February 17, 2006.
5. D. Kupfer, M. First, and D. Regier, *A Research Agenda for DSM-V* (Arlington: APA, 2002); D. Kupfer and D. Regier, "Neuroscience, Clinical Evidence, and the Future of Psychiatric Classification in DSM-5," *AJP*, 168 (2011), 672–674.
6. Gordon Parker, "Retrospective: Pursuing Melancholia: The Australian Contribution," *Australian & New Zealand Journal of Psychiatry*, 51 (2017), 7–8.
7. American Psychiatric Association, *Diagnostic and Statistical Manual of Mental Disorders*, 5th ed. (DSM-5) (Arlington VA: APA, 2013), 155.
8. " Ivan" [Goldberg], comment, *1BOM*, May 16, 2012, 3.
9. Kupfer and Regier, "Neuroscience, Clinical Evidence, and the Future," *AJP*, 168 (2011), 672–674.
10. Allen Frances, "DSM-5 Field Trials Discredit APA," *Psychology Today*, October 30, 2012.
11. Donald Klein to correspondents, August 27, 2016.
12. Joel Paris, *An Evidence-Based Critique of Contemporary Psychoanalysis* (New York: Routledge, 2019), 149.

Index

For the benefit of digital users, indexed terms that span two pages (e.g., 52–53) may, on occasion, appear on only one of those pages.

AACAP (American Academy of Child and Adolescent Psychiatry), 151–52, 216
Aarhus University, 37, 174–75
Abbott, 79, 294–95
Abilify (aripiprazole), 146, 281, 292, 296
Abrams, Richard, 103
acetylcholine, 32–33
ACNP (American College of Neuropsychopharmacology), 39, 48–49, 134, 193, 204, 221–22, 276, 305, 314–15, 317–18
ADAMHA (Alcohol, Drug Abuse, and Mental Health Administration), 103
Adderall, 196–97
ADHD (attention-deficit/hyperactivity disorder), 53, 62, 116, 121, 149–50, 196–97, 250, 292, 294
Adkison, Claudia, 157
adrenaline, 31
advertising. *See* industry and commerce; marketing and advertising
affect-laden paraphrenia, 116–17
Aghajanian, George, 314–15
Alcohol, Drug Abuse, and Mental Health Administration (ADAMHA), 103
Alexander, Leo, 64, 252
Allan Memorial Institute, 44
allopregnanolone, 252–53
alprazolam (Xanax), 191–92, 239, 244
Alzheimer's disease, 200
AMA. *See* American Medical Association
Amberson, J. Burns, 167
amentia, 65
American Academy of Child and Adolescent Psychiatry (AACAP), 151–52, 216
American Association for the Advancement of Science, 43, 172
American Association of Manufacturers of Medicinal Products, 22
American Board of Psychiatry and Neurology, 27

American College of Neuropsychopharmacology (ACNP), 39, 48–49, 134, 193, 204, 221–22, 276, 305, 314–15, 317–18
American Cyanamid, 80
American Drug Manufacturers Association, 23, 90–91
American Home Products, 80
American Journal of Geriatric Psychiatry, 217
American Journal of Pharmaceutical Education, 209
American Journal of Psychiatry, 49, 159–60, 187, 214–15, 226–27, 272
American Medical Association (AMA)
    Bureau of Investigation, 10
    Council on Pharmacy and Chemistry, 9, 10, 21–22
    Section on Nervous and Mental Diseases, 19
American Neurological Association, 78
American Pharmaceutical Manufacturers Association, 22, 23, 90–91
American Psychiatric Association (APA), 27, 35, 43, 105, 106, 107, 111, 115, 120, 122, 140–41, 144, 155, 160, 198, 204–6, 215–16, 219, 284, 289, 324, 325
American Psychiatric Press, 271
American Psychopathological Association, 13, 60, 113–14, 215–16
amitriptyline, 82, 135, 177
    Elavil, 54–55, 91, 255
    Triavil, 54–55
amoxapine (Asendin), 91, 177
amphetamines, 7, 23, 27–28, 73, 258, 319
Amsterdam, Jay, 52–53, 83, 94, 159, 160–61, 193, 197, 225–27, 228, 248–49, 259–60, 287, 291, 292, 313, 316–17, 320
Amytal (sodium amytal), 28, 50–51, 133–34
Anafranil (clomipramine), 163, 320–21
Andreasen, Nancy, 108–9, 121, 318–19
Angell, Marcia, 94–95, 226–27, 265–66
Angrist, Burton, 37

Angst, Jules, 179, 249, 276
antidepressants, 3–4, 20–21, 23, 39–40, 53–54,
    55–57, 59, 82–83, 92, 117–18, 121, 124–25,
    127–28, 135–36, 145, 159–60, 161, 177,
    178, 185, 187, 189, 193, 202, 226, 235, 243–
    63, 291, 313, 314, 315. See also depression;
    major depressive disorder; names of
    specific antidepressants
    administering sedatives with trial
        antidepressant , 193
    dangers of depression, 244–45
    imipramine, 179
    major depressive disorder, 250–54
    Paxil and Sally Laden, 265–74
antipsychotics, 3–4, 5, 7, 10, 11, 30, 43–44, 45,
    47, 48, 51, 52, 53–54, 55–57, 59, 68, 121,
    153–54, 196, 198, 199, 200, 202, 216, 224,
    228, 232–33, 275, 323. See also atypicals;
    names of specific antipsychotics
Antonuccio, David, 193
Anttila, Verneri, 62
anxiety, 30–31, 33–34, 46, 55–56, 93, 121–22,
    172, 247, 291, 296
    mixed depression-anxiety, 57–58, 60
    sedation threshold, 133–34
    SSRIs, 256–57
APA (American Psychiatric Association), 27,
    35, 43, 105, 106, 107, 111, 115, 120, 122,
    140–41, 144, 155, 160, 198, 204–6, 215–16,
    219, 284, 289, 324, 325
Archer, Neil, 211–12
Archives of General Psychiatry, 49, 213
aripiprazole, 228, 297
    Abilify, 146, 281, 292, 296
    Maintena, 146–47
Armstrong, Jay, 249
Armstrong, M. D., 31
Arvanitis, Lisa, 192, 282–83
A/S Syntetic, 53
ascorbic acid, 168
Asendin (amoxapine), 91, 177
aspirin, 77
Astra, 86, 246, 282, 285
Astra-Hässle Research Laboratories
    (Hässle), 86
AstraZeneca, 86–87, 89, 128, 140, 141, 156, 192,
    200, 211, 214, 216, 218, 281–82, 283–85,
    308–9. See also Zeneca
Atarax (hydroxyzine), 195, 282
Ativan (lorazepam), 116, 120, 191–92, 236,
    239, 281–82
atomoxetine (Strattera), 292

attention-deficit/hyperactivity disorder
    (ADHD), 53, 62, 116, 121, 149–50, 196–97,
    250, 292, 294
atypical depression, 73–74
atypicals, 275–97, 307, 323
    billion-dollar drugs, 285–87
    clozapine, 276–80
    effectiveness of, 287–90
    eldercare market, 293
    origin of term, 281
    pediatric market, 293–95
    schizophrenia and, 290–91
    scrambling for indications, 291–92
    Seroquel, 282–85
    TMAP, 299–303
    treatment-resistant depression, 295–97
Auburn University, 102
autism, 65, 121, 291–92, 294
AV/MD, 205
Axelrod, Julius (Julie) 31, 49
Ayd, Frank, 33, 78, 82, 201, 204, 226, 236–
    37, 278

Baker, Robert, 211
Baldessarini, Ross, 131, 324
Balint, Michael, 5–6
Ball, Richard (Dick), 175
Balt, Steve, 255
Baltimore–District of Columbia Society for
    Psychoanalysis, 106
Ban, Thomas, 47–48, 49, 66, 78, 79, 91, 92, 109–
    10, 116–17, 140, 250, 315, 320
Barber, Charles, 244
barbiturates, 20–21, 27–28, 39, 49, 52, 54,
    57, 85, 133, 243–44, 253, 258. See also
    names of specific barbiturates
Barondes, Samuel, 36
Baruk, Henri, 29
Batstra, Laura, 115–16
Baumeister, Alan, 278
Bayer Pharmaceuticals, 77
Bayer Veronal, 20–21
Bayh-Dole Act, 156
Baylor University, 43
Beasley, Charles, 83, 211
Beaumont, George, 314
Bellafante, Gina, 38
Bellevue Hospital, 37, 167, 259, 293–94
Benadryl (diphenhydramine), 307, 313
Bente, Dieter, 134
Benzedrine, 23, 87, 142, 171
benzene ring, 77

benzodiazepines, 7, 12, 32–33, 39, 54, 57–58, 73, 85, 116, 121–22, 179, 191–92, 193, 199, 204, 239, 243–44, 245, 247, 256, 261, 282, 310. *See also names of specific benzodiazepines*
Berger, Frank, 13–14, 208, 312
Berger, Hans, 133
Bergesio, Bartolomeo, 18
Bernard, Claude, 18
Best Pharmaceuticals for Children Act (BPCA), 236
Beth Israel Medical Center, 113
Biederman, Joseph, 149, 153, 154–55, 246–47, 291–92
Biological Psychiatry, 144, 161, 271, 272
bipolar depression, 229
bipolar disorder, 40, 62, 75, 102–3, 116, 117–18, 119, 121, 148–55, 158–59, 198, 200, 203, 206–7, 250, 256, 272, 283–84, 286, 291–92, 294, 300, 309
Black, Bob, 88, 89
Black Dog Institute, 254–55
Blackwell, Barry, 5, 71, 72, 77, 126, 212, 309, 317–18
Blashfield, Roger, 102
Blatnik, John, 220
Bleuler, Eugen, 62–63, 64, 75
Bleuler, Manfred, 318
BMJ (British Medical Journal), 223, 228, 310, 316, 319–20
Bobon, Jean, 84
Bodkin, J. Alexander, 254
Bogeso, Klaus, 89–90
BOLDER project, 284
Boston City Hospital, 165, 305
Boston Globe, 154, 265–66
Boston State Hospital, 55–56, 64, 142, 173, 252
Boston University Medical School, 319
Bowden, Charles, 70
Boyer, Francis, 87
BPCA (Best Pharmaceuticals for Children Act), 236
Brady, Joseph, 32
Brando, Marlon, 148
Brecher, Martin, 217
Breier, Alan, 83, 210–11, 286
Brenner, Ronald, 217
brexpiprazole (Rexulti), 146–47, 191
Brezis, Mayer, 321
Brill, Henry, 33, 43, 105
Brill, Steven, 84
Brintellix (vortioxetine), 226

Bristol-Myers Squibb, 92, 146, 200, 228, 281, 292. *See also* Squibb
British Journal of Psychiatry, 160, 305–6
British Medical Journal (BMJ), 223, 228, 310, 316, 319–20
Broad Institute, 62
Broadhurst, Alan, 169, 175
Brodie, Bernard, 31, 88, 130
Brody, Benjamin, 185
Brody, Bernard, 32–33
Bromo-Seltzer, 78
Brooks, George, 65
Brown, Richard J., 206
Brown, Walter, 275
Brown University, 142, 145, 213–14, 222, 265, 275
Bruins, John, 151
bulimia, 256
Bullard, Dexter, 35
Bumke, Oswald, 63
Bunney, William (Biff), Jr., 45–46
Burden Neurological Institute, 135
Bureau of Medicine, FDA, 164
Burger, Alfred, 312
Burris, Boyd, 106
Burroughs Wellcome, 9–10, 90
buspirone (BuSpar), 92

caffeine, 258
Calcibronat, 85
California State University, Northridge, 213–14
Cambridge Medical Communication Ltd., 191
Cambridge University, 89, 126–27, 202
Canadian Department of Health and Welfare, 173–74
Cancro, Robert, 7–8, 132
Cardiff Insane Hospital, 168
Carey, Benedict, 294–95
Carlat, Daniel, 156–57, 158
Carlson, Gabrielle, 215–16
Carlsson, Arvid, 86, 92–93, 130, 212, 307, 312
Carpenter, Daniel, 299–300
Carpenter, William, 66, 288, 290–91
Carroll, Bernard (Barney), 4, 34, 35, 49, 61, 74, 86–87, 105, 108, 112–13, 114, 118, 124, 125, 127, 136–37, 144, 148, 157, 161, 179, 181, 186, 191–92, 196, 197, 201, 218, 219, 224, 228, 243, 249, 251–52, 253, 257–58, 261–62, 274, 286, 295, 296, 297, 309–10, 311, 316
Carson, Stan, 269
Carter Wallace Pharmaceuticals, 52
Case Western University, 147, 214–15, 277

Castoria, 78
catatonia, 33–34, 40, 50–51, 62–63, 64, 66–67, 116, 120
catecholamines, 31, 45–46, 123, 125, 132
catechol-*O*-methyltransferase (COMT), 31
Cathell, Daniel, 20, 243
CATIE (Clinical Antipsychotic Trials of Intervention Effectiveness), 136, 287–88, 290, 294–95
Celexa (citalopram), 123–24, 184, 227, 255
Cenerx, 156
Center for Evaluation of Drug Research (CDER), FDA, 232–33
Central Islip Hospital, 43
Chakos, Miranda, 281
Charles University, Prague, 131
Charney, Dennis, 144, 161, 271, 272, 278, 321
chemical imbalances, 123–25
Chemistry of the Brain (Page), 30
Chestnut Lodge, 35, 36, 37
Children's Hospital, Boston, 149
chloral hydrate, 19–20, 261, 281–82
chlordiazepoxide (Librium), 30–31, 38, 39, 54–55, 57, 85, 201, 204, 243–44, 247, 310
chlorpromazine, 7, 24, 27–28, 29, 30–31, 32–33, 35, 39–40, 41, 43–44, 45, 46–47, 51–52, 59–60, 66, 78, 95, 134, 169–70, 172, 174, 180, 189, 275, 277–78
    chlorpromazine-procyclidine, 59–60
    Largactil, 87
    Thorazine, 10, 36, 51, 53, 71, 87, 173, 199, 210, 320–21
chlorprothixene (Taractan), 52
chronic fatigue syndrome, 258
Chronicle of Higher Education, 161
Ciba, 40, 46, 52, 55, 56, 60, 77, 78, 80, 85, 124, 127–28, 172
Ciba-Geigy, 85, 88, 89, 209–10, 321. *See also* Geigy
CINP (International College of Neuropsychopharmacology), 29–30, 47–48, 78, 80, 85, 88, 134, 147, 206, 215–16, 276–77, 318
Cipramil (citalopram), 246
citalopram
    Celexa, 123–24, 184, 227, 255
    Cipramil, 246
City College of New York, 156
Clare, Anthony, 29
Clayton, Paula, 101, 111
Clinical Antipsychotic Trials of Intervention Effectiveness (CATIE), 136, 287–88, 290, 294–95

Clinical Neuropharmacology Research Center, 44–45, 91
clinical research organizations (CROs), 185–86, 187–88, 192, 311–12
clinical trials, 21, 163–76. *See also* placebo-controlled trials; randomized controlled trials
    administering sedatives with trial antidepressants, 193
    approaches, 164–65
    cutting corners, 191–93
    delegating, 180
    depression, 177
    in Europe, 174–75
    evolution of, 165–67
    exclusion criteria, 183–85
    industry takeover of, 189–93
    recruitment through newspaper ads, 185–87
    statistical significance, 181–83
    treating fantasy patients for fantasy diseases, 177–88
    in UK, 167–71
    in US, 171–74
clomipramine (Anafranil), 163, 320–21
clozapine, 85, 187, 189, 257, 276–80, 281, 282, 285–86, 287–88, 289, 301, 308
    Clozaril, 57, 85, 276, 289
CME (continuing medical education), 140–41, 143, 144, 197, 217, 219–20, 283–84
CNS Spectrums, 159–60
cocaine, 23
Cochrane, Archie, 165, 166, 181
Cohen, Jay, 257–58
Cohen, Mandel, 35, 101–2
Cohen, Robert, 37, 44–45, 91
Cohen, Sidney, 53–54
Cole, Jonathan, 32, 36, 41, 45, 53, 95–96, 164
Columbia University, 18, 27, 46, 72, 105, 106, 139–40, 142, 165, 217, 221, 263, 267, 300, 313
commerce. *See* industry and commerce
Community Mental Health Center, Denver, 189
Compazine (prochlorperazine), 71
COMT (catechol-*O*-methyltransferase), 31
Coniglio, Diane, 156–57, 271, 272
Connecticut Mental Health Center, 289
Console, A. Dale, 128, 139, 239
Consta (injectable Risperdal), 308
Consultant X, 144
continuing medical education (CME), 140–41, 143, 144, 197, 217, 219–20, 283–84
Cook, Leonhard, 28–29, 87–88, 92, 310–11
Coppen, Alec, 86, 124, 245

Corcept Therapeutics, 157
Cornell University, 177, 185, 208–9
coronavirus, 38
Correll, Christoph, 146
cortisol, 120, 126
Coryell, William, 117–18
Cosgrove, Lisa, 226
COSTAR, 214
Couerbe, Jean-Pierre, 18
counter-detailing, 151–52, 247, 309–10
Cramp, Arthur, 10
Creighton University, 89
Crichton Royal Hospital, 133
Crocker, Benjamin, 261
CROs (clinical research organizations), 185–86, 187–88, 192, 311–12
Crout, Richard, 143
Current Medical Directions, 218–19
Current Therapeutic Research, 224, 225–26
Curtis, George, 34
Curzon, Gerald, 315
Cushing Hospital, 239
Cyberonics, 144, 157, 218
Cymbalta (duloxetine), 202, 219, 308
Czech psychopharmacology association, 48

Danziger, Phoebe, 253
Darkness Revisited (Styron), 74
Davies, David Lewis, 170
Davies, E. Beresford, 202
Davis, John, 46, 48–49, 106, 199, 320
DBDs (disruptive behavioral disorders), 152
DBSA (Depression and Bipolar Support Alliance), 271
de Boor, Wolfgang, 47–48
de Haen, Paul, 54
Deacon, Brett J., 258–59
Decker, Hannah, 101–2
Delaware State Hospital, 27–28, 36, 179
Delay, Jean, 29–31, 47, 51, 84
DelBello, Melissa, 141, 158
Dell Medical School, 158
dementia, 18, 283, 293
Denber, Herman (Hy), 43, 44, 47, 135, 215
Deniker, Pierre, 51, 279
Depakote (semisodium valproic acid), 309
depression, 24, 30–31, 35, 48–49, 51, 52–53, 55–56, 82, 92, 93, 94, 102–3, 173, 183, 206–7, 215, 227, 233, 238, 265–74, 283, 286, 291, 294, 311, 315, 316. *See also* antidepressants; *names of specific drugs*
   atypicals and treatment-resistant depression, 295–97

as backbone of psychiatry, 59, 75
chemical imbalances, 124–25
danger of, 244–45
"depression awareness" campaigns, 221
diagnosing, 59–62
diagnostic and classification difficulties, 70–75
diagnostic criteria, 101–2, 105
DSM vs. RDC, 105–6
DSM-III and, 103–5
mixed depression-anxiety, 57–58, 60
NIMH and, 45–46
Paxil and Sally Laden, 265–74
pediatric depression market, 265–66
psychoneuroses, 119
trials treating fantasy patients, 177–80
Depression and Anxiety, 160
Depression and Bipolar Support Alliance (DBSA), 271
depressive neurosis, 113
DESI (Drug Efficacy Study Implementation), 199
desipramine, 123, 189
desoxycortone acetate, 168
Detre, Thomas, 244, 305
Dewan, Naakesh, 299–300
dexamethasone suppression test (DST), 12, 70, 120, 149, 311, 316–17
Dexamyl, 54, 87
Dexedrine, 23
DHEW (US Department of Health, Education and Welfare), 95–96
Diagnostic and Statistical Manual of Mental Disorders (DSM), 4, 7, 37, 59, 60, 62, 67–68, 69, 148
consensus-based diagnoses, 108–10, 120
decline of psychopharmacology and, 119–22
dimensional vs. categorical diagnostic system, 233
dominance of, 116
DSM-II, 37
DSM-III, 37, 57–58, 65, 69, 73, 74–75, 101–22, 130, 187, 203–4, 234, 235, 250, 255, 295
DSM-III-R, 115, 117, 203–4
DSM-IV, 37, 112, 117, 121, 148–49, 154, 178, 203–4, 299, 325
DSM-5, 74, 112, 117–18, 121–22, 154, 203–4, 287, 319–20, 324, 325
major depressive disorder, 110–13, 114, 250, 255
medical model and, 102
melancholia, 117
micro-diagnoses, 113–14

Diagnostic and Statistical Manual of Mental Disorders (DSM) (*cont.*)
  nosology vs. statistical classification, 105–7
  origin of, 101–8
  pediatric bipolar disorder, 148–49, 154
  prevalence of mental illness and, 118–19
diazepam (Valium), 54, 57, 199, 236, 240, 243–44, 247, 281–82
diphenhydramine (Benadryl), 307, 313
disruptive mood dysregulation disorder, 121
Docherty, John, 299–300
Dodson, William W, 196–97
DOJ (US Department of Justice), 197–98, 267, 285, 293
Domenjoz, Robert, 88
Domino, Edward, 145–46
dopamine, 124–25, 130–32, 137, 257, 278, 281, 289, 312, 313–15, 319
double-blind studies, 185, 189
Douglas Hospital, 30, 49, 91
doxepin (Sinequan), 135
Drachman, David, 55, 261
Drazen, Jeffrey, 225–26
Drexel University College, 157
Drug Efficacy Study Implementation (DESI), 199
DSM. *See Diagnostic and Statistical Manual of Mental Disorders*
DST (dexamethasone suppression test), 12, 70, 120, 149, 311, 316–17
Duby, Lauren, 284
Duff, David, 274
Duke University, 4, 66–67, 114, 115–16, 127, 156, 299
duloxetine (Cymbalta), 202, 219, 308
Dupont Company, 310
dysphoria, 8
dysthymic disorder, 113

Early Clinical Drug Evaluation Unit (ECDEU), 45
EBM (evidence-based medicine), 129–30, 145, 306
ECDEU (Early Clinical Drug Evaluation Unit), 45
ECNP (European College of Neuropsychopharmacology), 211, 216, 268
ECT (electroconvulsive therapy), 12, 56–57, 78–79, 107, 116, 133, 134, 171, 173, 175, 183, 245, 258, 260, 295, 301
Edronax (reboxetine), 246
EEG. *See* electroencephalography
Effexor (venlafaxine), 127, 221, 246, 308

Eisdorfer, Carl, 123
EKS (Expert Knowledge Systems), 299–300, 301
Elavil (amitriptyline), 54–55, 91, 255
electroconvulsive therapy (ECT), 12, 56–57, 78–79, 107, 116, 133, 134, 171, 173, 175, 183, 245, 258, 260, 295, 301
electroencephalography (EEG), 113–14, 120
  pharmaco-EEG, 133–37, 190, 317
  quantitative EEG, 135, 136
  SSRIs, 257
Eli Lilly, 145, 150, 209, 308. *See also* Lilly
Elkes, Charmian, 32–33, 44, 170
Elkes, Joel, 3, 19, 29–30, 32–33, 44–45, 46, 48, 49–51, 91, 170
Ellenberger, Henri, 74–75
Elliott, Kimberly, 144
Elvehjem, Conrad, 18
Emerson Drug Company, 78
Emory University, 4, 28, 56–57, 94–95, 140, 144, 155, 156, 157, 158, 159, 161, 222, 270–71, 296, 306
Endicott, Jean, 105–6, 109
endocrine system, 70, 126, 149, 316
epinephrine, 137
Equanil (meprobamate), 40
ER Squibb & Sons 56, 128, 139, 204. *See also* Bristol-Myers Squibb
escitalopram (Lexapro), 159–60, 206, 227, 245, 246, 260, 307
Escobar, Javier, 261
Eskay Neuro Phosphates, 87
Esquirol, Etienne, 166–67
European College of Neuropsychopharmacology (ECNP), 211, 216, 268
Evans, Dwight, 159, 161, 271, 272
Every-Palmer, Susanna, 306
evidence-based medicine (EBM), 129–30, 145, 306
Excerpta Medica, 214–15, 217–18, 301
Expert Knowledge Systems (EKS), 299–300, 301

Fairleigh Dickinson University, 89
Falret, Jean-Pierre, 165–66
Fanapt (iloperidone), 288
Farley, Robert, 290
Fava, Giovanni, 145, 247
Fawcett, Jan, 35, 319
Fawver, Jay, 219
FDA. *See* Food and Drug Administration
FDA Act, 164, 232
FDA Modernization Act, 182, 265
Feather, Kenneth, 143–44, 161–62, 225

Federal Proceedings, 31
FeedBlitz, 154–55
Feighner, John, 101–2, 103, 257–58
Feinstein, Alvan, 181
fenfluramine, 135
fentanyl, 84
Ferriar, John, 59
Fibiger, Christian, 308
Findling, Robert, 214–15, 227
Fink, Max, 34–35, 40, 49, 53–54, 59–60, 71–72,
    78–79, 94, 113–14, 117–18, 120, 132–33,
    134–35, 136–37, 145, 155, 174, 190–91,
    221–22, 257, 258, 317, 323
First World Congress of Psychiatry, 27
Fischelis, Robert, 22, 78
Fish, Frank, 62
Fishbein, Morris, 22, 237–38
Fisher, Ronald Aylmer, 169
Fisher, Seymour, 185
Fishman, Mark, 308–9
Flügel, Fritz, 47
fluoxetine, 226
    Prozac, 73, 83, 90, 94, 112–13, 116–18, 123–
        24, 127, 191, 193, 202, 203, 206–7, 221,
        240, 243, 245–48, 249, 250, 252–54, 255,
        256–57, 258–59, 261, 262, 263, 292, 295,
        306, 307, 309–10
    Sarafem, 256
fluphenazine (Prolixin), 173
Food and Drug Administration (FDA), 11,
    21–22, 45–46, 51, 52, 55–56, 63, 80, 83, 87,
    88, 90–91, 97, 103, 136–37, 143, 146–47,
    152, 153, 154, 163, 179, 187–88, 190, 191,
    192, 195, 203, 207, 213–14, 215, 225–26,
    227, 244–45, 246, 258–59, 268–69, 275–76,
    277–78, 283, 290, 293, 295, 312,
    314, 320
    Cardiorenal Division, 110
    clinical trials, 164–65
    Division of Drug Advertising, 161–62,
        220, 225
    Division of Neuropharmacological Drug
        Products, 57–58, 165, 198
    Division of Neuropharmacology, 180,
        233, 235–36
    Division of Psychiatry Products, 260
    expanding indications for
        prescription, 198–99
    gaming trials, 238–40
    labels (package inserts), 240
    major depressive disorder, 234
    origin of, 22
    placebo-controlled trials, 235–37

Psychopharmacologic Drugs Advisory
    Committee, 55, 63, 81–82, 93, 103, 123,
    127–28, 186, 187, 190, 199, 231–32, 233,
    234, 236, 244, 260, 261, 279, 280, 281–
    82, 320
    relationship to industry, 231–40
    statistical significance, 182, 183
    testing for efficacy, 237–38
Forbes, 321
Forest Laboratories, 159–60, 184, 227, 228,
    246, 260
Fort Sam Houston, 34
Fouts, Paul, 83
Fox News, 232–33
Frances, Allen, 115–16, 121, 126, 154, 177, 203–
    4, 299–300, 325
Francis, Jennifer, 278
Frank, Jerome, 251–52
Freedman, Daniel X. (Danny), 49
Freedman, Robert (Bob), 49
Freedom of Information Act, 239–40
Freeman, Walter, 19
Freud and Freudianism, 27, 61, 71–72, 102–3,
    106–8, 326
Freudenberg, Rudolf Karl, 27
Freyhan, Fritz, 27–28, 36, 39–40, 44, 51–52,
    179, 202
Fromm-Reichmann, Frieda, 36

gabapentin (Neurontin), 309
Gaddum, John, 50
Galen, 315
Garattini, Silvio, 47–48, 289
Gardos, George, 55–56
Garnier, Jean-Pierre, 256–57
Garrett, Floyd, 229–30
GB-94 (mianserin; Tolvon), 135–36
Geigy Pharmaceuticals 52, 54, 77, 85, 88, 94,
    139, 145, 169, 175, 189, 314. *See also*
    Ciba-Geigy
Gelenberg, Alan, 279
Geodon (Ziprasidone), 294
George Washington High School, 156
Gerard, Ralph, 9, 32, 36, 37, 168
Gerard, Warren, 64–65
Gershon, Sam, 86, 134, 154, 185–86, 256, 293–
    94, 315
Ghaemi, S. Nassir, 102–3, 116, 201, 284
ghostwriting, 94, 141, 146–47, 155–57, 159,
    160–61, 213–19, 258, 265–66, 267, 270,
    271, 272, 301
Gibson, Melvin, 209
Gilmartin, Raymond, 89

Glaxo Wellcome Pharmaceuticals, 150
GlaxoSmithKline (GSK), 82–83, 87–88, 90, 157, 158–59, 160–61, 197–98, 215–16, 238, 256–57, 263, 265–66, 267–68, 269, 270–71, 272, 273, 274, 308–9. *See also* Smith, Kline & French; SmithKline; SmithKline Beecham
Glenmullen, Joseph, 96
Goddard, James, 232
Gold, Harry, 185
Goldberg, Ivan, 229, 292, 323, 324
Goldberg, Terry, 288
Goldberger, Joseph, 18
Golden, Robert N., 270
Goldman, Eric, 87–88
Goldstein, Burton, 185
Goldstein, Jeffrey, 128
Gonzalez, John P., 284
Good Morning America, 159–60
Goodrich, William, 207
Goodwin, Donald, 67–68, 102
Goodwin, Frederick, 17
Göpfert, Michael, 148
Gordon, Joshua, 313–14
Gorman, Jack, 159–60, 226–27, 269
Gorsky, Alex, 89, 151, 285–86
Gottlieb, Jacques, 28–29
Gottschalk, Louis, 68
Grassley, Charles, 96, 153, 158, 161
Green, Francis, 167–68
Greenberg, Gary, 121
Greenberg, Roger, 5–6, 185, 243–44
Greenspan, Andrew, 220
Gregory, John, 305
Griesinger, Wilhelm, 60–61
Grinker, Roy, Sr., 36
GSK (GlaxoSmithKline), 82–83, 87–88, 90, 157, 158–59, 160–61, 197–98, 215–16, 238, 256–57, 263, 265–66, 267–68, 269, 270–71, 272, 273, 274, 308–9. *See also* Smith, Kline & French; SmithKline; SmithKline Beecham
Guislain, Joseph, 253
Guze, Sam, 67–68, 102, 105, 107
Gyulai, Laszlo, 159, 160–61

Haase, Hans-Joachim, 47
Hadassah University Hospital, 149
Halcion (triazolam), 191–92, 213
hallucinogens, 30–31, 39
haloperidol (Haldol), 52, 84, 180, 210, 223, 279, 281–82, 287, 289, 308
Hämatoporphyrin (Photodyn), 18

Hamburg, David, 44–45
Hamilton, Max, 20–21, 32, 49, 248
Hamilton Rating Scale—Depression (HRSD; HAM-D), 178, 180, 184, 186, 193, 235, 244, 260, 267–68, 297
Harding, Courtenay, 65
HARKing (Hypothesizing After the Results are Known), 267
Harvard Business School, 89, 310
Harvard University, 27, 35, 39, 46, 48–49, 62, 96, 101–2, 103, 104, 124–25, 153, 154, 214–15, 222, 279, 281–82, 296, 318
hashish, 23
Hässle (Astra-Hässle Research Laboratories), 86
Hawkins, Zachary, 274
Hayes, Thomas, 103–4
Health Care Renewal, 213–14
Healy, David, 32, 44, 47–48, 65–84, 90, 92–93, 119, 121, 128, 129, 131, 140, 163, 179, 180, 183, 205, 214, 218, 223, 229, 233–34, 246–47, 248, 252, 255, 256, 261, 263, 279–80, 310, 313
hebephrenia, 67, 70
Hebrew University of Jerusalem, 182
Hecker, Ewald, 67
Heller, Abraham, 189
Helmer, O. M., 83
Henn, Fritz, 101
Hill, Austin Bradford (Tony), 169
Hillside Hospital, 34–35, 53–54, 59–60, 72, 94, 134, 145, 174, 277, 279
Hillside–North Shore Long Island Jewish Health System, 146
Hillside–North Shore Long Island Jewish Health System (Zucker-Hillside), 146–47, 288
Hippius, Hanns, 85, 276–77
Hoagland, Hudson, 47
Hoch, Paul, 128, 180
Hoechst Pharmaceuticals, 234
Hoechst-Roussel Pharmaceuticals, 100
Hoegstedt, Johan, 140, 284
Hoenig, Julius, 105
Hoff, Hans, 16, 64
Hoffmann-La Roche, 52–53, 85, 89, 168, 310. *See also* Roche
Hofmann, Albert, 50
Hollender, Marc, 116–17
Hollister, Leo, 13–14, 29–30, 43, 45, 66–67, 84, 95, 171–73, 178, 179–80, 236–37, 240, 275, 276, 289, 314–15
Hopkins, Claude, 195–96
Hornykiewicz, Oleh, 131

Horwitz, Alan, 60
Houston, William, 19
Houston Press, 301
HPA axis, 70, 126
HRSD (Hamilton Rating Scale—Depression; HAM-D), 178, 180, 184, 186, 193, 235, 244, 260, 267–68, 297
Humphrey, Hubert, 39–40
Hunter, Richard, 12–13, 15, 61
Huxley, Aldous, 39–40
hydroxyzine (Atarax), 195, 282
hyoscine (scopolamine), 20
Hypothesizing After the Results are Known (HARKing), 267

ICI (Imperial Chemical Industries), 86, 282
iloperidone (Fanapt), 288
imipramine (Tofranil), 30–31, 41, 46–47, 52, 53, 54, 59–60, 94, 134, 139, 145, 158–59, 171, 173, 174, 175, 189, 190, 202, 229, 254, 258, 261–62, 266
Imperial Chemical Industries (ICI), 86, 282
Imperial College London, 289–90
Indianapolis General Hospital, 83
industry and commerce, 19–21, 77–97. *See also names of specific companies and pharmaceuticals*
    abandonment of psychopharmacology, 308–9
    academic–industrial complex, 145–48, 197
    beginnings of, 77
    conflict between research and marketing, 127–29
    continuing medical education, 219–20
    convincing doctors to keep prescribing drug after patent expiration, 204–7
    defending against investigations, 212–14
    "depression awareness" campaigns, 221
    DSM-III and, 103–4, 119
    end of psychopharmacologic era, 108
    executives from non-marketing background, 88–89
    expanding indications for prescription, 198–99
    FDA and, 231–40
    gentleman's club-like culture, 89–90
    ghostwriting, 214–19
    hard marketing, 196–98
    historical overview of, 77–80
    industry–academy collaboration, 90–97
    journals, 223–30
    Key Opinion Leaders, 139–62
    major depressive disorder, 112–13
    marketing and advertising, 195–222
    mergers and bankruptcies, 80
    patent medicines, 9–10, 21–22
    promoting off-label indications, 200
    sales reps, 207–10
    science-based competition, 80–88
    takeover of clinical trials, 189–93
    targeting symptoms, 201–4
    trumping science, 306–8
    Zyprexa weight-gain problem, 210–12
InfoScriber, 291–92
Insel, Thomas, 126–27, 161, 203–4, 305, 319–20
INSERM (National Institute of Health and Medical Research), 29
Institute for Early Life Adversity, 158
Institute for Psychosomatic and Psychiatric Research and Training, 35
Institute of Psychiatry, London, 29, 40–41, 130–31, 170
insulin therapy, 35, 134
International College of Neuropsychopharmacology (CINP), 29–30, 47–48, 78, 80, 85, 88, 134, 147, 206, 215–16, 276–77, 318
International Consensus Group on Depression and Anxiety, 270
International Journal of Risk & Safety in Medicine, 224–25
International Pharmaco-EEG Group, 136
International Psychiatric Association, 216
iproniazid (Marsilid), 52–53
isocarboxazid (Marplan), 173
Istanbul University, 134
Itil, Turan, 132–33, 134, 135–36, 257, 317
Iversen, Leslie, 92, 131–32, 253
Ives Laboratories, 93

J&J (Johnson & Johnson), 84, 89, 150–52, 153, 155, 217–18, 220, 238, 276, 285–86, 293, 299–300, 301–3. *See also* Janssen
JAACAP (Journal of the American Academy of Child and Adolescent Psychiatry), 270
Jackson, Hughlings, 66
Jacobi, Walter, 17
JAMA (Journal of the American Medical Association), 231, 237
JAMA Psychiatry, 70, 136, 228
Janssen, 52, 62–63, 84, 89, 96, 97, 141, 157–58, 192, 197, 200, 202–3, 210, 214–15, 216, 224, 280, 281, 285–86, 290, 293, 294, 296, 308–9, 314. *See also* Johnson & Johnson
Janssen, Paul, 62–63, 84, 180, 279
Janssen, Wallace, 90
Jaspers, Karl, 61

Johns Hopkins University, 9–10, 27, 28, 33–34, 120, 163, 172–73, 214–15, 251–52, 263, 313
Johnson, Robert Wood, II, 84
Johnson & Johnson (J&J), 84, 89, 150–52, 153, 155, 217–18, 220, 238, 276, 285–86, 293, 299–300, 301–3. *See also* Janssen
Jones, Allen, 290, 302
Jones, Tone, 197, 202–3, 303
Josiah Macy Jr. Foundation, 47
Journal of Affective Disorders, 228
Journal of Child and Adolescent Psychiatry, 265–66
Journal of Clinical Psychiatry, 224, 270
Journal of Clinical Psychopharmacology, 228
Journal of Medicinal Chemistry, 312
Journal of the American Academy of Child and Adolescent Psychiatry (JAACAP), 270
Journal of the American Medical Association (JAMA), 231, 237
Journal of the Royal College of Physicians, 306
journals, 223–30. *See also names of specific journals*
Jureidini, Jon, 227, 228

Kahn, Cara, 221
Kahn, David, 299–300
Kahn, René, 66–67
Kahneman, Daniel, 182
Kali-Duphar Laboratories, 142
Kane, John, 146, 277–78, 280
Kansas University, 267
Karolinska Institute, 325
Kartzinel, Ronald, 198, 233
Kasper, Siegfried, 216
Katon, Wayne, 193
Katz, Martin, 104–5, 135–36
Keats, Matt, 287
Keefe, Richard, 66–67
Kefauver, Estes, 195, 208–9, 213, 225
Kefauver Committee, 79, 90, 128, 213, 216, 225
Kefauver-Harris drug act amendments, 80, 164, 189, 195, 227, 232, 237
Kekulé, August, 77
Keller, Martin, 215–16, 265–66, 268, 269, 270
Kelsey, Frances, 45–46
Kendell, R. E., 103
Kennedy, Ted, 239
Kessler, David, 153, 156–57
Kessler, Linda, 244
Kessler, Robert M., 69
ketamine, 231, 314–15
Kety, Seymour, 32, 44–45, 47, 91

Key Opinion Leaders (KOLs), 7, 80, 87, 94, 128, 130, 139–62, 197, 203–4, 206–7, 208, 211, 213, 217, 218, 257–58, 260, 261–62, 265–66, 273, 283–84, 295–96, 297, 302, 309–10, 311–12, 318
    academic–industrial complex, 145–48
    Biederman and pediatric bipolar disorder, 148–55
    categories of, 140–41
    defined, 4, 139
    money and, 142–44
    Nemeroff, 155–61
    rise of, 139–42
Kiloh, Leslie Gordon, 175
Kings County Hospital, 7–8
Kinnier, Bill, 215–16
Kinross-Wright, Vernon, 43, 44
Kirsch, Irving, 184, 258–59
Klein, Donald, 27, 34–35, 37, 41, 53–54, 59–60, 69, 73–74, 93, 94, 104–5, 106, 109, 112, 113, 114, 115, 145, 174, 183, 203–4, 236–37, 252–53, 259, 313, 325–26
Klein, Rachel, 174, 267–68
Klerman, Gerald, 48–49, 102, 103, 105, 266, 318
Kline, Nathan, 6–7, 39, 43, 44, 50, 56, 215, 277, 317
Kocsis, James, 91, 177
Kohn, Melvin, 132
Kohut, Heinz, 49
KOLs. *See* Key Opinion Leaders
Korn, David, 127
Kornetsky, Conan, 319
Kraepelin, Emil, 24–25, 55, 59, 61, 62–63, 64, 65, 69, 71–72, 74, 75, 101, 102–3, 114, 121–22
Kraepelinian (medical) model, 24–25, 102, 120
Kramer, Mark, 5, 73, 82, 89, 93–94, 116, 129, 130, 143, 178, 186, 189, 192, 222, 229, 250, 254, 295, 307, 311, 321
Kramer, Morton, 60
Kramer, Peter, 258–59, 262
Kuhn, Roland, 88, 139, 179, 184–85
Kupfer, David, 324
Kurland, Albert, 41

Lacasse, Jeffrey, 125
lactate infusion test, 120
Laden, Sally, 157, 159–60, 218, 226–27, 243, 266, 267–73
Lader, Malcolm, 16, 40–41, 179
Laehr, Heinrich, 16

Lambert, Bruce, 211
Lambert, Carl, 170
Lambert Pharmaceutical Company, 78
Lancet, 74, 289–90
Lapin, Ira (Slava), 124–25
Largactil (chlorpromazine), 51
Lasagna, Louis, 32, 163, 165, 171–73, 175–76, 182, 231
LaSalle University, 265, 269
Laughren, Thomas, 232–33, 238, 277–78
Lawrence, Richard, 192, 282
Lazarsfeld, Paul, 139–40
L-dopa, 45–46, 307
Leary, Timothy, 39
Leber, Paul, 57–58, 63, 87, 163, 165, 175, 180, 183, 231–32, 233, 234, 235–37, 244–45, 278, 279–80, 320
Lederle Laboratories, 91, 177
Lee, Hillary, 234
Lee, Philip R., 51
Leech, Paul Nicholas, 10
Lehmann, Heinz, 6, 30, 44, 50, 91
Leo, Jonathan, 125
Leonhard, Karl, 69–70, 102–3, 116–17
Lesch, John E., 81
Lespinasse, Julie de, 37
Lettvin, Jerome, 165
Leucht, Stefan, 289–90
Lewin, Louis, 21
Lewis, Aubrey, 170
Lexapro (escitalopram), 159–60, 206, 227, 245, 246, 260, 307
Library of Congress, 213
Librium (chlordiazepoxide), 30–31, 38, 39, 54–55, 57, 85, 201, 204, 243–44, 247, 310
Lidone (molindone), 294–95
Lilly (Eli Lilly and Company), 49, 53, 77, 83, 124, 129, 147, 151–52, 156, 165, 191, 193, 200, 201, 202, 203, 207, 208, 210–12, 219, 221, 240, 245, 246–47, 256–58, 261, 279, 280–81, 283, 286, 301, 308. *See also* Eli Lilly
Lilly Research Laboratories, 79, 83, 245
Listening to Prozac (Kramer), 262
Listerine, 78
lithium, 44, 48, 51, 78–79, 158–59, 174–75, 189, 231, 261–62, 297, 309–10, 323
London Hospital Medical School, 190
London School of Hygiene, 169
Longview Hospital, 68, 171
Lorazepam (Ativan), 116, 120, 191–92, 236, 239, 281–82
Lorich, Reinhard, 28

Losec (omeprazole), 86
Louisiana State University, 278
LSD (lysergic acid diethylamide), 30–31, 32, 39, 49, 50, 85
Lucas, Steve, 196
Ludiomil (maprotiline), 60, 85, 127–28
Luminal (phenobarbital), 20, 39, 51, 54
Lundbeck Pharmaceuticals, 52, 89–90, 146–47, 191, 246
Lydia E. Pinkham's Vegetable Compound, 10
Lyons, Fred W., Jr., 88, 89
lysergic acid diethylamide (LSD), 30–31, 32, 39, 49, 50, 85

Maastricht University, 218
Macalpine, Ida, 12, 15
Macfadden, Wayne, 284–85
Macht, David, 28
MacIntyre, Roger, 284
Mackay, Charles, 177
Madhusoodanan, Subramoniam, 217
MADRS scale, 297
Maintena (aripiprazole), 146–47
Maj, Mario, 256
major depressive disorder (MDD), 40, 73, 75, 102–3, 105–6, 110, 114–16, 119, 121, 191, 198, 255, 272, 287, 305–6. *See also* antidepressants; depression; *names of specific pharmaceuticals*
    DSM-III, 110–13, 114
    FDA and, 234
    sharp decline in treatment progress, 318–19
    SSRIs, 250–54
Maldonado, Sam, 236
Malitz, Sidney, 46–47
Mallick, Heather, 263
Manchester Infirmary and Lunatic Asylum, 59
Manhattan State Hospital, 43, 215
mania, 51, 198
MAO (monoamine oxidase), 31
Mao, C. Gloria, 270
MAOIs (monoamine oxidase inhibitors), 52–53, 54, 73–74, 112–13, 116–18, 136, 171, 173, 229, 254–55, 259–60, 287, 309–10, 317–18, 323. *See also names of specific MAOIs*
maprotiline (Ludiomil), 60, 85, 127–28
Maraviglia, Theodore, 239
Marburg University, 185
Mario Negri Institute, 289
Marion Laboratories, 89
Marion Merrell Dow, 88, 89

marketing and advertising, 195–222. *See also* industry and commerce
　academic–industrial complex, 197
　continuing medical education, 219–20
　convincing doctors to keep prescribing drug after patent expiration, 204–7
　defending against investigations, 212–14
　"depression awareness" campaigns, 221
　expanding indications for prescription, 198–99
　ghostwriting, 214–19
　hard marketing, 196–98
　promoting off-label indications, 200
　sales reps, 207–10
　targeting symptoms, 201–4
　Zyprexa weight-gain problem, 210–12
Marks, Harry, 163
Marplan (isocarboxazid), 173
Marshall University, 92
Marsilid (iproniazid), 52–53
Maryland Psychiatric Research Center, 288
Massachusetts General Hospital (MGH), 149, 150, 151–52, 153, 154–55, 159, 172–73, 246–47
Massachusetts Mental Health Center, 50, 67
Massachusetts State Lunatic Hospital, 8–9
Masserman, Jules, 106
"Mathematical Theory of Affective Psychoses, A" (Lettvin and Pitts), 165
Mattes, Jeffrey, 208
Maudsley, Henry, 16
Maudsley Hospital, 34, 40–41, 71, 110–11, 168, 170, 175
Maurer, Christopher, 283
May, Charles, 221
May and Baker, 170
Mayer-Gross, William (Willi), 29, 30–31, 65, 133
McCafferty, James, 215–16, 265, 269, 270
McCowan, Peter, 168
McEvoy, Joseph, 299
McGill University, 44, 46–47, 49, 110–11, 125, 133–34, 316, 326
McHenry, Leemon, 213–14, 224–25, 226–27, 228
McHugh, Paul, 33–34
McKeen, John Elmer, 196
McLean Hospital, 36, 67–68, 131, 254
McNeil Laboratories, 84
McQuillan, Rufus, 208–9
MDD. *See* major depressive disorder
Medawar, Charles, 121
Medicaid, 292, 295, 302

medical (Kraepelinian) model, 24–25, 102, 120
Medical Research Council (MRC), 166, 167–68, 169, 170–71, 245
Medical World News, 225
Meduna, Laszlo, 64
melancholia, 12, 15, 17–18, 33–34, 40, 71–72, 74, 75, 82, 111, 112, 115, 116, 117, 120, 234, 254–55, 324
Mellaril (thioridazine), 53–54, 173, 275, 280
Meltzer, Herbert Y. (Herb), 49, 187, 277–78, 279
Mencken, Henry L. (H L), 20
Mendels, Joseph, 103, 124
Menninger, Karl, 107
Mental Health Surveillance Survey, 118
mepazine (Pacatal), 169–70
mephenesin (Tolserol), 172–73
meprobamate, 12, 37, 43–44, 201
　Equanil, 40
　Miltown, 13–14, 30–31, 39, 40, 52, 53, 57, 208
MER-29, 239
Merck & Company, 5, 54–55, 77, 79, 81–83, 86–87, 89, 92, 93, 129, 131–32, 143, 178, 186, 222, 229, 237, 246, 253, 307, 308–9, 311, 321
Merck Sharp and Dohme, 81
Merck, George, 129
Merck Institute for Therapeutic Research, 79, 81
Merck Neuroscience Research Centre, 82–83
Merck Research Laboratories (MRL), 81
Merital (nomifensine), 183, 234
Merlis, Sidney, 43
Merrell Dow Pharmaceuticals, 89, 150
methylphenidate (Ritalin), 53, 54, 55, 121, 309–10
methyprylon (Noludar), 53
Metropolitan State University, 129
Meyer, Alfred, 120
Meyer, Gerald, 88
MGH (Massachusetts General Hospital), 149, 150, 151–52, 153, 154–55, 159, 172–73, 246–47
mianserin (GB-94; Tolvon), 135–36
Michael Reese Hospital, 35–36
mifepristone (RU 486) 157
Miltown (meprobamate), 13–14, 30–31, 39, 40, 52, 53, 57, 208, 243–44, 312
mirtazapine (Remeron), 136
Missouri Institute of Psychiatry, 317
MIT, 62, 135
Mitchner, Natasha, 227
Modell, Walter, 208–9
Mojtabai, Ramin, 263
molindone (Lidone), 294–95

Molitor, Hans, 81
Monase, 62
monoamine oxidase inhibitors (MAOIs), 52–53, 54, 73–74, 112–13, 116–18, 136, 171, 173, 229, 254–55, 259–60, 287, 309–10, 317–18, 323. *See also names of specific MAOIs*
monoamine oxidase (MAO), 31
Monsanto Company, 80
mood disorders, 35, 51, 55, 69, 70–71, 93, 102–3, 189, 259, 309, 317
Moreau, Jacques-Joseph, 18
morphine, 19–20, 30–31
Mother Jones, 159–60
MRC (Medical Research Council), 166, 167–68, 169, 170–71, 245
MRL (Merck Research Laboratories), 81
Mt. Sinai Hospital, 144
Murray, Robin, 130–31
Musso, Giuseppe, 18
Myerson, Abraham, 142

narcotics, 85
Nardil (phenelzine), 53, 116–17, 171, 173
Nardo, John M. (Mickey), 3–4, 5–6, 7, 8, 12–13, 16–17, 39, 56–57, 75, 94–95, 104, 106, 107–8, 109, 111–12, 117, 129, 130, 140, 142–43, 144, 146, 154–55, 156, 160, 178, 187, 191, 201, 203–4, 209, 216, 218, 222, 223, 224, 237, 250, 252, 255, 265, 270, 271, 272, 283, 294–95, 296, 297, 303, 305, 306, 311–12
Nasrallah, Henry, 211, 212, 217
National Center for Health Statistics, 152–53, 251
National Heart Institute, 32–33, 130
National Hospital for Neurology and Neurosurgery (Queen Square, London), 12, 19, 61
National Institute of Health and Medical Research (INSERM), 29
National Institute of Mental Health (NIMH), 17, 35, 37, 44–46, 49, 60, 67, 68–69, 83, 91, 104–6, 126–27, 131–32, 135–36, 141, 146–47, 158, 161, 203–4, 210, 251, 257, 294–95, 305, 313–14, 319–20, 325
    Adult Psychiatry Branch, 46
    Early Clinical Drug Evaluation Unit, 45
    New Clinical Drug Evaluation Unit, 215–16
    Psychopharmacology Research Branch, 45, 48–49
    Psychopharmacology Service Center, 32, 36, 45, 95–96, 164, 173, 325
    Section on Clinical Neuropharmacology, 124

National Institutes of Health (NIH), 31, 44–45, 79, 81, 88, 95–96, 158
National Schizophrenia Guidelines Development Group, 287
National Survey of Psychotherapeutic Drug Use, 251
Nature Neuroscience, 157
NEJM (New England Journal of Medicine), 94–95, 154, 213, 218–19, 220, 225–27, 265–66
Nelson, J. Craig, 296
Nemeroff, Charles, 144, 155–58, 161, 224, 246–47, 266, 270, 271, 272, 296
neurasthenia, 71, 73
neurochemistry, 18, 32–33, 46, 126
neurokinin-1 receptor antagonist (NK1RA) antidepressants, 129
neuroleptics, 38, 47
Neurologic Drugs Advisory Committee, 198
neuronal reuptake, 31, 32–33, 88, 123, 126, 127–28
Neurontin (gabapentin), 309
Neuropsychobiology, 136
Neuropsychopharmacology, 144, 157–58, 272
neurosciences, 32–33
neurotransmitters, 127–28, 130–33, 136–37, 278, 312–16, 319. *See also names of specific neurotransmitters*
New and Nonofficial Remedies (AMA), 21–22
New England Journal of Medicine (NEJM), 94–95, 154, 213, 218–19, 220, 225–27, 265–66
New York Academy of Medicine, 128
New York Academy of Sciences, 43–44
New York Medical College, 46, 49
New York State Mental Hospital system, 46, 60
New York State Psychiatric Institute (PI), 13, 41, 46–47, 70, 93, 102, 104–5, 106, 107, 109, 128, 180, 254
New York Times, 38, 132, 141, 144, 153, 155, 157, 158, 159–60, 196–97, 206–7, 209, 218–19, 225–26, 262, 294–95, 302
New York University, 132, 293–94
Newell, Audrey, 101
Newman, Thomas, 257
Newport, D. Jeffrey, 270–71
Newsweek, 263
Nichols, John, 167
nicotinic acid, 83
NIH (National Institutes of Health), 31, 44–45, 79, 81, 88, 95–96, 158
NIH (Not Invented Here) problem, 92–93
NIMH. *See* National Institute of Mental Health
NIMH RAISE-ETP study, 146–47

NK1RA (neurokinin-1 receptor antagonist) antidepressants, 129
NNH (Number Needed to Harm), 182–83
NNT (Number Needed to Treat), 182–83, 254, 267–68, 297
Noludar (methyprylon), 53
nomifensine (Merital), 183, 234
nonbarbiturate sedatives, 53
Nordmark Company, 18
norepinephrine (noradrenaline), 31, 45–46, 123, 124–25, 126, 127–28, 130–31, 132, 312, 313–14, 315
Norristown State Hospital, 28
Northampton State Hospital, 19–20
nortriptyline (Pamelor), 254, 259, 308
Nostrums and Quackery and Pseudo-Medicine (Cramp), 10
Not Invented Here (NIH) problem, 92–93
Novadel, 156
Novartis Pharmaceuticals, 84, 85, 89, 150, 192, 209–10, 285–86, 308–9, 315
nucleotides, 173–74
Number Needed to Harm (NNH), 182–83
Number Needed to Treat (NNT), 182–83, 254, 267–68, 297

O'Brien, James, 108, 306, 324
obsessive-compulsive disorder (OCD), 48, 149, 150, 256, 320, 321
Ohio State University, 60, 215–16, 217
olanzapine (Zyprexa), 83, 96, 97, 151–52, 195, 196, 201, 202, 203, 206–7, 210–12, 256, 279, 280–81, 282, 283, 286, 287–88, 294–95, 300–1, 309
olanzapine and fluoxetine (Symbyax), 256
Olfson, Mark, 263
omeprazole (Losec), 86
Omnicare, 293
One Flew Over the Cuckoo's Nest (film), 107
1 Boring Old Man blog, 4, 115, 160, 262
oneirophrenia, 64
opioids, 316
opium, 15, 18, 25, 258
Orap (pimozide), 280
Organon, 135, 136
Osler, William, 9–10
Östholm, Ivan, 86
Ostroff, Robert, 296
Oswald, Ian, 213
Otago Medical School, 306
Otsuka, 146–47, 191, 292
Out of Darkness (TV movie), 221

outcome switching, 267
Overall, John, 66–67, 104, 234
oxazepam (Serax), 57
Oxenkrug, Gregory, 124–25
Oxford University, 46
Oxycontin, 27

Pacatal (mepazine; perazine), 169–70
Page, Irvine, 30, 83
Pamelor (nortriptyline), 254, 259, 308
Pande, Atul, 308–9
Pandina, Gahan, 151–52
panic disorder, 120, 174, 185, 273
Parexel Medical Marketing Services, 140, 284–85
Paris, Joel, 326
Paris World Congress, 43–44
Parisian School of Pharmacy, 18
Parke, Davis & Company, 9–10, 209
Parker, Gordon, 71–72, 117–18, 182, 254–55, 259, 324
Parkinson's disease, 200, 307
Parnate (tranylcypromine), 52–53, 73–74
paroxetine
    Paxil, 87, 123–24, 125, 156–57, 158–61, 197–98, 215, 223, 226–27, 233, 238, 245, 246–47, 251, 256–57, 265, 266, 267–68, 269–72, 273–74, 309
    Seroxat, 246–47
Pasamanick, Benjamin, 60
Pascal, Constantine, 23
patent medicines, 9–10, 21–22
Paul, Steven (Steve), 49
Paxil (paroxetine), 87, 123–24, 125, 156–57, 158–61, 197–98, 215, 223, 226–27, 233, 238, 245, 246–47, 251, 256–57, 265, 266, 267–68, 269–72, 273–74, 309
Payne Whitney Clinic, 91
PDAC (Psychopharmacologic Drugs Advisory Committee), 55, 63, 81–82, 93, 103, 123, 127–28, 186, 187, 190, 199, 231–32, 233, 234, 236, 244, 260, 261, 279, 280, 281–82, 320
PDR (*Physicians' Desk Reference*), 199
Pedersen, Vagn, 90
pellagra, 18, 83
pentobarbital, 172–73
perazine (Pacatal), 169–70
perphenazine (Trilafon), 54–55, 287–88
Perris, Carlo, 124
Pertofrane (desipramine), 123
Petersen, Melody, 206
peyote, 23

Pfizer, 77, 79, 80, 135, 150, 190, 196, 218–19, 231, 239–40, 245, 258, 262, 301, 308–9, 321
Phantastica (Lewin), 21
Pharmaceutical Executive, 140, 216
Pharmaceutical Manufacturers Association (PMA), 23
Pharmaceutical Research and Manufacturers Association (PhRMA), 191
Pharmacia, 80
pharmaco-EEG, 49, 133–37, 190, 317. *See also* electroencephalography
Pharmacological Basis of Therapeutics, The (Goodman and Gilman), 278
Pharmacopsychiatry, 213
phenaglycodol (Ultran), 53
phenelzine (Nardil), 53, 116–17, 171, 173
phenobarbital (Luminal), 20, 39, 51, 54
phenothiazines, 40, 45, 52, 53–54, 71, 275. *See also names of specific phenothiazines*
phobic anxiety depersonalization syndrome, 116–17
Photodyn (Hämatoporphyrin), 18
PhRMA (Pharmaceutical Research and Manufacturers Association), 191
PHS (Public Health Service), 95–96
Physicians' Desk Reference (PDR), 199
PI (New York State Psychiatric Institute), 13, 41, 46–47, 70, 93, 102, 104–5, 106, 107, 109, 128, 180, 254
Pick, Ernst Peter, 16
Pickering, George, 171
Pilgrim State Hospital, 33
pimozide (Orap), 280
Pink Sheet, The, 207, 256–57
Pinkham, Lydia E., 10
Pinsker, Henry, 113
piperazine, 282
placebo-controlled trials, 166–67, 172–73, 174–75, 189, 235–37, 281–82
placebos, 20, 24, 92, 166–67, 187, 193
Pletscher, Alfred, 88, 126
PMA (Pharmaceutical Manufacturers Association), 23
Poffenberger, Albert, 18
Polatin, Phillip, 46
Pope, Alfred, 30
Pope, Harrison, 67–68
Poses, Roy, 141, 145, 213–14, 318
post traumatic stress disorder (PTSD), 33–34, 252, 270, 291, 296
potassium bromide, 19–20
Potter, William, 81–82
Powers, John E., 195–96

Praag, Herman Van, 120–21
Prange, Arthur J. (Art), 52
premenstrual dysphoric disorder, 121, 292
Prevention & Treatment, 259
PricewaterhouseCoopers, 180
Princeton University, 47, 87–88, 208
Pringle, Evelyn, 260
prochlorperazine (Compazine), 71
Prolixin (fluphenazine), 173
promazine (Sparine), 45
propanediols, 52
Propublica, 212
Prozac (fluoxetine), 73, 83, 90, 94, 112–13, 116–18, 124, 127, 191, 193, 202, 203, 206–7, 221, 240, 243, 245–48, 249, 250, 252–54, 255, 256–57, 258–59, 261, 262, 263, 292, 295, 306, 307, 309–10
PSC (Psychopharmacology Service Center), 32, 36, 45, 95–96, 164, 173, 325
Psychiatria Polska, 227
Psychiatric Research Institute, 30, 83
Psychiatric Times, 255
psychiatry
  age of psychopharmacology, 10–11
  biological approaches to, 16, 17, 32, 102
  biological vs. social, 11–14
  causation and treatment cycles, 8–10
  degradation and derailment of, 4–5, 7
  development of psychopharmacology, 15–25
  early European, 16–18
  effectiveness of, 5–6, 7–8
  end of psychoanalysis, 33–37
  experimental psychiatry, 46–47
  increasing disability rate, 58
  medical model and, 12, 24–25
  neurochemistry, 18
  neurology and, 19
  postwar developments in, 6–7
  prevalence of mental disorders, 11
  science in, 17–19
  shifts and cycles of, 107–8
  therapeutic alliance, 5–6, 7–8
PsychNet, 159
psychoanalysis, 27, 30–31, 33–37, 40–41, 48–49, 105, 106, 107–8
Psychology Today, 325
psychoneurosis, 73
Psychopharmacologic Drugs Advisory Committee (PDAC), 55, 63, 81–82, 93, 103, 123, 127–28, 186, 187, 190, 199, 231–32, 233, 234, 236, 244, 260, 261, 279, 280, 281–82, 320

psychopharmacology. *See also* clinical trials;
industry and commerce; marketing and
advertising; *names of specific companies
and pharmaceuticals*
academia's abandonment of, 317–18
biological approaches to, 48–50, 316–17
commerce in, 19–21
culture of, 37–40
defined, 4
deinstitutionalization, 56–57, 72–73
development of, 15–25, 43–50
drug classifications, 55–56
endocrinological approach, 126
evidence-based medicine, 129–30
experimental psychiatry, 46–47
failure of drug discovery, 309–12
fall of, 305–21
golden age of, 10–11, 23–24, 51
hospital clinicians and industry, 43–47
industry's abandonment of, 308–9
journals, 223–30
linking drugs to behavior, 21
neurotransmitters, 126, 130–33, 312–16
NIMH, 44–47
origin of terminology, 28–30
patent medicines, 21–22
pharmaco-EEG, 133–37
recommended solutions, 325–26
rise of, 27–41
science in psychiatry, 17–19
science of, 30–32, 47, 123–37
science trumped by commerce, 306
Psychopharmacology, A Review of Progress
(ACNP and NIMH), 48–49
Psychopharmacology Bulletin, 157,
270–71
Psychopharmacology Service Center (PSC), 32,
36, 45, 95–96, 164, 173, 325
psychosis, 52, 55–56, 63
Psychosomatic Medicine, 28–29
psychotherapy, 247, 326
Psychotropic Drugs (Garattini), 47–48
PTSD (post traumatic stress disorder), 33–34,
252, 270, 291, 296
Public Health Service (PHS), 95–96
Purdue Pharma L.P., 27

quantitative EEG (QEEG), 135, 136
Queen Charlotte's Hospital, 31
Queen Square, London (National Hospital for
Neurology and Neurosurgery),
12, 19, 61
Queen's University, 139

quetiapine (Seroquel), 86, 128, 141, 183, 192,
200, 201, 214, 216, 218, 278, 281, 282–85,
296, 300–1
QVX Communications, 146–47

Rafaelsen, Ole, 257–58
Ramón y Cajal, Santiago, 17
randomized controlled trials (RCTs), 24, 44, 83,
129, 157, 164, 167, 169, 171–76, 180, 181,
183, 187, 188, 189, 193, 226, 229, 232, 235,
258, 259, 261, 265, 276, 287, 296, 316–17.
See also clinical trials
randomized withdrawal studies, 188
ranitidine (Zantac), 263
Rankin, William, 164
Rapaport, Mark, 296
rapid eye movement latency (REM latency), 12
Rasmussen, Nicolas, 81, 142
RCTs (randomized controlled trials), 24, 44, 83,
129, 157, 164, 167, 169, 171–76, 180, 181,
183, 187, 188, 189, 193, 226, 229, 232, 235,
258, 259, 261, 265, 276, 287, 296, 316–17.
See also clinical trials
RDC (St. Louis Research Diagnostic Criteria),
105–6, 110–11
REACH Program, 283–84
reboxetine (Edronax), 246
*Recognition and Treatment of Psychiatric
Disorders* (Nemeroff and Schatzberg),
156–57, 271, 272
Recognizing the Depressed Patient (Ayd), 82
Rees, Linford, 30, 168, 170, 175
Rees, Thomas P., 64
Regier, Daryl, 324
Régis, Emmanuel, 64
Reidy, Jamie, 262
Relman, Arnold, 154–55, 220
REM latency (rapid eye movement latency), 12
Remeron (mirtazapine), 136
remoxipride (Roxiam), 82, 86–87
Repp, Ed, 284
reserpine (Serpasil), 40, 43–44, 46, 52, 56, 85,
170, 172
Restoril, 191–92
Rexulti (brexpiprazole), 146–47, 191
Rhône-Poulenc SA, 28
Richards, Alfred N., 81
Rickels, Karl, 47, 93, 139
Rifkin, Arthur, 93
Rinkel, Max, 50
Rising, Kristin, 227
risperidone (Risperdal), 84, 89, 96, 97, 141,
150–51, 152, 153, 157–58, 200, 203, 210,

214–15, 216, 217–18, 232–33, 280, 281, 285–86, 288, 293, 294–95, 296, 299–303, 306, 308, 314
Ritalin (methylphenidate), 53, 54, 55, 121, 309–10
Robert Wood Johnson Foundation, 299
Roberts, Dick, 172
Robins, Eli, 35, 67–68, 101–2, 103, 104–6
Robinson, Donald S., 92
Robinson, Valerie, 210
Roche (F Hoffmann-La Roche AG), 32–33, 38, 52–53, 57, 84, 85, 88, 89, 205–6. *See also* Hoffmann-La Roche
Rockefeller Foundation, 29, 168
Rockefeller Institute, 83
Rockefeller University, 255
Rockland State Hospital, 43, 56, 215, 277, 319
Roerig (division of Pfizer), 79, 195
Romankiewicz, John, 160, 266, 267, 268
Rosenbaum, Jerrold, 246–47
Rosenheck, Robert, 290
Roth, Martin, 44, 116–17, 133
Rothlin, Ernst, 47–48, 78, 80, 88
Rothman, David, 150–51, 217, 300, 301
Rothman, Theodore, 48, 180
Roxiam (remoxipride), 82, 86–87
Royal Society of Medicine, 61, 77
RU 486 (mifepristone) 157
Rubin, Robert, 15, 157, 161
Rupniak, Nadia, 92
Rush, A. John, 144, 193, 299, 300, 301
Ryan, Neal, 265, 268

Sabshin, Melvin (Mel), 35, 205, 219
Sachs, Gary, 159
Sackler, Arthur, 27
Sadusk, Joseph, 232
Sainz, Tony, 44
Salpêtrière Hospital, 166–67
Salzman, Carl, 240, 281–82
SAMSHA (Substance Abuse and Mental Health Services Administration), 118
San Francisco State University, 89
Sandler, Merton, 31, 72
Sandoz, 32, 47–48, 50, 53–54, 77, 78, 80, 85, 88, 89, 168, 205, 209–10, 221, 275, 276–78
Sanocrysin, 167
Sanofi SA, 308–9
Sarwer-Foner, Gerald, 43–44
Saskatchewan Hospital, 173–74
Schatzberg, Alan, 156–57, 246–47, 271, 272
Schildkraut, Joseph, 46, 48–49, 69, 104, 124–25, 312

schizophrenia, 12, 17, 24–25, 30–31, 32, 35, 36, 40, 45, 48–49, 52, 62–70, 82, 83, 119, 121–22, 146–47, 153, 168, 172, 173–74, 191, 198, 201, 214, 231–32, 233, 235, 250, 282, 283, 287, 288, 289, 294, 295–96, 305–6, 315
atypicals and, 275, 277–78, 279–81, 290–91
as backbone of psychiatry, 59, 75
chemical imbalances, 124–25
consensus-based diagnoses in DSM-III, 108–9
diagnostic and classification difficulties, 59–70, 75
diagnostic criteria, 105
dopamine hypothesis, 130–32, 278, 314–15, 319
medication, 68
positive and negative symptoms, 66–67
psychosis at core of, 66–68
sedation threshold, 133–34
sharp decline in treatment progress, 318–19
TMAP, 299, 300–1, 303
unitary concept vs. components, 62–66, 108–9
Schneider, Kurt, 71–72, 74, 116–17
Schou, Mogens, 44, 51, 174–75
Schumacher, Martin, 295, 315
Schuster, Bob, 49
Scientific Therapeutics Information (STI), 156–57, 159, 160, 161, 217, 266, 267, 268, 270, 271, 274
Scolnick, Edward, 81
scopolamine (hyoscine), 20
Scrip, 82–83, 245
SDAs (serotonin-dopamine antagonists), 280
secobarbital (Seconal) 172–73
Second International Congress of Psychiatry, 30, 31
second-generation antipsychotics (SGAs), 7, 11, 30, 66–67, 275–76. *See also* atypicals
sedation threshold, 49, 133–34, 316, 317
sedatives, 193
Seeman, Philip, 131–32, 314
selective serotonin reuptake inhibitors (SSRIs), 7, 11, 12, 30, 39, 54, 58, 73–92, 94, 107, 110, 112–13, 117–18, 119, 121, 123–24, 125, 127, 135, 158–60, 168–69, 177, 178, 184, 202, 214, 216, 224, 235–36, 243–44, 245–47, 248–49, 274, 291, 295–96, 305–6, 307, 309–10, 311–12, 313, 314, 319–20, 321, 323. *See also names of specific SSRIs*
lack of effectiveness, 257–62
major depressive disorder, 250–54
NNT, 183, 254
pediatric depression market, 265, 267
scrambling for indications, 256–57
TCAs vs., 254–55

semisodium valproic acid (Depakote), 309
Sequenced Treatment Alternatives to Relieve Depression (STAR*D) study, 136, 184, 295
Serax (oxazepam), 57
Seroquel (quetiapine), 86, 128, 141, 183, 192, 200, 201, 214, 216, 218, 278, 281, 282–85, 296, 300–1
serotonin, 50, 86, 123–25, 130–31, 132, 137, 245, 257, 270, 289, 312, 313–15
serotonin and norepinephrine reuptake inhibitors (SNRIs), 127, 246, 323
serotonin antagonists, 135
serotonin-dopamine antagonists (SDAs), 280
Seroxat (paroxetine), 246–47
Serpasil (reserpine), 40, 43–44, 46, 52, 56, 85, 170, 172
sertraline (Zoloft), 123–24, 125, 190, 218–19, 239–40, 245, 246, 247, 258, 262, 309, 321
Servier Laboratories, 315
SGAs (second-generation antipsychotics), 7, 11, 30, 66–67, 275–76. See also atypicals
Shader, Richard, 119
Shagass, Charles, 49, 133–34, 316
Shapin, Stephen, 90
Shaw, Daniel, 168–69
Shaw, K. N. F., 31
Sheller, Stephen, 232–33
Shepherd, Michael, 34, 110–11, 170–71, 175
Sheps, Mindel, 168
Shire PLC, 196–97
shock treatment, 23
Shon, Steven, 301–2
Shopsin, Baron, 259
Silveira, Raza, 270
Silverman, Edward, 272
Simmons, George, 9, 10–11
Simon, Pierre, 279
Simpson, George, 44, 192, 247, 277, 289, 319
Simpson, Pippa, 190
Sinequan (doxepin), 135
Sismondo, Sergio, 139, 140–41, 216
SKB (SmithKline Beecham), 87–88, 158–60, 245, 246–47, 251, 256, 265, 266, 267, 268–70, 271, 273, 274, 310. See also GlaxoSmithKline
Skrabanek, Peter, 204
Slater, Eliot, 19, 64
Smith, Kline & French (SKF), 28, 40, 71, 78, 87–88, 91, 95, 142, 173, 206, 321. See also GlaxoSmithKline
Smith, Richard, 223, 228

SmithKline, 40, 41, 52–53, 54, 71, 92, 95, 156–57, 160–61, 233, 275. See also GlaxoSmithKline
SmithKline Beecham (SKB), 87–88, 158–60, 245, 246–47, 251, 256, 265, 266, 267, 268–70, 271, 273, 274, 310. See also GlaxoSmithKline
Smithsonian Institution, 91–92, 181
Smythies, John R., 126–27
SNRIs (serotonin and norepinephrine reuptake inhibitors), 127, 246, 323
Snyder, Laurie, 302
Snyder, Solomon, 131–32, 313, 314
sodium amytal (Amytal), 28, 50–51, 133–34
Sollmann, Torald, 15, 23–24
Solomon, Harry, 50
Solomon, Philip, 305
Solvay Pharmaceuticals, 150
Soul of Brutes (Willis), 62
Sourkes, Theodore, 32, 44
Sparine (promazine), 45
Spartase, 62
Spence, Des, 129–30
Spielmans, Glen I., 129, 258–59
Spitzer, Robert (Bob), 37, 73, 103, 104–7, 108, 109, 110–12, 113, 114, 115, 117
Springfield State Hospital, 41
Squibb Institute for Medical Research, 79
SSRIs. See names of specific SSRIs; selective serotonin reuptake inhibitors
St. Bartholomew's Hospital, 30, 168
St. Elizabeths Hospital, 32, 44–45, 91
St. John's Episcopal Hospital, 217
St. Louis Research Diagnostic Criteria (RDC), 105–6, 110–11
St. Louis State Hospital, 134
St. Mary's Hospital, 19, 171
St. Pete Times, 290
Stablon (tianeptine), 315
Stadtroda Mental Hospital, 17
Stanford University, 156–57, 158, 185, 222, 255
Stanley Foundation, 150
Stanton, Alfred, 36
STAR*D (Sequenced Treatment Alternatives to Relieve Depression) study, 136, 184, 295
Starr, Victoria, 200
State University of New York, Stony Brook, 71–72, 103, 215–16, 258
State University of New York, Syracuse, 185
Ste. Anne mental hospital, 29, 52
Steingard, Sandra, 125
Stelazine (trifluoperazine), 53, 71
STEP-BD study, 136

Stephansfeld Asylum, 17
Stephens, Malcolm R., 237–38
Stevenson, Ian, 220
STI (Scientific Therapeutics Information),
    156–57, 159, 160, 161, 217, 266, 267, 268,
    270, 271, 274
Stille, Günther, 85, 276–77
stimulants, 142, 196–97, 243. *See also names of
    specific stimulants*
Stockbridge, Lisa, 314
Stowe, Zachary, 270–71
Strattera (atomoxetine), 292
Strauss, Israel, 72
Strauss, John, 66
streptomycin, 169
Strober, Mike, 215–16
Strömgren, Eric, 37
strychnine, 23
Styron, William, 74
Substance Abuse and Mental Health Services
    Administration (SAMSHA), 118
Sugarman, Michael, 253
Sullivan, Michael, 253
Surgeon General's Catalogue, 16
Surmontil (trimipramine), 93
Sutleffe, Edward, 123
Swartz, Conrad, 120
Sykes, Richard, 90
Symbyax (olanzapine and fluoxetine), 256
Szasz, Thomas, 57

Tait, Ian, 20
Talbot (pseudonym), 139–40, 213
Tamminga, Carol, 280
Taractan (chlorprothixene), 52
Taurel, Sidney, 202
Taylor, Michael Alan, 33, 67, 71–72, 94, 103,
    104, 120, 122, 182, 195, 204–5, 238–39
Taylor Manor Hospital, 33, 78
TCAs (tricyclic antidepressants), 7, 46–47, 53,
    72, 91, 93, 107, 112–13, 123, 127, 135, 171,
    177, 189, 245, 251, 253, 257–58, 259–60,
    274, 295, 308, 310, 323
Technical University, Munich, 289–90
Temple, Robert (Bob), 110, 143, 182, 187, 188,
    190, 235–36, 238, 248, 260, 275–76
Temple University, 93
Texas Department of Mental Health, 300,
    301, 302–3
Texas Medical Algorithm Project (TMAP), 141,
    150–51, 184, 197–98, 202–3, 210, 290,
    299–303
Texas v. Janssen, 96–97

thalidomide, 45–46, 95, 225
The Medicine Group (TMG), 269
therapeutic alliance, 5–6, 7–8
thiopental, 133
thioridazine (Mellaril), 53–54, 173, 275, 280
thioxanthenes, 52
Third World Congress of Psychiatry, 134
Thompson, W. Furness, 71
Thompson, W. Leigh, 165, 245
Thorazine (chlorpromazine), 36, 51, 53,
    71, 210
Thorndike Laboratory, 83
Thorner, Melvin Wilfred, 28
Thouret, Michel-Augustin, 18
Thuillier, Jean, 29, 38, 51
tianeptine (Stablon), 315
Times Literary Supplement, 12
TMAP (Texas Medical Algorithm Project), 141,
    150–51, 184, 197–98, 202–3, 210, 290,
    299–303
TMG (The Medicine Group), 269
Tofranil (imipramine), 30–31, 41, 46–47, 52, 53,
    54, 59–60, 94, 134, 139, 145, 158–59, 171,
    173, 174, 175, 189, 190, 202, 229, 254, 258,
    261–62, 266
Tollefson, Gary, 246–47, 261
Tolserol (mephenesin), 172–73
Tolvon (mianserin; GB-94), 135–36
topiramate (Topamax), 238
Toronto Star, 186
tranquilizers, 34, 38, 39–40, 52, 53, 54, 71, 195,
    199, 275–76. *See also names of specific
    tranquilizers*
tranylcypromine (Parnate), 52–53, 73–74
Triavil (amitriptyline and perphenazine),
    54–55
triazolam (Halcion), 191–92, 213
tricyclic antidepressants (TCAs), 7, 46–47, 53,
    72, 91, 93, 107, 112–13, 123, 127, 135, 171,
    177, 189, 245, 251, 253, 257–58, 259–60,
    274, 295, 308, 310, 323
trifluoperazine (Stelazine), 53, 71
Trilafon (perphenazine), 54–55,
    287–88
trimipramine (Surmontil), 93
Trintellix (vortioxetine), 226
Tufts University, 116, 119, 201, 284
Tulane University, 124
Tumas, John, 214
Turner, Eric, 314
Tversky, Amos, 182
tyramine, 31, 72
Tyrer, Peter, 289–90, 305–6

UCLA (University of California, Los Angeles), 135, 215–16, 219, 269
UK General Practice Research Data Base, 211
Ulett, George, 134
Ultran (phenaglycodol), 53
Umea University, 124
UNC (University of North Carolina), 52, 156
University Medical School of Buenos Aires, 149
University of Basel, 88
University of Birmingham, 44, 50–51, 91–92
University of Bologna, 247
University of Bonn, 88
University of California, Los Angeles (UCLA), 135, 215–16, 219, 269
University of California, San Francisco, 36, 227
University of Cincinnati, 141, 158, 211
University of Connecticut, 184, 261, 267
University of Erlangen-Nuremberg, 134
University of Florida, Gainesville, 159
University of Georgia, 19
University of Groningen, 115–16
University of Homburg/Saar, 88
University of Illinois, 106, 120, 320
University of Iowa, 27, 28–29, 117–18, 121, 217, 318–19
University of Jena, 133
University of Kansas, 67–68
University of London, 72
University of Louisville, 13–14
University of Maryland, 280, 290–91
University of Massachusetts, 55, 261
University of Miami Miller Medical School, 158
University of Michigan, 4, 21, 27, 32, 34, 49, 64–65, 71–72, 74, 89, 94, 101, 112, 145–46, 182, 186
University of Minnesota, 111
University of Nevada School of Medicine, 193
University of New South Wales, 259
University of North Carolina (UNC), 52, 156
University of Pennsylvania, 27–28, 47, 52–53, 81, 83, 93, 159, 160–61, 197, 259, 272, 292, 313, 317
University of Pittsburgh, 168, 244
University of Sydney, 71–72
University of Texas, 215–16, 227, 269, 299
University of Toronto, 314
University of Vermont, 65
University of Vienna, 131
University of Virginia, 220, 312
University of Washington, 123, 193
University of Wisconsin, 18
University of Zurich, 179
Upjohn Company, 62, 80, 191–92, 213, 239, 244

Upjohn, W. E., 77
Upstate University Hospital, 5–6, 243–44
US Department of Agriculture, 22
US Department of Health and Human Services, 158
US Department of Health, Education and Welfare (DHEW), 95–96
US Department of Justice (DOJ), 197–98, 267, 285, 293
US Patent Office, 90
US Public Health Service, 18
USV Pharmaceutical Corp., 123

VA (Veterans Administration), 43, 45, 53–54, 66, 161, 171–72, 173, 179–80, 184–85, 187
Vagelos, Roy, 79, 81–82, 89
vagus nerve stimulation (VNS), 157, 218, 272
Valium (diazepam), 54, 57, 199, 236, 240, 243–44, 247, 281–82
Van Norman, James, 288
van Os, Jim, 218
van Praag, Herman, 71–72
Vanda Pharmaceuticals, 288
Vanderbilt Clinic, 46–47
Vanderbilt University, 109–10, 116–17, 140
venlafaxine (Effexor), 127, 221, 246, 308
Vere, Duncan, 190
Vermont State Hospital, 65
Veterans Administration (VA), 43, 45, 53–54, 66, 161, 171–72, 173, 179–80, 184–85, 187
Viagra, 309
Ville-Evrard asylum, 23
Vinar, Oldrich, 48, 131
vital depression, 71–72, 74, 116–17
VNS (vagus nerve stimulation), 157, 218, 272
Vorster, Johannes, 17
vortioxetine (Brintellix; Trintellix), 226
Vossenaar, Jack, 135–36

Wade, Owen, 91–92
Waelsch, Heinrich, 46
Wagner, Karen, 197–98, 215–16, 227
Wall Street Journal (WSJ), 152–53, 157, 209–10, 219
Wallace Laboratories, 40, 53
Walter, Grey, 135
Wander Pharma GmbH, 85, 276–77, 278
Warawa, Edward, 282
Wardell, William, 182, 231
Ward's Island asylum, 171
Warner-Lambert, 80
Washington University, St. Louis, 35, 67–68, 101, 102, 104–5, 106, 134

Watson, Douglas G., 88, 89
Wayne State University, 185–86, 190
Weber Shandwick Communications, 227
Weiden, Peter, 299
Weill Medical College, 185
Weinberger, Daniel, 17, 65, 67
Weinstein, Haskell, 79, 195, 204, 215, 225
Weller, Elizabeth, 215–16
Wells Health Care Communications, 216
Wendt, Henry, 87–88
West London Hospital, 16
West Park Hospital, 124, 245
Westaway, Jackie, 268–69
Western Psychiatric Institute, 265
Western Reserve University, 15
Whitaker, Robert, 58, 125, 259
Whitehouse, Peter, 147–48
WHO (World Health Organization), 15, 38, 49, 243
Wiesel, Benjamin, 68
Wildgust, Hiram, 211
Wilens, Timothy E., 153
William S. Merrell Company, 239
Willis, Thomas, 62
Willstätter, Richard, 30
Winkler, Helmut, 17
Winson Green Hospital, 50–51, 170
Woodruff, Robert, 106
Woodward, Samuel, 8–9
Worcester Foundation for Experimental Biology, 47
Work, Henry, 205–6
World Health Organization (WHO), 15, 38, 49, 243

WPP PLC, 206
WSJ (Wall Street Journal), 152–53, 157, 209–10, 219
Wyeth Laboratories, 40, 57, 62, 80, 127, 168, 191–92, 221, 236, 239

Xanax (alprazolam), 191–92, 239, 244

Yale University, 27, 48–49, 65, 83, 103, 105, 181, 210, 290, 296, 314–15
Yale-Brown Obsessive-Compulsive Scale (Y-BOCS), 163
Yonkers, Kimberly, 270
Young, Albert, 21
Young, Muriel, 159

Zalesky, Ed, 270
Zantac (ranitidine), 263
Zelmid (zimelidine), 86, 246
Zeneca Pharmaceuticals, 86, 89, 282. See also AstraZeneca
Zenner, Patrick, 88, 89
zimelidine (Zelmid), 86, 246
Ziprasidone (Geodon), 294
Zoloft (sertraline), 123–24, 125, 190, 218–19, 239–40, 245, 246, 247, 258, 262, 309, 321
Zubin, Joseph, 13, 106
Zucker-Hillside (Hillside–North Shore Long Island Jewish Health System), 146–47, 288
Zurich Cantonal Psychiatric Hospital, 75
Zyprexa (olanzapine), 83, 96, 97, 151–52, 195, 196, 201, 202, 203, 206–7, 210–12, 256, 279, 280–81, 282, 283, 286, 287–88, 294–95, 300–1, 309

CPSIA information can be obtained
at www.ICGtesting.com
Printed in the USA
BVHW030350131122
651491BV00001B/2